D1647784

THE YOGA SUTRAS DESK REFERENCE

Also by Nicolai Bachman

BOOKS

The Path of the Yoga Sutras: A Practical Guide to the Core of Yoga

The Language of Yoga: Complete A-to-Y Guide to Asana Names, Sanskrit Terms, and Chants

AUDIO PROGRAMS

The Yoga Sutras: An Essential Guide to the Heart of Yoga Philosophy

THE YOGA SUTRAS DESK REFERENCE

A Comprehensive Guide to the Core Concepts of Yoga

NICOLAI BACHMAN

sounds true
BOULDER, COLORADO

Sounds True
Boulder CO 80306

© 2010, 2021 Nicolai Bachman

Sounds True is a trademark of Sounds True, Inc.

All rights reserved. No part of this book may be used or reproduced in any manner without written permission from the author and publisher.

Cover design by Lisa Kerans
Book design by Rachael Murray & Meredith March

All Sanskrit translations by the author. The chanting notations of the *Yoga Sūtra-s* as presented in Part 4 are based on a system designed and taught by T. K. V. Desikachar. This method of chanting the *Yoga Sūtra-s* is the sole copyright of T. K. V. Desikachar. No part of this system of notation may be used/recorded for any commercial purpose without prior written permission from the copyright holder.

Printed in South Korea

BK06229

Library of Congress Cataloging-in-Publication Data

Names: Bachman, Nicolai, author. | Patañjali. Yogasūtra. English.
Title: The Yoga Sutras desk reference : a comprehensive guide to the core concepts of Yoga / Nicolai Bachman.
Description: Boulder : Sounds True, 2021. | Includes bibliographical references. | In English; includes Sanskrit Text with meaning and commentary in English.
Identifiers: LCCN 2020048027 (print) | LCCN 2020048028 (ebook) | ISBN 9781683648031 (paperback) | ISBN 9781683648048 (ebook)
Subjects: LCSH: Patañjali. Yogasūtra. | Yoga–Early works to 1800. | Yoga–Philosophy. | Hindu philosophy–Early works to 1800.
Classification: LCC B132.Y6 B269 2021 (print) | LCC B132.Y6 (ebook) | DDC 181/.452–dc23
LC record available at https://lccn.loc.gov/2020048027
LC ebook record available at https://lccn.loc.gov/2020048028

10 9 8 7 6 5 4 3 2 1

When the stains from old habits are exhausted, the original light appears, blazing through your skull, not admitting any other matters. Then you can reside in the clear circle of brightness. Open-mindedly sparkling and pure, they are like a mirror reflecting a mirror, with nothing regarded as outside, without capacity for accumulating dust.

—ZEN MASTER HONGZHI

Contents

Preface

The *Yoga Sūtra-s* is an ancient text that, more than any other, defines what yoga is and how it can be practiced. Written in Sanskrit, the mother tongue and sacred language of India, the *Yoga Sūtra-s* consists of 195 concise aphorisms called *sūtra-s* that function as seeds of knowledge, each a plethora of information condensed into a tiny space. The author, Patañjali, made sure his presentation was not limited to geography, culture, religion, or even time period. Universal principles such as nonviolence and truthfulness, along with a focus on self-development and clarification of the heart-mind, make the application and pursuit of yoga good for all people and for society as a whole.

I came to study this text from a background in yoga āsana, meditation, and Sanskrit. At first it felt daunting to me: almost two hundred tiny sūtra-s written in such a way as to require at least one commentary to comprehend what each one is trying to convey. If no guidance is available, studying this text can be an exercise in "the blind leading the blind." After reading several different translations and still not feeling comfortable with my understanding, I sought out qualified teachers who had themselves studied the *Yoga Sūtra-s* over many years with their teachers and had applied the principles and practices to their lives. For me this was the key that unlocked the door. There is no substitute for having a good teacher.

Each time I revisited the sūtra-s, over the course of many years of study and life experience, additional subtleties and applications revealed themselves. Each time I came upon a different translation of a sūtra, my understanding expanded and deepened. Integrating yoga philosophy into my life was also absolutely necessary. Yoga is meant to be experiential, not just intellectual. Yet it was asking questions of my primary teachers that caused the proverbial lightbulbs to brighten my understanding.

I personally appreciate the *Yoga Sūtra-s* as much for its masterful design as for its universality and emphasis on personal growth. Each individual sūtra is a wonderful gem of wisdom, while the entire collection offers unique and powerful tools for inner development and outer poise. Learning the concepts and implementing the practices of yoga is a lifelong pursuit that is bound to create outer joy and inner happiness.

The ability to catch myself before acting unconsciously based on past habitual patterning, then deciding to change course and act in a beneficial and positive way, makes me appreciate the usefulness and profundity of the *Yoga Sūtra-s*. Every time I am able to listen to all sides of an argument, or see another person as a manifestation of the radiant light of awareness that we all share, I am reminded of how powerful and transformative Patañjali's practices are.

THIS APPROACH TO THE *YOGA SŪTRA-S*

The *Yoga Sūtra-s* of Patañjali has been translated and commented upon for thousands of years. In the past twenty years numerous English interpretations have been written, each giving a slightly different perspective, from the very orthodox, with precise translation from the original Sanskrit and strict Vedic interpretation, to quite New Age, with much more liberal translation. The vast majority of translations present the text in its original order and take you through the sūtra-s from beginning to end.

This interpretation differs in several ways. First, it is focused on learning in depth certain key concepts embedded in the sūtra-s and building a working vocabulary of the Sanskrit terms for each concept. Each section focuses on a core principle or practice of yoga, providing thoughts and empowerments that can be meditated upon and applied to everyday life. Second, the sounds of the sūtra-s are emphasized, as they contain their life-force (prāṇa). Third, color illustrations provided in appendix F show many of the concepts in flowchart and table form for additional reference.

This course will allow you to truly understand yoga philosophy by focusing on core principles and acquiring a working conversational vocabulary wherein you can refer to real Sanskrit words instead of their diluted and inevitably inaccurate English correlates.

Yoga is primarily concerned with the transformation of our field of consciousness, which consists of our heart-mind complex. I have chosen to refer to this field, called *citta* in Sanskrit, as the "heart-mind" throughout this program to most accurately represent it. Yoga practice involves shifting our attention from outer/external/superficial interests to inner/internal/deeper parts of ourselves.

HOW TO USE THIS BOOK

This reference book has been designed to focus on fifty-one key concepts from the *Yoga Sūtra-s*. This approach not only cultivates an understanding of core principles, but it builds a working vocabulary of important Sanskrit terms that have no direct equivalents in English or other languages. Rather than gleaning pieces of each concept by moving through the text in a linear way, we can instead focus on the idea and see its various aspects across the entire text.

A single sūtra that either defines or represents the term appears at the top. Then the concept is explained in detail, with references to all related sūtra-s. This is where you can dive into the idea, find its esoteric aspects, understand its practical applications, and dissect the Sanskrit word all the way down to its root.

The terms, when first mentioned in each commentary, appear in bold/italic to make them stand out. If a word appears in italics only, it is being emphasized in the sentence. Because the original Sanskrit script has no capital letters, Sanskrit terms are presented in lowercase. To conform to English standards, if the Sanskrit term is a proper name, it is capitalized.

The introduction provides background information including history, and discusses key overriding concepts that apply to the study of yoga as a whole. Part 3 shows a full translation of the entire text, to be referenced when desired. Part 4 shows the entire text in large type with tonal marks, designed to be practiced orally.

part 1

OVERVIEW AND FOUNDATIONAL CONCEPTS

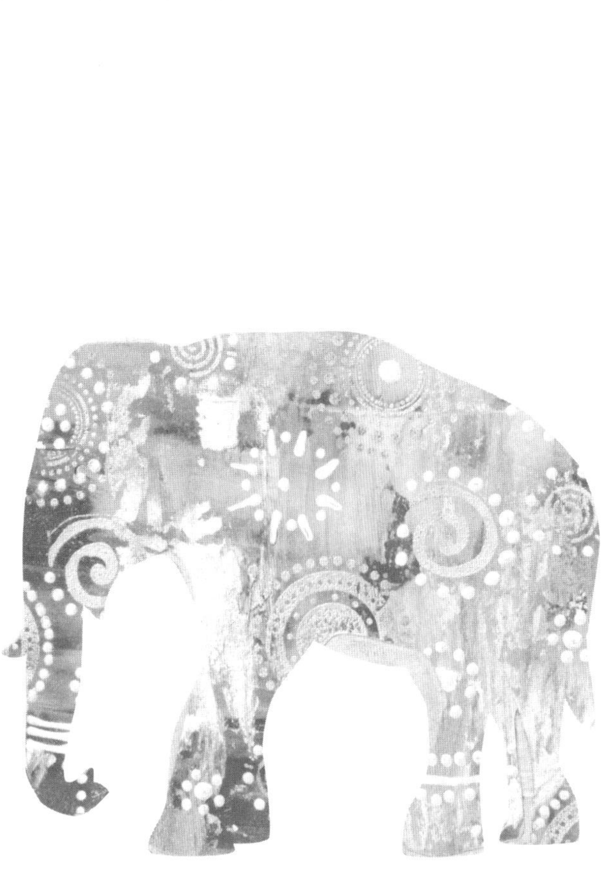

Gaṇeśa Gāyatrī Mantra

To remove obstacles and promote auspiciousness.

तत्पुरुषाय विद्महे	tat puruṣāya vidmahe
वक्रतुण्डाय धीमहि ।	vakratuṇḍāya dhīmahi,
तन्नो दन्तिः प्रचोदयात् ॥	tanno dantiḥ pracodayāt.

May we all know that inner light of awareness.
May we all meditate upon the one with the curved trunk.
May that tusked one guide us.

What Is Yoga?

Yoga is an unassuming word with deep and broad interpretations. Many equate yoga with physical postures or stretching exercises, which captures only a tiny fraction of its true identity. According to the text at hand, the *Yoga Sūtra-s*, "yoga is the stilling of fluctuations in the heart-mind field of consciousness" (1.2). Yoga is a set of tools for refining and stabilizing our body, breath, heart, and mind, which allows our attention to turn inward to discover our own true nature, our quiet inner light of awareness. The term yoga is also used to describe the state of mind in which our thoughts and emotions do not distract our attention, again enabling our innate radiance to shine forth.

The dictionary lists a variety of meanings for yoga, including joining, uniting; union, junction, combination; contact, touch, connection; employment, application, use; mode, manner, course, means; a yoke; and a conveyance, vehicle. Various texts define yoga in a similar way, yet all are slightly different. According to the *Kaṭha Upaniṣad*,

> They consider holding the senses steady as the state of yoga.
> Then one becomes vigilant. Yoga is indeed subject to growth
> and decay. (2.3.11)

The *Śvetāśvatara Upaniṣad* states

> By practicing the yoga of meditation, they saw
> the power of the divine self hidden by its own effects. (1.3)

The *Bhagavad-Gītā*, one of the most important texts on yoga, defines yoga as

> equanimity (2.48)
> skill/welfare/well-being in actions (2.50)
> not eating too much, not absolutely not eating, not the habit of
> sleeping too much, and not staying awake either (6.16)
> separating from the bondage of suffering (6.23)

According to the *Caraka Saṃhitā*, a text on Āyurveda (East Indian Medicine),

> Happiness and suffering proceed from contact with the self, sensory organs, mind, and sense objects. When the mind is steadily resting in the self, both happiness and suffering cease due to not engaging the sensory organs, and complete control (of the heart-mind) arises in the person. This state is known as "yoga" by the expert sages. (Śarīrasthānam 1.138-139)

Yoga can take on several different yet overlapping forms. The list below is not necessarily all-inclusive.

rāja	"king"	Yoga according to the *Yoga Sūtra-s*
bhakti	"devotion"	Connecting through pure devotion, complete surrender to the divine
jñāna	"knowledge"	Study and contemplation
karma	"action"	Service to others, self-practice
mantra	"sacred chanting"	Chanting a mantra repeatedly
nāḍa	"resounding"	Hearing the inner sounds, inaudible to our outer sense of hearing
haṭha	"force, will"	Purification, awakening the kuṇḍalinī-śakti

A BRIEF HISTORY OF YOGA

The source texts for yoga philosophy are the four *Veda-s: Ṛg, Sāma, Yajur,* and *Atharva.* Both *Sāma-Veda* and *Yajur-Veda* derive heavily from the original *Ṛg-Veda*. "Veda" means "knowledge," from the root "vid," meaning "to see, find," the origin of the English words "vision" and "video." It is said that all four *Veda-s* were channeled from a divine source through ṛṣi-s (sages/poets) into Sanskrit sounds. The Sanskrit language itself is considered to be of divine origin. The *Upaniṣad-s,* written much later, are considered "Vedānta," which literally means "end of the *Veda-s.*" They are extrapolations of the *Veda-s,* often couched in story format and more accessible and easier to understand than the *Veda-s.* Both the *Veda-s* and *Upaniṣad-s* are classified as "śruti," meaning "heard," a class of knowledge accorded to divine origin. All other texts are classified as "smṛti," meaning "remembered," and are considered to be of human origin. The *Yoga Sūtra-s* is considered "smṛti" because it was written by a man (Patañjali) and does not reference the *Veda-s* directly.

All the *Veda-s* have been preserved orally by means of Vedic chanting. In fact, they are still memorized by families in India, and the oral rendition is usually considered the most accurate. At some point in history they were written down on palm or banana leaves. When the leaves dried up, they were rewritten based on the chanting, not copied from the old leaves. Thus, the earliest written text does not date the true origin of the *Veda-s*. The *Ṛg-Veda* is the oldest of all the *Veda-s*, its written form dating back to at least 1500 BCE, with some traditions placing it at 3000 BCE or earlier.

Yoga philosophy existed long before the *Yoga Sūtra-s* was written. The *Yoga Sūtra-s* were compiled between 500 and 200 BCE, much later than the *Veda-s* in which yoga is mentioned. There are six classical darśana-s, "views" that are rooted in the *Veda-s*. (See below.) The *Yoga Sūtra-s* is considered to be the primary text of what is called yoga-darśana. Sāṅkhya-darśana is its pair, providing a foundational theory of creation for yoga-darśana.

SIX VIEWS
(Ṣaḍ-Ḍarśana-s)

There are six "views" of Vedic thought, called ṣaḍ-ḍarśana-s, that are like branches of the same tree. These are six different perspectives on the same underlying Vedic principles. The Sāṅkhya perspective delineates the components of existence (the twenty-five tattva-s) and how they emerge to form the manifest world. This view provides a foundational structure for Patañjali's yoga, which describes in detail how the human psyche works. Patañjali mentions several tools for living a kind, civil life; refining the body, mind, and sense organs; and turning attention inward to understand the true nature of one's inner Self.

NAME OF VIEW	SĀṄKHYA	YOGA	PŪRVA-MĪMĀṂSĀ	UTTARA-MĪMĀMSĀ, OR VEDANTA	NYĀYA	VAIŚEṢIKA
MEANING OF NAME	Enumeration	Application/ union	Early investigation	Later investigation	"That by which the mind is led to a conclusion"	Particularization
PRIMARY TEXT	*Sāṅkhya Kārikā*	*Yoga Sūtra-s*	*Mīmāṃsā Sūtra-s*	*Vedānta/ Brahma/ Śārīraka Sūtra-s*	*Nyāya Sūtra-s*	*Vaiśeṣika Sūtra-s*
FOUNDER	Kapila	Hiranyagarbha	Jaimini		Gotama	
AUTHOR(S)	Īśvarakṛṣṇa	Patañjali	Jaimini	Bādarāyaṇa	Gotama	Kaṇāda/ Kāśyapa
APPROX DATES	700–600 BCE, 200–300 AD	500–200 BCE	400 BCE	500–200 BCE	300–200 BCE	300–200 BCE
COMMENTATORS	Vācaspati Miśra	Vyāsa	Śabara	Śaṃkara, Rāmānuja, Madhva	Vātsyāyaṇa	Śaṃkara Miśra
DESCRIPTION	Seer and seeable meet and manifest into the twenty-five tattva-s, guṇa-s	Psychological map of consciousness with tools and practices to reach samādhi	Ritual, worship, ethical conduct, sound, mantra	Nondual—all is Brahman; anything that appears to exist is only a projection of Brahman	Logic, the basis for scientific inquiry and philosophical debate	Everything is made up of individual atomic particles; physics, chemistry

SĀṄKHYA-DARŚANA

The Philosophy Behind the Yoga Sūtra-s

Underlying the experiential practice of yoga is a philosophy that provides a blueprint for the manifest world. Sāṅkhya means "enumeration" and refers to a theory of creation and dissolution that consists of twenty-five "tattva-s," components of the manifest world. Some say that only twenty-four of them are actually tattva-s and the twenty-fifth (Puruṣa) is not really a tattva since it is not part of the manifest world per se.

According to the *Sāṅkhya-Kārikā,* the primary text of this philosophy, objects come into existence from subtle to gross. Puruṣa is the unmanifest, conscious witness that pervades Prakṛti, the manifest universe. (See draṣṭṛ and dṛśya.) If Puruṣa is a magnet, Prakṛti is the iron filings. When in close proximity, Puruṣa causes Prakṛti to stir. Prakṛti, the manifest world, has three qualities, called guṇa-s: sattva (intelligence, purity, balance), rajas (activity, stimulation), and tamas (inertia, stagnation). (See below.) Sāṅkhya theory describes how matter is formed into specific products, including the five elements (solids, liquids, fire, gases, and space). (See appendix F, figure 1.)

THE GUṆA-S
Sattva, Rajas, and Tamas

Guṇa means attribute, quality, property, or characteristic. In Sāṅkhya philosophy, there are three guṇa-s: sattva, rajas, and tamas. Each represents a set of qualities that, taken together, comprise all qualities present in the natural, manifest world, called Prakṛti. Guṇa also means rope, string, or cord, so the guṇa-s can be likened to three strands of a rope that bind the individual's spirit (Puruṣa) within his or her body (part of Prakṛti). There are two ways to view the guṇa-s: cosmic or psychological.

The Sāṅkhya philosophy provides the cosmic view, where every substance in the manifest world contains all three guṇa-s in various proportions. Tamas, the grossest and densest guṇa, represents inanimate matter, which does not require an embodied being. The five gross elements (space, air, fire, water, and earth) and corresponding subtle elements (sound, touch, form, taste, and smell) arise from tamas. Rajas, the energy of activity, is responsible for change and movement. Sattva, a balance of the positive aspects of tamas and rajas, is present in animate matter, which requires an embodied being. The outer mind (manas), buddhi, five sense organs, and five motor organs arise from sattva. From this point of view, tamas and rajas have positive and negative attributes. Tamas is matter; rajas is the heat and energy necessary to transform; and sattva is the purity, intelligence, and light of knowledge.

The *Yoga Sūtra-s* and Āyurveda both refer to the guṇa-s in the psychological sense, as qualities of the individual heart-mind. Ideally, sattva leads and rajas and tamas follow. Relative to the field of sattva in the heart-mind (citta), rajas and tamas appear unhealthy and negative. The physical body is inherently tamasic; the prāṇa is rajasic; and the spirit is sattvic. Chapters 14 and 17 of the *Bhagavad-Gītā* describe the triguṇa in detail, with sattva regarded as positive and helpful while rajas and tamas are negative and harmful. Yoga and Āyurveda advocate a heart-mind that moves toward sattva and away from rajas and tamas, which are considered detrimental to one's spiritual progress.

Sūtra 2.18 refers to these guṇa-s not by name but by adjectives describing the main property of each: brightness (sattva), activity (rajas), and inertia (tamas). One stage leading up to kaivalya is a realization of the difference between a sattvic heart-mind and the seer (4.25). A sattvic heart-mind is indeed an advanced stage, but not the end. Sattva is like a golden chain. Although its qualities are all positive and helpful, it is nevertheless a guṇa, binding our spirit to impermanent manifest existence. The last sūtra in chapter 4 (4.34) equates kaivalya with going inward to the point at which one returns to the source of the guṇa-s and can distinguish between the changing guṇa-s of Prakṛti and the unchanging inner light of Puruṣa.

Generally we want the qualities of our heart-mind to progress from tamas and rajas toward sattva. Tamas and rajas can counteract each other for the eventual good of the individual. For example, if we are stuck in tamas, rajas can act as motivation to loosen up the inertia and start practicing. On the other hand, if we are too nervous or agitated or cannot slow down (too much rajas), tamas can help ground and stabilize our heart-mind. Sattva can be viewed as a balance of the positive qualities of tamas and rajas. For example:

Water

Ice = tamas—immobile, rigid crystals; slow to melt
Steam = rajas—fast moving particles; hot and energetic
Liquid = sattva—flowing gently

Direction

Veering to right = rajas
Veering to left = tamas
Centering = sattva

According to Āyurveda, our physical constitution (called Prakṛti) is governed by three doṣa-s (vāta, pitta, and kapha), and our mental constitution (manas-prakṛti) by the three guṇa-s. The individual heart-mind field of consciousness (citta, specifically the buddhi) is innately transparent, a characteristic of sattva. When the dark veil of ignorance is lifted, the citta becomes clear, which allows the inner light of knowledge to shine through for us to experience.

SATTVA	RAJAS	TAMAS
Love, compassion, wisdom, intelligence, truthfulness, radiance, purity, clarity, peace, harmony, equilibrium/balance, nonviolence. Know when and how to act for the greater good, how stable to be, etc. Blend best of both sides = balance	Dynamic movement, desire, motivation, direction, competition, aggressiveness, kinetic energy, turbulence, agitation, change	Inertia, solidity, dullness, darkness, veiling, coarseness, resistance to change, laziness, destructive nature, violence, dizziness, sleepiness
Virtue, appropriateness	Activity, stimulation	Inertia, stagnancy
Light	Color	Darkness
Light	Energy	Matter
Knowledge, wisdom	Too intellectual	No interest in knowledge
Adaptable, appropriate change	Quick to change	Slow to change, resists change
Positivity, optimism		Negativity, pessimism
Truthfulness	Deceit	Untruthfulness, lying
Pure, clean, neat	Disorderly	Impure, dirty, sloppy
Nonviolence	Angry violence	Perverse violence
Vegetarian, fresh foods, easy to digest, promote a clear mind, nutritious	Stimulating foods like coffee (caffeine), cayenne, peppers	Stale, leftover, fried, or canned foods
Not attached to actions. Don't talk about them, just do	Intent to harm, unclear speech and action, easily affected by pairs of opposites	Postpones action, ineffective, indirect, cannot find best way to handle situations
Steady, does not give up if fails unless there is no hope	Ever seeking happiness: What can I get?	Lack of belief in higher force, depressed, gives up easily

YOGA-DARŚANA

As Sāṅkhya shows evolution happening from the subtlest and innermost to the grossest, outermost level, yoga provides the means for involution, going in reverse from the grossest external to the subtlest internal state. Spiritual development involves conscious change and refinement, replacing one's unconscious, negative habitual patterns with conscious, positive, helpful practices that dissolve attachments and lead to a healthier, happier being.

The purpose of yoga is purification of the heart-mind (citta-prasādana). Yoga, working from outer to inner, focuses on how to connect to the inner light of awareness, our inner self, called Puruṣa or Ātman. Yoga is a preparation for Vedānta, which works from inner to outer and focuses on the question "What is Ātman?"

YOGA AND YOGA-DARŚANA

There is a distinction to be made between yoga in a broad sense and yoga-darśana. Patañjali did not create yoga. He brilliantly compiled its essence, entitled *Pātañjala-Yoga-Darśanam,* meaning "view of yoga according to patañjali" and known in the West as the *Yoga Sūtra-s.* Yoga existed long before Patañjali. In the initial sūtra, the term "anuśāsana" indicates this teaching follows (anu) a long tradition of teachings (śāsana). The Patañjali yoga tradition is a later expression of older, vedic teachings originally founded by Hiraṇyagarbha, and as such occurs in the context of a broader yoga-darśana. As mentioned previously, the term "yoga" is defined in the *Kaṭha* and *Śvetāśvatara Upaniṣad-s.* The *Mahābhārata,* the huge Indian epic that includes the *Bhagavad-Gītā,* refers to yoga numerous times. The *Bhagavad-Gītā* itself, each chapter of which is called a "yoga," is considered one of the primary ancient yoga śāstra-s.

Many texts exist on yoga-darśana, listed below in chronological order.

NAME	DATE	AUTHOR	NOTES
Bhagavad-Gītā	600–200 BCE	Veda Vyāsa	18 chapters, 700 verses, part of the *Mahābhārata*
Pātañjala-Yoga-Darśana	500–200 BCE	Patañjali	4 chapters, 195 sūtra-s
Yoga-Yajñavalkya	200–400 CE	Yajñavalkya	12 chapters, 462 verses, teaching to Gargi, a woman
Yoga-Vasiṣṭha	800–900 CE	Vasiṣṭha	29,000 verses, taught by Vasiṣṭha to Rāma

NAME	DATE	AUTHOR	NOTES
Haṭha-Yoga-Pradīpikā	1300–1400 CE	Swātmarāma	4 chapters, 389 verses, primary āsana text
Śiva-Saṃhitā	1650–1750 CE	Unknown	5 chapters, 517 verses
Gheraṇḍa-Saṃhitā	1650–1750 CE	Gheraṇḍa	7 chapters, 346 verses, primary āsana text
Yoga-Upaniṣad-s	Broad range	Many	Not well known

OVERVIEW OF THE *YOGA SŪTRA-S* (PĀTAÑJALA-YOGA-DARŚANAM)

The *Pātañjala-Yogadarśanam* is an exercise in philosophy, "love of wisdom"; ontology, "study of existence"; and psychology, "study of the psyche." It describes human consciousness in detail and provides tools and practices for self-development and refinement. Even if the ultimate goal of emancipation (kaivalya) is not attained, the process of studying and learning the *Yoga Sūtra-s* serves to make one a better, happier, kinder person.

The *Yoga Sūtra-s* has four chapters with approximately 195 sūtra-s (some versions have one more or less). Keep in mind the circularity of Indian thought when viewing the organization of this text. In the West, we typically read a book from the beginning to the end. This particular book does not necessarily work that way. Pāda means "part," which here translates to "chapter."

CHAPTER	# SŪTRA-S	MEANING
1 Samādhi Pāda	51	Absorption
2 Sādhana Pāda	55	Practice
3 Vibhūti Pāda	55	Extraordinary Power
4 Kaivalya Pāda	34	Freedom

Chapter 1, entitled Samādhi Pāda, is meant for students already steeped in yoga practice. It jumps right into the various fluctuations present in the heart-mind, then provides ways to quell those distracting thoughts. Samādhi, an advanced stage of yoga practice, is discussed in detail.

Chapter 2, called Sādhana Pāda, is the most practical. It describes numerous tools and practices for purifying the body, breath, and heart-mind in preparation for the journey inward. It is said that a beginner should start in the middle of this chapter, with the mention of the eight limbs of yoga and description of the first five outer limbs. The practices in chapter 2, needed for one who is still involved in worldly matters, are preparations for chapter 1.

Chapter 3, Vibhūti Pāda, describes the last three inner limbs (collectively called saṃyama, focusing inward) and their side effects. The powers accrued during deep meditation are extraordinary and not to be shown off or abused; they are merely to be noticed and then ignored, since they can sidetrack one's focus away from the final goal of yoga, described in chapter 4.

Chapter 4, Kaivalya Pāda, describes the heart-mind (citta) and the changes that occur during the journey inward culminating in absolute freedom (kaivalya).

Patañjali consistently lists concepts in deliberate order, most often from outer/external/superficial to inner/internal/deep, and also in sequence, one leading to the next. It is interesting to note that the first real word of the text is yoga (the word "atha" is equivalent to "the Beginning"), and the last real word is śakti (the final word "iti" is equivalent to "the End"). Given the circular nature of Indian thought, it is fair to say that yoga is directly related to śakti (power or ability). This relationship is discussed further in "The Power of Attention," below.

SŪTRA WRITING FORMAT

The *Pātañjala-Yoga-Darśanam* is written in sūtra format, one of several possible formats for recording information. Sūtra format, described in the verse below, is the most concise way of presenting information, and is meant to be used as a mnemonic device. Since sūtra-s are so terse, a written or live commentary is necessary to understand them. Traditionally one memorizes them via chanting, then a teacher expounds on their meaning. Because the sound of the sūtra is associated in memory with its expanded commentary, it becomes easy to recall vast amounts of information by mnemonic association.

Alpākṣaram

Qualities of a Sūtra

अल्पाक्षरमसंदिग्धं	alpākṣaram asandigdhaṃ
सारवत् विश्वतो मुखम् ।	sāravat viśvato mukham,
अस्तोभ्यमनवध्यं च	astobhyam anavadhyaṃ ca
सूत्रं सूत्रविदो विदुः ॥	sūtraṃ sūtravido viduḥ.

Those who know sūtra know that a sūtra is:
very brief (small-worded), unambiguous,
full of depth (fertile, like a seed),
broad (multifaceted), fact, not fiction (not fancy),
and dignified.

PRĀṆA

Prāṇa, the life-force, is the energetic link that carries sensory information in and action impulses out of the human system. It lives in and around the nervous system and blood, and can emanate from the body when one concentrates one's attention. Prāṇa is the single most important part of yoga. The state of yoga cannot occur unless prāṇa flows quietly, smoothly, and without obstruction.

Life itself is defined by the existence of prāṇa, which means "life-force" or "breath." When a baby is born, everyone waits for the newborn's first breath or utterance, an indication that his or her individual life apart from the mother is beginning. After a person's last breath, at the time of death prāṇa leaves the body. One is not declared dead until the heart stops, the breath stops, and the pupils of the eyes are dilated and unresponsive. Prāṇa is not just oxygen, for if so, an oxygen tank would be filled with life, and plants would not be considered alive.

Individual prāṇa in the human body has five forms, called vāyu-s (winds), some of which are mentioned in the sūtra-s (3.39–40). These "winds" are responsible for all active movement in the body. The term prāṇa can refer to all vāyu-s or specifically to the first one, depending on the context.

VĀYU	MEANING	DIRECTION	FUNCTIONS
Prāṇa	"Lead breath," "Forward breath"	Inward	Ingestion, sensory perception, thought emanation
Udāna	"Upward breath"	Upward	Speech, effort
Samāna	"Equalizing breath"	Centripetal (toward the center)	Digestion, homeostasis
Vyāna	"Pervasive breath"	Centrifugal (away from the center)	Circulation
Apāna	"Outward breath," "Downward breath"	Outward, downward	Excretion, menstruation

In the macrocosmic sense, cosmic prāṇa (called spanda-tattva) is the energy of prāṇa outside the body, the eternal pulsation and "life" of the universe. This includes planetary movement, gravitational forces, the movement of time, and indeed all motion in the manifest world. It is the vibration between Puruṣa (seer) and Prakṛti (seeable).

Where individual prāṇa meets cosmic prāṇa, at the threshold between microcosm and macrocosm, there is a stillness. Some say it exists twelve finger-widths from the nose. This gap exists between thoughts as well. The empty space between inhalation and exhalation, or between thoughts, is a moment when time seems to stop, and is a powerful place on which to focus one's meditation.

The heart cakra (pronounced "chakra") is the center of the seven-cakra system, and its element is air (vāyu). Its yantra (geometrical shape) is composed of two interlaced triangles. One points upward, representing the masculine energy of fire (agni); the other points downward, representing the feminine energy of water (soma). In the center is the primary seed sound of "yam" that is the expression of vāyu or prāṇa. The inner light of awareness, the basis for life itself, rests in the heart area, like a soft, cool flame in a windless place (prāṇa rests here, unmoving and still).

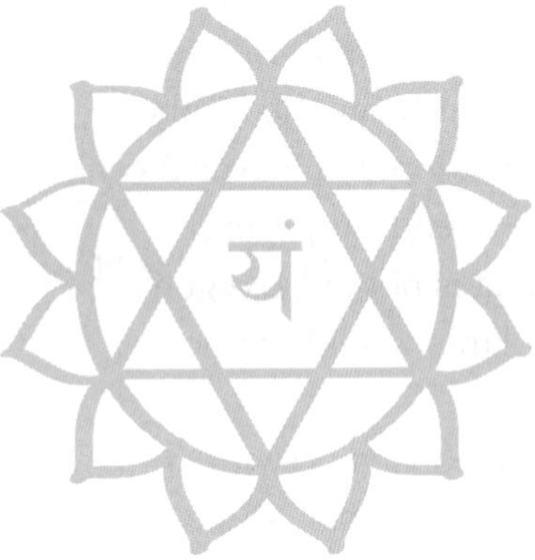

Prāṇa is the living force connecting all aspects of perception. Wherever the mind goes, the prāṇa follows. In other words, wherever the attention is directed, our life-force is projected there, adding śakti to that place. (See "The Power of Attention" on the next page.)

The layer (kośa) consisting of prāṇa (prāṇa-maya-kośa) lies between the physical layer and the layer of the mind. (See appendix F, figure 2.) The mind influences the body through prāṇa and vice versa; both work through the nervous system, the breath, and the subtle energy channels (nāḍī-s). Prāṇāyāma is meant to calm the nervous system by means of breathing exercises that control and regulate the breath. Irregular breathing patterns and restlessness indicate blockages to the flow of prāṇa and result from the nine obstacles (antarāya-s) to practice. Prāṇāyāma balances and slows down the breath, which helps clarify the heart-mind (citta-prasādana) and prepare it for the journey inward (saṃyama). Understanding what prāṇa is and how it works is vital to practicing yoga in its truest sense.

THE POWER OF ATTENTION

Śakti, literally "power" or "ability," is the energy of the universe, a generic term that can be applied even to electricity. Prāṇa is a type of śakti that exists in living creatures. Kuṇḍalinī is a kind of śakti that sleeps coiled up at the base of the spine, waiting for its potential energy to activate through haṭha-yoga. Śakti, like electricity, is amoral, meaning it will go wherever it is directed, independent of good or bad. Wherever the attention goes, there the śakti known as prāṇa follows.

Focusing attention is central to the practice of yoga. In order to progress, attention must be paid to setting aside time to practice—whether our practice involves doing physical postures (āsana), breathing exercises (prāṇāyāma), or sitting quietly in meditation (saṃyama). Being good to others (yama-s) and to ourself (niyama-s) also requires attention. Yoga involves learning about ourself and how we interact with other people, then refining our behavior to reduce pain and suffering. A heart-mind purified and calmed by the fire of yoga develops an ability to focus the attention on a single place, leading to inner contentment and a sense of freedom.

When we pay attention to someone, they receive our śakti. More attention generates more śakti, and vice versa. Simply looking at someone gives him or her some power. An infant who receives plenty of loving attention will grow up feeling more secure and content, compared to one who grows up neglected and then craves attention as a teenager or adult.

Outer beauty or charisma attracts attention and draws śakti from others. A supermodel walking down the street will cause heads to turn. An evangelist preacher in the throes of a fiery sermon receives power from his congregation. Even an unattractive rock star is able to enthrall an audience with his charisma.

Outer adornments like beautiful clothes, pretty makeup, and a stylish haircut attract attention as well.

Inner beauty or charisma can have the same effect. A spiritual guru quietly delivering gems of wisdom captivates his or her followers. Have you ever noticed that when you feel really good about yourself, others find you more attractive? On the other hand, feeling depressed or sad, and thus unattractive, can have the opposite effect.

In a romantic relationship, sometimes one person (A) is more drawn toward the other (B), because of B's outer and/or inner beauty/charisma, or her not being attentive to A. In this case, A craves attention from B. Meanwhile B, who is receiving more attention than she wants, tends to become more aloof from A and give less attention to him. If this goes on, neither party in the relationship feels good. If A can withdraw attention from B, or B can deliberately throw attention toward A, the balance of power can be restored. Withdrawing or increasing attention can be as simple as looking at or listening to the other person, either more or less.

The power of prayer to alleviate or cure an illness is well documented. When we direct our śakti toward a single goal, it can often be achieved.

Practicing yoga involves directing our attention toward the refinement of our body, breath, and heart-mind. Moving from external to internal, our attention is gradually focused inward as we come to understand who we really are. Through committed practice over a long period of time, we can guide the outer and inner śakti toward personal transformation and true happiness.

THE PROCESS OF LEARNING

Learning occurs through repetition, like forming a habit. A child will perform the same operation over and over or repeat a new word or phrase incessantly. Each instance etches it deeper into her consciousness, until it is utterly part of her being, "in her bones," so to speak. A song we hear numerous times becomes embedded in our consciousness, never to be forgotten. The heart-mind is programmed by the sensory stimuli received and the thoughts, words, and actions issuing forth.

All sensory perception is recorded, even if ever so slightly, in our heart-mind field of consciousness (citta). We are constantly learning, whether we are aware of it or not. These stored impressions are called saṃskāra-s. With each repetition, the saṃskāra strengthens and its very own groove forms in the heart-mind. A habitual pattern develops. Over time our heart-mind is programmed with these saṃskāra-s, which shape and form our personality, likes, and dislikes.

For example, as water flows over the land, it carves out a path for itself. The more intense the current, the deeper the furrow becomes. Over time an arroyo forms. At this point, the water is *directed by* the arroyo. In order to divert the flow, another arroyo just as deep or deeper must be formed. The water will flow in whatever arroyo offers the path of least resistance.

The water represents the flow of sensory inputs and action outputs. The arroyo is the groove in our heart-mind called a saṃskāra. When it reaches a certain depth it determines our course of action. The intensity of the flow corresponds to the intensity of the impression. A trauma can be so intense as to have a lifelong effect on one's behavior. As diverting water requires the formation of a new channel, redirecting a habitual tendency necessitates forming a better, healthier one that will supersede the unhelpful pattern.

Mantra is a yogic technique to reprogram the heart-mind field. The power of a mantra requires thousands upon thousands of recitations (japa) to energize its effectiveness. This can "brainwash," in a helpful sense, the heart-mind, cleaning out old, negative patterns and replacing them with fresh, positive impressions.

This course has been designed for gradual, step-by-step learning, allowing the ideas to percolate into your bones one at a time. With enough repetition and patience, what yoga really *is* will unfold over time.

Ācāryāt Pādamādatte

A Student's Four Parts of Learning

आचार्यात् पादमादत्ते	ācāryāt pādamādatte
पादं शिष्यः स्वमेधया ।	pādaṃ śiṣyaḥ svamedhayā
पादं सब्रह्मचारिभ्यः	pādaṃ sabrahmacāribhyaḥ
पादं कालक्रमेण च ॥	pādaṃ kālakrameṇa ca

A student receives
1/4 part (of their learning) from a teacher,
1/4 part from (their) own intelligence,
1/4 part by means of fellow students,
and 1/4 part with the course of time.

part 2

The Concepts

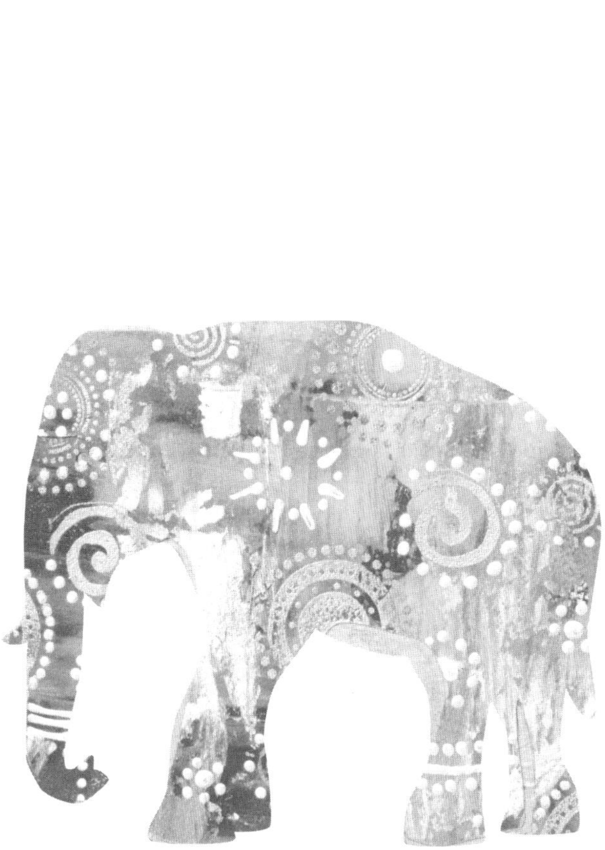

Each concept has one primary sūtra (shown at the top of its page) and several related sūtra-s that are referenced in the commentary. The full translation of the primary sūtra is shown with the commentary. To see a full translation of any related sūtra, please refer to the complete translation of the sūtra-s in part 3. When a reference is made to a specific sūtra, it is shown with the chapter number, then the sūtra number, in parentheses. For example, (2.2) refers to chapter 2, sūtra 2.

Each commentary is presented with the following parts:

Original Sanskrit of the Sūtra

This shows the sūtra in its original form, written in Sanskrit Devanāgarī script.

Transliteration of the Sūtra

This shows the Sanskrit sūtra using Roman letters with diacritical marks. Transliteration allows us to sound out the sūtra without knowing how to read the original Sanskrit script, called Devanāgarī. A key showing how to pronounce each letter is given in appendix E.

Simple Translation of the Sūtra (shown in italics)

This shows what the sūtra means, as interpreted by the author.

Commentary

This is a full explanation of the Sanskrit term, referencing all related sūtra-s, progressing from easy and practical to more advanced and abstract. The commentary is a detailed elucidation of the concept, including what it means, how it relates to other concepts, any practical applications of it, and how the term was derived from its root.

Complete Translation

Line 1 Sūtra in the Romanized transliteration, representing the original exactly

Line 2	Sūtra words before the sounds are joined together. Dashes indicate that the words are part of a compound phrase.
Line 3	Individual words with their meanings

At the end:

1. Literal translation of the sūtra
2. More readable and understandable translation of the sūtra

See appendix E if you want more information about Sanskrit endings and grammar.

Derivation of Terms

Prefix	Any prefix and its meaning
Original Root	Original root from which the word was derived
Prefixed Root	Prefixed root, which may alter the meaning of the original root
Word	Some terms are combinations of one or more words
Literal Meaning	Meaning based on prefix(es) and root only
Dictionary	Relevant meanings from the dictionary
Translation Here	Author's translation in the context of this and surrounding sūtra-s
Other Translations	If applicable

Related Sūtra-s

This is a list of sūtra-s in which the term appears or that relate in some way.

Contemplations

Here are questions to ask yourself related to this concept. These are to be reflected upon and meant to provoke you into applying the concept in your life.

KEY PRINCIPLES

There are certain key principles that are important to understand up front. These concepts form the bedrock on which further study depends, and are mentioned throughout the *Yoga Sūtra-s*. The first term, "atha," represents a state of student preparedness and commitment. "Citta," or the heart-mind, is the field in which yoga as a process or state happens, and understanding it early on is necessary. Next are explained the seer, our inner light of awareness, and the seen, the changeable world that is watched by the seer. They are the most basic principles that underlie yoga. The next three terms are fundamental requirements for the practice of yoga: keen discernment (viveka-khyāti), diligent practice (abhyāsa), and nonattachment to external objects (vairāgya). These lead in to yoga and nirodha, the silencing of the heart-mind. The final three concepts also pervade the text. The infinite storehouse of knowledge known as Īśvara is tapped every time we learn. Karma and its effects of creating habitual tendencies known as saṃskāra-s are central to how the process of perception works in the heart-mind. Finally, change itself (pariṇāma) is viewed according to Patañjali, the author of this brilliant work.

Yogena Cittasya

To Patañjali, author of the Yoga Sūtra-s

योगेन चित्तस्य पदेन वाचां	yogena cittasya padena vācāṃ
मलं शरीरस्य च वैद्यकेन ।	malaṃ śarīrasya ca vaidyakena,
यो ऽपाकरोत्तं प्रवरं मुनीनां	yo 'pākarottaṃ pravaraṃ munīnāṃ
पतञ्जलिं प्राञ्जलिरानतो ऽस्मि ॥	Patañjaliṃ prāñjalirānato 'smi.
आबाहुपुरुषाकारं	ābāhu puruṣākāraṃ
शङ्खचक्रासिधारिणम् ।	śaṅkha-cakrāsi-dhāriṇaṃ,
सहस्रशिरसं श्वेतं	sahasra-śirasaṃ śvetaṃ
प्रणमामि पतञ्जलिम् ॥	praṇamāmi Patañjalim.
श्रीमते अनन्ताय नागराजाय नमो नमः	Śrīmate anantāya nāgarājāya namo namaḥ

I am a deep bow with hands folded to Patañjali,
the most excellent of sages, who removed
impurity of consciousness through yoga,
impurity of speech through word (grammar), and
impurity of the body through medicine (Āyurveda).

In the form of a man up to the shoulders,
holding the conch (divine sound), discus (wheel of time),
and sword (discrimination),
thousand-headed, white,
I bow respectfully to Patañjali.

To the magnificent endless one, the king of the nāgas,
salutations, salutations.

ATHA
Readiness for Yoga

अथ योगानुशासनम् ॥ १.१ ॥

1.1 atha yogānuśāsanam
Here begins the instruction of yoga.

Commentary

This first sūtra begins as many instructional texts begin, with the word ***atha***. Atha does not literally mean "now" as in "right now" but a "now" in sequence, following something else. When used at the beginning of a book, it means "here begins . . ." and is considered an auspicious way to initiate a text. The initial letter "a" is the first letter of the Sanskrit alphabet and the first part of the sound Om (aum), the genesis of the manifest world. Atha is considered a saṃkalpa (decision, promise, or vow) to study diligently and devote a significant amount of time in order to understand yoga thoroughly.

Atha implies that the teacher and student are ready, and adhikāra, the prerequisite preparation of the student, is in place. Traditionally only students who had shown dedication to their studies and respect for their teacher were permitted to learn the deeper and more powerful aspects of yoga. A teacher can determine a student's readiness by assessing his or her current level of knowledge and eagerness to learn. Once teaching commences, the student's ability to learn and integrate what he or she has received is observed.

Where a student begins depends upon his or her current knowledge of the subject matter—here, yoga philosophy. For someone with little or no knowledge (stage 1), 2.29 (the eight limbs) is the most appropriate place to begin because it describes the easiest, most concrete practices and tools to develop the body and heart-mind. If someone is already practicing yoga (not just āsana), including the eight limbs, then 2.1 (kriyā-yoga) allows him to refine his knowledge further (stage 2). One who has already integrated the eight limbs with kriyā yoga, and whose heart-mind is calm and steady, can enter chapter 1 (samādhi: going deeper into the eighth limb) immediately (stage 3).

1.	Āruruksu	starting yoga, desirous of growth
2.	Yuñjāna	practicing yoga, in the process of developing
3.	Yogarūḍha	"grown in yoga"; has already achieved results of the eight limbs and kriyā-yoga

Sūtra 1.22 mentions three levels of practice, which can be applied to a student's eagerness to learn and frequency of practice. Keep in mind that a person can be extremely excited to learn yoga, but may not have the discipline to follow through with the practices. On the other hand, practicing often but in an inattentive way will also hamper progress.

LEVEL	MEANING	EAGERNESS	FREQUENCY
Mṛdu	Soft, mild	Weak	Seldom
Madhya	Medium	Medium	Medium
Adhimātra	Extraordinary	Strong	Often

A heart-mind that is fresh and open will absorb information like a sponge. Repetition reinforces the knowledge learned by creating a pattern in the heart-mind. Young children are a perfect example. Not only do they have less in their minds to interfere with perception, but they will repeat something over and over to themselves until it leaves a lasting impression in their memory. Over time a person accumulates obstacles to learning in the form of physical limitations, emotional scars, and intellectual or spiritual rigidity. Cultivating a "beginner's mind" during our studies allows us to truly grasp the profound depths of yoga. (See "The Process of Learning" in part 1.)

Whereas Western philosophy can be linear, logical, and appealing to our intellect, Indian philosophy is circular and filled with apparent paradoxes because it focuses on that which is beyond the intellect and difficult to explain. These paradoxes resolve themselves as the inner light of awareness reveals itself and is understood on a subtle level.

Yoga is the topic of this text. Studying and practicing the methods described herein create beneficial saṃskāra-s (habitual impressions) that are fresh and serve to recondition the heart-mind toward personal health, happiness, and spiritual connection.

Anuśāsanam implies a teaching that has been followed and is to be followed. The prefix "anu" means "after, following" and śāsana means "teaching." With humility, the author Patañjali acknowledges that these teachings are not his but come from a continuous transmission of knowledge.

A teacher is necessary to understand yoga. There are four steps to following a teaching:

1. adhyāyanam	mechanical learning, chanting the text so it becomes part of us
2. bodhanam	meaning is given and explained according to student's level and situation
3. ācaraṇam	put into practice, observing through experience
4. pracāram	teaching what has been learned and experienced

Complete Translation

1.1 atha yogānuśāsanam

atha yoga-anuśāsanam

atha	now (in sequence, not at this moment)
yoga	process of calming the fluctuations in the heart-mind; topic of this text
anuśāsana	the following teaching

1. Now, the teaching of yoga.
2. Here begins the instruction of yoga.

Related Sūtra-s

1.22

Contemplations

Am I ready and committed to pursue the practice of yoga, beyond physical postures?

Am I open to accept what I may learn about myself?

Can I apply what I learn to improve myself?

CITTA

Heart-Mind Field of Consciousness

तदुपरागापेक्षित्वाच्चित्तस्य वस्तु ज्ञाताज्ञातम् ॥ ४.१७ ॥

4.17 taduparāgāpekṣitvāccittasya vastu jñātājñātam
We visually know an object based on the color of light reflected off it. If no reflection is there, we do not see it and therefore it is unknown to us.

Commentary

Citta is our individual consciousness that is conditioned by our experience. It is our heart-mind field that accepts sensory input from outside, processes it, integrates it into us, remembers, ruminates, and directs our thoughts, words, and actions. This heart-mind complex stores our experiences in memory, including emotions, and over time constructs an identity with this information that defines who we think we are. The citta acts as a middleman between the external world and our pure inner light of awareness. A critical aspect of yoga is clarifying the citta so external objects are perceived accurately and truthfully. (See appendix F, figures 4 and 6.)

The citta is composed of three distinct entities: manas, ahaṅkāra, and buddhi. This triad is also called "antaḥ-karaṇa," meaning "inner instrument." Memories are stored in the citta in the form of outer memories and deeper habitual patterns known as saṃskāra-s. Activities (thoughts and emotions) in the citta that distract us and scatter our attention are called vṛtti-s. A vṛtti presently directed toward an object is called a pratyaya. During dhyāna (meditation) this is the only vṛtti active.

Citta has three functions:

1. Cognition/recognition/perception
2. Will, direction
3. Retention (memory)

Citta has two properties:

1. Pratyaya (conscious thought/feeling in the form of vṛtti-s)
2. Samskara (unconscious, latent impressions formed into a tendency)

In terms of perception, manas is the instrument that processes sensory input; buddhi is the agent that decides on a course of action; and ahaṅkāra uses both, along with memory, to construct an individual's self-image.

Manas (Outer Mind)

Root	man, "think, believe, suppose, imagine; consider, deem; know, understand, perceive"
Dictionary	"mind, heart, understanding, perception, intelligence; internal organ of perception and cognition"
Translation Here	"outer mind"

Manas consists of the sensory organs, motor organs, and all voluntary and involuntary action that takes place in the body. It is responsible for accepting in sensory perceptions and issuing out thoughts, words, and actions. Thus, it takes care of the outer operations of our body and mind. Manas includes likes and dislikes, pleasure and pain, emotions, etc. Because it is so active, manas is the part of citta in which rajas, the quality of activity, predominates.

Ahaṃkāra (Ego)

Word	aham, "I"
Suffix	kāra, "doer, maker, producer"
Dictionary	"egotism, sense of self, self-love; pride, self-conceit; the conception of individuality"
Translation Here	"ego"

Ahaṃkāra is what makes us think that we are our body and mind. Asmitā, "I am-ness," can be a synonym, and is also the affliction (kleśa) of egotism. This component of citta consolidates everything that appears to it through the outer mind into one, unified sense of "I." The ahaṃkāra is responsible for piecing together our complicated experiences into a single, unified "me." It is the tamasic part of citta, since it holds one's identity together.

Our ego likes to be the master, not the slave. When ahaṅkāra calls the shots, our higher, inner mind (buddhi) takes a back seat, which usually results in some form of suffering. The ego can become attached to its position of power, afraid that relinquishing control will somehow mean the beginning of the end of the individual. This fear, caused by ignorance (avidyā), limits the influence of the impartial buddhi on thoughts and actions, and spans all five deep afflictions (kleśa-s) that torment our psyche.

BUDDHI (INNER MIND)

Root	budh, "know, understand, comprehend; notice, recognize; consider; reflect; awaken; advise"

Dictionary "perception, comprehension; intellect, intelligence; knowledge; discrimination, judgment, discernment"

This aspect of citta is the gateway to our pure, inner light of awareness, the Puruṣa. The purpose of buddhi is to figure out the truth. Buddhi presents its interpretations to the seer, which illuminates it and watches what is displayed on the screen of citta. The buddhi is the sattvic part of citta, inherently transparent and clear. It is the citta's decision maker, the piece that discerns and contemplates and generates new ideas and connections. Outwardly the buddhi acts as our intellect, distinguishing between names and forms, time, space, etc. Inwardly the power of viveka distinguishes between the outer names/forms and the inner consciousness. Viveka-khyāti then further discriminates between the sattvic buddhi, in which the qualities of openness, intelligence, virtue, etc., predominate and the seer. (See Puruṣa.)

In terms of perception and action, manas is the instrument and buddhi is the agent. A traditional example, mentioned in the *Kaṭha Upaniṣad* (3.3–4), is riding a chariot. The road represents sense objects, the horses are the sensory organs, the reins are the dual-natured mind, the chariot driver is the buddhi, and the chariot master is the ātman/Puruṣa. If the driver lets the horses run wild, chaos results. When a discerning intellect (driver) listens to the higher self (master) it can guide the outer mind (reins) in the desired direction, with the sensory organs (horses) following the reins.

CIT AND CITTA

Cit is our unconditioned heart-mind field of consciousness, equivalent to the unchanging inner light of awareness, called Puruṣa. Interestingly, it is also used as a suffix in Sanskrit to create an "indefinite pronoun." Cit represents something indefinable and incommunicable.

Citta is conditioned cit and becomes conditioned over time as we experience the world. This conditioning can distort our perception, causing us to act without an accurate understanding of external objects.

Purification and clarification of citta (citta-prasādana) is the primary goal of yoga and leads us to connect with our divine inner awareness. All perception and action create impressions in our memory that can affect our subsequent perception and action. (See karma and saṃskāra.) Deep patterns cause our citta to become biased in one direction or another and distracted by the resulting chatter happening there (vṛtti-s).

The individual's heart-mind field of consciousness (citta, specifically the buddhi) is innately sattvic (see guṇa-s), having the ability to become transparent to allow the inner light of knowledge to shine through for us to experience. Citta is the medium through which the ātman manifests its light. (See appendix F, figure 4.) The ego (ahaṅkāra) part of citta makes us identify ourselves as our thoughts, emotions, and body, yet the citta is not limited to these things. Citta can be focused on anything at all and can take on the characteristics of whatever it is focused on. The presence of distracting activities in the heart-mind (vṛtti-s) in the form of thoughts, ideas, baggage, etc., is what blocks us from experiencing the inner light of Puruṣa.

The ahaṃkāra (ego) is responsible for piecing together our complicated experiences into a single, unified "me" (4.4). Those around us influence our personality, so our individual identity is molded by other individual identities that we come in contact with. Conversely, our heart-mind can influence other heart-minds through motivation (4.5). A strong, charismatic personality can get others to follow along, even if doing so is unhealthy or harmful. A citta polished by meditation produces only positive, sattvic influences that leave no karmic residue behind (4.6).

When an object is experienced, the sensory signals pass through every component of the heart-mind, including the outer mind (manas), ego (ahaṃkāra), and intellect (buddhi). (See appendix F, figure 4.) Each person has a set of filters that can distort the reality of an object, resulting in a less-than-perfect perception of what the object is (4.17). When the components are clear, the object is perceived accurately and truthfully. It is the programming of each individual citta that causes the same object to appear differently to different citta-s (4.15). Objects are independent from any individual citta (4.16). The Puruṣa, resting in stillness, witnesses the operations in the heart-mind (4.18) with its unique, inherent self-luminosity. Relative to the Puruṣa, the citta is an object that is not self-luminous (4.19). So the Puruṣa illuminates its object, the citta, and the citta perceives external objects. The citta cannot perceive itself and its object simultaneously (4.20), for so doing would lead to a recursive cycle of perception and confusion of memories (4.21). When an object is reflected in the citta, the Puruṣa is aware of the change (4.22). The citta is the middleman between external objects and the Puruṣa, the medium through which perception passes and on which the inner light of awareness shines (4.23). This is why clarification of the citta is the primary process of yoga. This heart-mind complex contemplates, coordinates, and collaborates all the multifarious aspects of perception and action for the primary purpose of experiencing the inner light of awareness, the Puruṣa (4.24).

Complete Translation

4.17 taduparāgāpekṣitvāccittasya vastu jñātājñātam

tad-uparāga-apekṣitvāt cittasya vastu jñāta-ajñātam

tad	that
uparāga	reflected color
apekṣitva	necessity
citta	heart-mind field of consciousness
vastu	object
jñāta	known
ajñāta	unknown

1. Because of the heart-mind being dependent on its reflected color, an object is either known or unknown.
2. We visually know an object based on the color of light reflected off it. If no reflection is there, we do not see it and therefore it is unknown to us.

Derivation of Terms

Root	cit, "to perceive, see, notice, observe; know, understand, be aware of"
Dictionary	cit, "heart, mind; soul, spirit"
Dictionary	citta, "observing; thought, attention; the mind; the heart; the reasoning faculty"

Related Sūtra-s

4.4–6, 4.15–16, 4.18–24

Contemplations

What do I favor more, my intellect or my emotions?

Can I catch myself when my ego exercises power over my intuition?

How does it feel when I act from a completely selfless place?

PURUṢA

Pure Inner Light of Awareness

तदा द्रष्टुः स्वरूपे ऽवस्थानम् ॥ १.३ ॥

1.3 tadā draṣṭuḥ svarūpe 'vasthānam

When the citta-vṛtti-s no longer cloud perception,
then pure awareness (Puruṣa) shines through
and is experienced within oneself.

Commentary

The ***Puruṣa*** is an individual's inner light of awareness, an inner spectator watching events unfold in the heart-mind. It only sees what the heart-mind presents to it. (See appendix F, figure 4.) Also known as the ātman, it is that underlying, conscious, changeless spirit that animates life and illuminates the truth.

Synonyms may broaden our understanding. Jīvātman means "having the nature of life" since the Puruṣa is the subtle essence that pervades life itself. It denotes one's individual spirit. Draṣṭā means "seer," as in the changeless entity that watches the activities taking place in the manifest world from behind the heart-mind, as if watching a movie.

The Puruṣa is the individual spirit that is part of the universal spirit. The greeting "namaste" literally means "salutations to you." On a deeper level it connotes honoring the Puruṣa that resides inside the other person. Seeing all beings as manifestations of the same light of awareness allows us to detach from outer labels, opinions, and judgments and act in a kinder and more compassionate way. Humans look different on the outside, but our basic inner nature is the same. The realization that all life forms share the same inner stuff of life encourages us to act toward others as if they are ourselves.

Puruṣa is difficult to explain in words or understand intellectually. The rational mind has trouble grasping anything that cannot be perceived by the sensory organs or constructed based on logic or hard evidence. As we turn our attention inward by introspection and meditation (saṃyama), the rational mind softens and opens to the experiences happening inside. Sometimes unanswerable questions, like the koans of Zen Buddhism or witnessing something inexplicable, serve to shock the logical mind and wake us up to new possibilities.

Large portions of the *Veda-s, Upaniṣad-s,* and the vast array of literature that followed are devoted to discussing the Puruṣa in great detail. Vedānta itself is primarily concerned with the question, "Who am I really?" and "What is the Puruṣa?" whereas yoga addresses "How can I experience the Puruṣa?"

It may be easier to understand Puruṣa in terms of its partner, Prakṛti. (See draṣṭṛ and dṛśya.) Essentially, Prakṛti represents the material world, which is considered unconscious and transient. Puruṣa is the underlying consciousness that pervades every atom of Prakṛti, yet is not affected by any of its changes. This background seer can influence our heart-mind in terms of decision-making. In fact one goal of practicing yoga is to reach the state in which our decisions and actions are based on perceiving our environment clearly and accurately, illuminated by the inner light of awareness, as opposed to functioning with clouded perception. (See appendix F, figure 6.)

The process of creation (2.19) begins when the spirit (Puruṣa, considered masculine) is attracted to nature (Prakṛti, considered feminine, like Mother Earth). This intimacy causes the guṇa-s (qualities of nature: sattva, rajas, and tamas) to stir, triggering a sequence of creation. (See draṣṭṛ and dṛśya.) The seer is not affected by the changing guṇa-s of nature, or by the thoughts or actions of an individual (2.20), and exists only to watch events unfold (2.21). As we can clearly perceive a situation when our heart-mind is quiet and objective, so the Puruṣa, quiet, still, and changeless, sees the activities in the heart-mind for what they are (4.18). When a person experiences kaivalya, a full awareness of the seer within (4.34), her body has fulfilled its purpose and in that state ceases to exist as a separate entity, even though other people around still perceive a body there (2.22).

Īśvara is a kind of Puruṣa that is universal and represents all knowledge known and to be known (1.25).

By focusing inward (saṃyama) and truly realizing that our own heart-mind, specifically the inherently sattvic buddhi, is distinct from the Puruṣa, knowledge of Puruṣa arises (3.35), leading to an intuitive flash, suprasensory perception, (3.36) and complete knowledge of the citta (3.49). (See saṃyama.)

Complete Translation

1.3 tadā draṣṭuḥ svarūpe 'vasthānam

tadā draṣṭuḥ svarūpe avasthānam

tadā	then
draṣṭṛ	the seer, the individual's witness state, Puruṣa
svarūpa	its own form
svasthāna	resting, dwelling

1. Then (in the state of yoga) the radiant seer (is seen clearly) resting in its own form.
2. When the citta-vṛtti-s no longer cloud perception, then pure awareness (Puruṣa) shines through and is experienced within oneself.

Derivation of Terms

Original Root	pṛ, "to fill; to sustain; to carry across"
Word	pur, "town, city"
Root	vas, "to reside, dwell" (changes to uṣa)
Dictionary	"person; the pupil of the eye; the passive, witnessing soul"
Literal Meaning	"resides in the city"
Translation Here	"pure light of awareness"

Related Sūtra-s

1.25; 2.19–22; 3.35–36, 49; 4.18, 34

Contemplations

Can I see through another's outer form, knowing that his pure light of awareness shines within him?

How can I practice "namaste" more often, without actually saying it?

How would it feel if someone else treated me with unconditional love?

DRAṢṬṚ AND DṚŚYA

Seer and Seen

तदर्थ एव दृष्यस्यात्मा ॥ २.२१ ॥

2.21 tadartha eva dṛṣyasyātmā
The manifest world exists only so the seer has something to perceive.

Commentary
The seer (***draṣṭṛ***) is our inner light of awareness, described fully in its own section (Puruṣa). ***Dṛṣya*** represents what the seer sees: the entire cosmic process, all matter and energy that encompass the changing, manifest world. Dṛṣya refers to Prakṛti, the more definitive term used in the Sāṅkhya philosophy. Prakṛti literally means "producing/acting forth," since it is always changing. Prakṛti also means "nature" and represents the original substratum of nature. The following table compares the seer with the seen:

SEER (DRAṢṬṚ/PURUṢA)	SEEN (DṚŚYA/PRAKṚTI)
Conscious	Unconscious
Inactive	Active
Permanent	Impermanent
Intelligent	Unintelligent
Unchanging	Changing
Unmanifest	Potential to manifest/gives rise to manifestation
Seer/Witness	Seeable/observable
Subject	Object
Independent	Dependent
Uniform	Composite
Absolute	Phenomenal

If the subject is the seer/observer and the object is the seeable/observable, then the citta (heart-mind field) is responsible for the act of seeing/observing. Again, citta is the middleman between the perceiver and what is perceived. From the perspective of Puruṣa, both the process of observing and the objects of observation are part of Prakṛti, the illusory and transient manifest world.

OBJECT	HEART-MIND	SUBJECT
Draśya (seeable/ observable)	Darśana (seeing/ observing)	Draṣṭā (seer/observer)
Prakṛti/māyā	Prakṛti/māyā	Puruṣa
Prameya (perceivable)	Pramāṇa (evaluating)	Pramatā (perceiver)

Distinguishing between the seer and seen is a major realization that is said to remove the dark covering of ignorance (avidyā) in the heart-mind, allowing the light of the seer to illuminate our heart-mind, which finally experiences its true nature. Thinking the seer and seeable are the same (see saṃyoga) is the basic blunder that prevents us from connecting with this inner light of awareness.

The universal dance known as "līlā" represents nature's dance, māyā, performed only for the seer, Puruṣa. Nature and its processes provide experience and a means to emancipation (2.18). The seer is not affected by the changing guṇa-s of nature, or by the thoughts or actions of an individual (2.20), and exists only to watch events unfold (2.21). When a person experiences kaivalya, a full awareness of the seer within, then his body has fulfilled its purpose and ceases to exist in his consciousness, even though other people around still perceive a body there (2.22).

Complete Translation

2.21 tadartha eva dṛṣyasyātmā

tad-arthaḥ eva dṛṣyasya ātmā

tad	(of) that (draṣṭṛ—the seer, observer)
artha	purpose
eva	only
dṛṣya	the seeable, seen, observed, manifest world
ātmā	nature

1. The nature of the seen exists only for the purpose of that (seer).
2. The manifest world exists only so the seer has something to perceive.

Derivation of Terms

Original Root dṛś "to see, look at, observe, behold; perceive; examine"

DRAṢṬṚ

Literal Meaning "seer, observer"

Dictionary "seer; judge"

DṚṢYA

Literal Meaning "seeable, observable; to be seen/observed"

Dictionary "to be seen/looked at; a visible object; the visible world"

Related Sūtra-s

2.18–22; 4.23

Contemplations

Can I recognize that everything changes, even things that do not seem to change?

Is it comforting to know that there exists a pure, unchanging awareness within all things?

How can I step back and watch events happening around me, as an objective and unaffected witness?

VIVEKA-KHYĀTI
Discriminating Perception

विवेकख्यातिरविप्लवा हानोपायः ॥ २.२६ ॥

2.26 vivekakhyātiraviplavā hānopāyaḥ
Mindful and continuous discriminating perception
is the way to the goal (kaivalya).

Commentary

Viveka-khyāti is a quality of the buddhi in which we knowingly and consciously discern one object from another. This is the opposite of avidyā. We make decisions and judgments all the time, every day, about things such as what to eat, how to dress, where to go, what to do, etc. Exercising clear judgment and taking into account what is helpful versus harmful can help avoid future suffering.

For example, an artist and a child can have the same perception of a painting, but the child will not see the painting as artistically significant because he or she has not developed discrimination. Both the realized yogi and the ordinary person have the same perception of the physical body, but the ignorant person identifies the body as herself, while the yogi sees the body as an instrument only, a formation of Prakṛti that her true nature has no connection with.

By distinguishing between what is permanent (seer) and what is transitory (seeable) we can overcome saṃyoga, the false superimposition of the seer onto the seeable. As we approach the stages leading up to kaivalya, we must discriminate between the sattvic buddhi and the Puruṣa, lest we prematurely think that a sattvic buddhi is the end in itself. When we see only the guṇa-s in objects and nothing else, kaivalya is imminent.

Discernment results from practicing the eight limbs, which remove impurities from the body and clean the dust (avidyā) off the mirror of the citta in order to let the inner light of knowledge shine through (2.28). Whenever our faculty of judgment (buddhi) listens to our clear, inner voice instead of our ego, we act selflessly.

In any action, it is important to know:

- Where/who we are (current state)
- Where we want to go (goal)
- Steps to get there (means)

After we have progressed through the preliminary stages (the eight limbs of yoga), eventually viveka-khyāti becomes continuous. When viveka-khyāti is continuously present at every moment, kaivalya is assured (2.26). At this point we are not interested in achieving anything more, and are showered with a raincloud of virtue, called dharma-megha-samādhi (4.29). Our focus is so strong that the extraordinary (powers: see saṃyama) gives way to the ordinary. This is the beginning of the now inevitable experience of kaivalya, absolute oneness. We have progressed from an outer orientation to an inner, simple state of stillness, a single flame of awareness.

The seven stages of insight from viveka-khyāti (2.27) are:

1. Recognize that there is pain or discomfort
2. Identify the cause of the pain and reduce it by weakening the kleśa-s (2.1, 2)
3. End the kleśa-s; nirodha/sabīja-samādhi is accomplished, (4.30) and we can now discern between seer and seeable (4.25)
4. The heart-mind is no longer occupied by practice; no more effort is needed (4.28)
5. The discriminating buddhi has finished its work (4.29)
6. The guṇa-s are known and do not affect our attention (4.32)
7. Nirbīja-samādhi or kaivalya: we are no longer limited by Prakṛti (4.34)

Complete Translation

2.26 vivekakhyātiraviplavā hānopāyaḥ

viveka-khyātiḥ aviplavā hāna-upāyaḥ

viveka	discrimination, discernment
khyāti	awareness, realization, understanding, identification
viveka-khyāti	identification with viveka; integration of viveka
aviplavā	flowing continuously, uninterrupted
hāna	end
upāya	way

1. Continuous viveka-khyāti is the way to the end (kaivalya).
2. Mindful and continuous discriminating perception is the way to the goal (kaivalya).

Derivation of Terms

VIVEKA

Prefix	vi, "separating, dividing"
Root	vic, "separate, sever; discriminate, distinguish, discern"

Prefixed Root	vivic, "separate, divide, remove from; discern; ascertain, judge"
Literal Meaning	"discernment"
Dictionary	"discrimination, judgment, discernment; consideration, investigation; power of distinguishing between the visible world and the invisible spirit"

KHYĀTI

Root	khyā, "to tell, communicate; to be named; to be made known"
Dictionary	"renown, fame, glory; knowledge"
Translation Here	"awareness, knowing"

VIVEKA-KHYĀTI

Dictionary	"right knowledge"
Translation Here	"knowing how to distinguish, discriminating awareness"

Related Sūtra-s

2.27–28; 3.52–54; 4.26, 29

Contemplations

Can I take more time before making an important decision?

How often do I submit to peer pressure when deciding on a course of action?

How can I maintain a continuous state of discriminating perception?

ABHYĀSA

Diligent, Focused Practice

तत्र स्थितौ यत्नो ऽभ्यासः ॥ १.१३ ॥

1.13 tatra sthitau yatno 'bhyāsaḥ
Diligent practice is the effort put forth to maintain a point of focus.

Commentary

Abhyāsa can be thought of as a core practice, one that is absolutely necessary to yoga. With viveka (wise discernment), it is the basis of all progress. Consistent and persistent effort toward a goal is bound to succeed. Here, the goal is complete understanding of and absorption in the chosen object (samādhi).

During an āsana practice, abhyāsa might be simply directing our mind to a particular body part that is stretching, or to our breath, or to the location of the gaze. Applied to a meditation practice (dhyāna), it is the effort exerted to maintain a point of focus.

Sūtra 1.14 describes how abhyāsa is to be accomplished. Abhyāsa is a disciplined, persistent effort at remaining focused, and is more subtle than sādhana, which involves specific physical, mental, and social practices. (See aṣṭāṅga and kriyā-yoga.) Yet abhyāsa is not as subtle as dhyāna, which is also defined as an uninterrupted focusing at a place (3.2). Whereas dhyāna is introspective meditation, abhyāsa is like a daily practice that can involve āsana (yoga posture), prāṇāyāma (breathing exercises), or even the focused act of playing a musical instrument or driving a car. As long as a yoga practice includes the qualities mentioned in 1.13 and 1.14 (see below) it can be considered abhyāsa:

- Effort of focusing on a point
- Over a long period of time
- Uninterrupted
- With sincerity
- Firmly grounded

Abhyāsa involves viveka and results in vairāgya (detached awareness). Both viveka and vairāgya are rooted in the yama-s and niyama-s. Abhyāsa and vairāgya are necessary for nirodha of the vṛtti-s (1.12). In the classical sense, there is no yoga practice without abhyāsa and vairāgya.

In the beginning, it can be difficult to establish a regular practice. Each time we practice, an impression is made in our subconscious heart-mind. Over time, the abhyāsa becomes a habit (saṃskāra) that eventually becomes stronger than other, less helpful habits. As the momentum of abhyāsa strengthens, practicing becomes easier and the beneficial results accrue. For example, we want to learn how to cook our own meals instead of eating at restaurants all the time. At first it takes a while to acquire the ingredients and follow the recipe. Each time we make the same dish, it becomes easier. Eventually a recipe that began as difficult and time consuming now seems simple and fast.

Abhyāsa on a single object can prevent or counteract the nine obstacles (antarāya-s) and their symptoms (1.30–32). Focusing on one object will reduce these distractions. It is important to stay on track and not give up, even when we want to.

Complete Translation

1.13 tatra sthitau yatno 'bhyāsaḥ

tatra sthitau yatnaḥ abhyāsaḥ

tatra	there
sthiti	staying, remaining
yatna	effort
abhyāsa	diligent, continuous practice, vigilance

1. Abhyāsa is the effort at remaining there.
2. Diligent practice is the effort put forth to maintain a point of focus.

Derivation of Terms

Root	abhyas, "to practice, exercise; repeat; learn by practice"
Dictionary	"repetition; repeated practice; habit; discipline"
Translation Here	"the effort put forth to maintain a focus"

Related Sūtra-s

1.12, 14, 32

Contemplations

Can I carve out time in my schedule when I am not interrupted during my practice?

Am I able to practice regularly and consistently over a long period of time?

Is my personality preventing me from accruing the momentum needed to keep my practice going?

VAIRĀGYA

Nonattachment to Sensory Objects

दृष्टानुश्रविकविषयवितृष्णस्य वशीकारसंज्ञा वैराग्यम् ॥ १.१५ ॥

1.15 dṛṣṭānuśravikaviṣayavitṛṣṇasya vaśīkārasaṃjñā vairāgyam
Vairāgya is a state of consciousness in which the mind no longer thirsts for objects perceivable by the senses, heard about or read.

Commentary

The state of ***vairāgya***, which can result from diligent, focused practice (abhyāsa), is characterized by an indifference to objects and a detachment from them. When an object is perceived it can produce an attraction, which can lead to an attachment. Over time the attachment may grow stronger, to the extent that we crave the object. This is the kleśa called rāga. Actions repeated over and over create deep patterns (saṃskāra-s) in our consciousness, which usually influence future action or reaction. Consciously directing our desires inward is different from attempting to restrict our outer desires.

Thirst (tṛṣṇa) is more intense than hunger and is commonly used to indicate a very strong craving. The "vi" prefix cuts the thirst into its opposite, vitṛṣṇa or noncraving. Vairāgya is to not allow our past action-patterns, addictions, or strong desires to affect our focus. Vairāgya is not a struggle with desires, but the result of an enduring abhyāsa that naturally leads to disinclination toward wordly desires. There is nothing inherently wrong with desiring something. But if we cannot fulfill that desire, can we let go of it or will we become upset? Vairāgya contains the ability to let go of unfulfilled desires.

The steps leading up to vairāgya are:

1. Trying not to succumb to desire, which over time makes it easier to resist temptation
2. Developing an attitude of nonattachment over time
3. Unattaching our sensory organs to objects (but the tendency for attachment remains in the mind)
4. Arriving at, finally, vairāgya = vaśīkāra-saṃjñā: there is no more effort or conflict, and desire for the object has gone away.

Vairāgya, with abhyāsa, is necessary for the quality of nirodha (silencing) to arise (1.12) and thereby render the vṛtti-s mute (1.2).

Eventually the nonclinging extends even to the guṇa-s themselves (1.16) and is termed paravairāgya, which is a higher, more subtle vairāgya. This state, where one's focus is not influenced by the operations of the guṇa-s or distracted by external objects (gross or subtle) only occurs in kaivalya (4.34), the ultimate state of connection with one's inner divinity. In 1.16, Patañjali takes the term for nonclinging (vitṛṣṇa) to a subtler level (vaitṛṣṇya) to accurately represent this higher level of nonattachment (paravairāgya).

Complete Translation

1.15 dṛṣṭānuśravikaviṣayavitṛṣṇasya vaśīkārasaṃjñā vairāgyam

dṛṣṭa anuśravika-viṣaya-vitṛṣṇasya vaśīkāra-saṃjñā vairāgyam

dṛṣṭa	seen
anuśravika	heard after
viṣaya	sensory object
vitṛṣṇa	nonclinging, noncraving (vi + tṛṣṇa)
vaśīkāra-saṃjñā	full knowledge of mastery
vairāgya	unattached awareness, noninvolvement, noninterference

1. Vairāgya is the complete mastery of nonclinging to sensory objects heard or seen.
2. Vairāgya is a state of consciousness in which the mind no longer thirsts for objects perceivable by the senses, heard about or read.

Derivation of Terms

Prefix	vi, "separating, cutting through, discerning"
Original Root	rañj, "to color, tinge; to be attached to; to be enamored of"
Prefixed Root	virañj, "to grow discolored or soiled, to be coarse or rough; to be disaffected"
Word	virāga, "change of color; change of disposition; disaffection; indifference to worldly attachments"
Literal Meaning	vairāgya, "having a disposition of disaffection or indifference"
Dictionary	vairāgya, "absence of worldly passions, indifference to the world"
Translation Here	"absence of clinging, nonattachment to external objects, noninvolvement"
Other Translations	"nonreaction, dispassion, disinterest"

Related Sūtra-s

1.16

Contemplations

How can I remain unattached to a situation and still experience emotion?

Am I aware when vairāgya is happening?

How strong is my desire for inner development?

YOGA AS NIRODHA
Silencing the Heart-Mind

योगश्चित्तवृत्तिनिरोधः ॥ १.२ ॥

1.2 yogaścittavṛttinirodhaḥ
Yoga is the process of calming down the heart-mind.

Commentary
Sūtra 1.2 provides the primary definition of yoga in this text, a process of thinning away or quieting the thoughts and emotions in our heart-mind. ***Nirodha*** results from the practices of yoga, especially a focused heart-mind. Sūtra 1.3 describes the state of yoga that results from the process of nirodha. Therefore yoga can be a means (process or practice) or an end (state).

As a process or practice, yoga connects our individual consciousness to the universal consciousness. Several yoga practices are mentioned in Patañjali's sūtra-s. The eight limbs of yoga (aṣṭāṅga-yoga) provide tools to refine ourselves and draw our attention inward. Kriyā-yoga, the synergistic triad of transformational practice, self-observation, and faith, is meant to weaken our deep afflictions (kleśa-s) and attain the state of complete attention (samādhi). We could say that saṃyama-yoga represents a subset of the eight-limbs that represents focusing inward and experiencing samādhi.

As a state (called niruddha, equivalent to samādhi), our attention is fully focused, resulting in the quelling of all distractions in the consciousness. Nirodha is a quality of citta resulting from the practice of yoga. Nirodha is not actively avoiding, suspending, or ending the vṛtti-s. It is present when all of our attention is focused in one direction, causing the vṛtti-s to submerge and the inner light of knowledge to emerge.

When we are in the state of yoga (1.3), our consciousness is quiet, and we experience the presence of our inner light of awareness, our true Self. This "seer" is resting in the perception of itself, and is experienced as clarity, understanding, compassion, and happiness. The citta is no longer tainted by the vṛtti-s or kleśa-s. We are unaware of our awareness because there is no separation between our individual self and our inner Self. This yoga is samādhi. Otherwise (1.4) we are in vṛtti-land, preoccupied, caught in the world of thoughts and memories that our individual ego erroneously identifies as our Self.

Nirodha of the vṛtti-s depends on two pillars of yoga: abhyāsa and vairāgya (1.12). The former, diligent and continuous practice, results in the latter, detached awareness, which in turn causes nirodha. As the business in the heart-mind slows down, the patterns become simpler and less distracting. As nirodha is practiced habitually, the fluctuations erode and a new, beneficial saṃskāra forms that eventually supersedes previous negative saṃskāra-s. This reprogramming of the heart-mind is the key to inner happiness.

Vyāsa describes certain states of mind leading up to nirodha:

- Kṣipta (restless)
- Mūḍha (stupified, infatuated, obsessed)
- Vikṣipta (distracted—calm at one time, restless at another, so changeable, up and down)
- Ekāgra (one-pointed, focused on a single thought continuously)
  - Leads to samprajñāta-yoga—vitarka, vicāra, ānanda, asmitā
  - Weakens the kleśa-s
  - Loosens bonds of karma
- Niruddha (the heart-mind is still, undistracted by any thoughts, emotions, or sensory input)

Complete Translation

1.2 yogaścittavṛttinirodhaḥ

yogaḥ citta-vṛtti-nirodhaḥ

yoga	connection, relationship, union, application
citta	heart-mind field of consciousness
vṛtti	fluctuation or activity in the heart-mind
nirodha	stilling, settling, calming, breaking

1. Yoga is quelling the fluctuations in the heart-mind field of consciousness.
2. Yoga occurs when we focus completely on a single object so that thoughts and emotions in our heart-mind field of consciousness do not distract us anymore.

Derivation of Terms

YOGA

Root	yuj, "to join, unite, attach, connect; to yoke; to use, apply; to concentrate our attention on"
Dictionary	"joining, uniting; union; connection; application; means"
Translation Here	"connection, relationship, harmonizing, developing composure"

NIRODHA

Prefix	ni, "down; into"
Original Root	rudh, "to obstruct, stop, arrest, impede; to conceal"
Prefixed Root	nirudh, "to obstruct, stop, oppose, block up; keep off; curb, restrain"
Dictionary	"confinement, locking up; enclosing, covering up; restraint, suppression, control"
Translation Here	"stilling, silencing, calming, dissolving, quelling"

Related Sūtra-s

1.3–4, 12

Contemplations

Has my yoga practice really calmed my heart-mind?

Am I conscious of the process of nirodha happening in myself?

When does my heart-mind fall into agitated or distracted states?

ĪŚVARA
Source of Knowledge

क्लेशकर्मविपाकाशयैरपरामृष्टः पुरुषविशेष ईश्वरः ॥ १.२४ ॥

1.24 kleśakarmavipākāśayairaparāmṛṣṭaḥ
puruṣaviśeṣa īśvaraḥ
Īśvara is a different kind of Puruṣa, unaffected by anything that happens in the manifest world.

Commentary

Īśvara is knowledge itself. Whereas our individual Puruṣa watches and is entertained by the manifest dance of Prakṛti, Īśvara exists as a universal source of knowledge. The individual Puruṣa, called the jīvātman, is bound in and by the body, while the universal (as opposed to the individual) Puruṣa, called paramātman or Īśvara, is not bound by time, space, or anything.

Īśvara is the seed of all knowledge (1.25) and can influence action if one taps into it. Actions coming from the place of Īśvara create beneficial (yogic) saṃskāra-s. In any given situation, a broader, more informed heart-mind allows us to see the whole picture, understand all points of view, and then act for the benefit of everyone. For example, a general contractor who has years of experience and a wide range of knowledge can anticipate and avoid potential pitfalls a novice would otherwise fall into.

Īśvara is best considered a teacher, and can bring about transformation just as a human teacher can catalyze inspiration and insight in a student's heart-mind by the transmission of knowledge. Some call Īśvara the original and eternal teacher (1.26), or ādiguru. All knowledge learned in the manifest world ultimately sprouts from the seed of Īśvara. Whether past, present, or future, this universal intelligence will always be available to those who seek to understand the truth.

Praṇava means "arising forth" and is the sound that began creation (1.27). Praṇava is the audio form of Īśvara, and so provides a direct link to Īśvara. By way of analogy:

ENTITY	EXPRESSION
Īśvara	Praṇava (like Om)
Meaning of a word	Sound of a word
Lamp	Light

Praṇava in other traditions may be different. Many religions have their own sound that connects the followers to the same divine source of knowledge, here named Īśvara. In India, that sound is typically Om, the Vedic expression of Īśvara.

Om, sometimes written "aum," has three component sounds. In Sanskrit, a + u becomes o. The first sound, "a," begins the Sanskrit alphabet and also represents the beginning of creation. The second sound, "u," represents preservation of creation. The third sound, "m," made by closing the lips, represents the end of creation, or dissolution. In the beginning was the sound, and that sound was Om. Om is the genesis of creation.

Japa (repetition) implies reciting a mantra over and over again. The more something is repeated, the more powerful its effect on our consciousness. Ritual holds power due to its repetition over many years. Repeating a praṇava links our consciousness to Īśvara. By repeating the praṇava we can feel the essence of Īśvara (1.28). If we mechanically and unattentively repeat this sound, our attention may drift elsewhere. In that case we are not truly practicing japa, which requires a focused heart-mind to experience the essence of praṇava's meaning, which is Īśvara.

Repeating praṇava draws our attention inward, and like pratyāhāra, automatically causes outer distractions like the antarāya-s to disappear (1.29). Sound has a way of reprogramming the consciousness and dissolving obstacles (1.30) like disease, doubt, etc.

Īśvara-praṇidhāna is surrendering and transferring the results of all action to Īśvara.

Īśvara can be worshipped through our iṣṭadevatā, "chosen deity," a manifestation of our personal source of devotion, a symbol that links us to Īśvara. In this sense some call Īśvara the personal God that resides in our heart. A common iṣṭadevatā in India is Gaṇeśa, the elephant-headed deity representing abundance and the clearing away of obstacles.

In terms of Sāṅkhya, the mahat is Īśvara's intelligence and the buddhi is the individual's intellect.

Complete Translation

1.24 kleśakarmavipākāśayairaparāmṛṣṭaḥ puruṣaviśeṣa īśvaraḥ
kleśa-karma-vipāka-āśayaiḥ aparāmṛṣṭaḥ puruṣa-viśeṣaḥ īśvaraḥ

kleśa	deep emotional affliction
karma	action
vipāka	ripening, fruition
āśaya	container, storehouse
aparāmṛṣṭa	not connected in any way, unaffected by, untouched by
puruṣa	the inner light of awareness, the observer
viśeṣa	special, distinct, separate
Īśvara	the teachings, universal teacher, eternal teacher, omniscience

1. Īśvara is a distinct (and separate) Puruṣa, in no way connected to the storehouse of ripened karma-s and kleśa-s (known as the karmāśaya, or here āśaya).
2. Īśvara is a different kind of Puruṣa, unaffected by anything that happens in the manifest world.

Derivation of Terms

ĪŚVARA

Original Root	īś, "to rule, master, govern, command; to have power; to allow"
Suffix	vara, "best, most precious, finest"
Literal Meaning	"most precious master"
Dictionary	"lord, master; king, ruler; supreme God"
Translation Here	"the universal teacher, all knowledge, the teachings themselves"

Related Sūtra-s

1.25–29

Contemplations

Do I pretend that I own certain knowledge?

Can I accept the presence of an eternal source of knowledge?

What would be appropriate for me as a praṇava?

KARMA AND SAṂSKĀRA
Action and Its Imprint

कर्माशुक्लाकृष्णं योगिनस्त्रिविधमितरेषाम् ॥ ४.७ ॥

4.7 karmāśuklākṛṣṇaṃ yoginastrividhamitareṣām
Actions of those who do not follow yoga are threefold: white (positive/good/right), black (negative/bad/wrong), or gray (neutral). The actions of a yogin (one who follows yoga) transcend good or bad, right or wrong.

Commentary

Karma means action or activity that produces some result. Any input via sensory perception or output via thought, word, or deed can be considered karma. This includes watching a movie, performing an act of kindness, focusing inward, etc. Every karma has consequences that may occur sooner or later and may be obvious or subtle. Karma is recorded in the memory of the heart-mind. When a perception or action is very strong or repeated many times, it becomes a deep impression in memory called a ***saṃskāra***, which is a habit or tendency that can influence future karma. These habitual patterns are stored in a place in memory called the karmāśaya, meaning "accumulation of actions."

Karma has the sense of retribution. As they say, "what goes around comes around." On an individual level, tradition teaches that the karmāśaya travels with a soul from death to rebirth, lifetime to lifetime, ad infinitum as long as a person stays in the cycles of birth and death, called saṃsāra. If a person evolves spiritually and acts in a sattvic way, without being attached to the results (see akarma on the next page), these actions do not accumulate in the karmāśaya, and eventually the previously incurred karma works itself out and the person is said to become enlightened, never to be reborn again.

Newton's third law of motion states: "For every action there is an equal and opposite reaction." On a cosmic level, the cause of an action contains its effects in subtle form. If you want to contribute the energy of kindness and compassion to the universe, act that way. Positive energy begets positive energy, and vice versa. For example, have you noticed how you feel around someone who is kind, generous, and happy? Does it make you feel more that way? On the other hand, when you are in the company of a negative, mean, pessimistic person, how does it make you feel?

Sūtra 4.7 implies four types of karma. The actions of non-yogins are good, bad, and neutral and will create impressions accordingly. The actions of a true yogin, on the other hand, are not based on value judgments, and so will only create or reinforce saṃskāra-s that serve to weaken distracting saṃskāra-s. Thus the yogin moves closer to a heart-mind connected to pure awareness.

There are action, inaction, and akarma. Action is white or black, as above. Inaction is the gray limbo of indecision, when one cannot decide what to do. Akarma, "not karma," is action directed by our inner awareness, not by saṃskāra-s, so we are not really the doer and thus do not create or reinforce any saṃskāra-s.

Every time we register an event (receive a sensory input or produce a thought, word, or deed), a subtle impression is recorded in the memory of our heart-mind. The more intense the event, or the more it is repeated, the stronger the impression. Eventually the impression forms a deep imprint, called a saṃskāra, which becomes part of who we are and influences our actions. "Neurons that fire together, wire together" is a neuroscience phrase based on research supporting this process. For example, if we glance at a squirrel on the road for a split second, it will leave a relatively weak impression. If we go through a painful, traumatic experience like a bad car crash, it will create a much stronger impression that may change how we drive in the future. If we hear a song over and over again, the sound imprints so deeply that we can sing it without even trying to remember it. (See "The Process of Learning" in part 1.) These deep impressions form habits and tendencies that affect our heart-mind. In contrast, "use it or lose it" explains how something learned or experienced, when not reinforced, loses its strength. Even a strong saṃskāra can be weakened over time by not allowing it to influence our actions.

For example, the more you exercise, the more habitual it becomes. As momentum builds, it gets easier and takes less effort to get up and go. If you stop for a while, the habit weakens and is possibly replaced by something else you begin doing more. When exercise is relegated to the back burner, your body weakens.

Negative or harmful saṃskāra-s can condense into kleśa-s, our deepest afflictions and causes of suffering. When our "buttons get pushed," an event has triggered these hurtful parts of ourselves that then arise from the depths of our memory and cause us to react in a negative way. For example, let's say you have sat in the same chair at the kitchen table for the past twenty years. Your son visits and sits in "your" chair for dinner. This may be uncomfortable for you, and you may become a little flustered at first. Some people would become angry and demand their son sit in another chair. Others may ask him politely to sit elsewhere. Either way, there is an underlying saṃskāra that is affecting your behavior, one that has been reinforced for many years, even though on the outside it seems quite unimportant.

Interestingly, saṃskāra is related to saṃskṛta, the word for Sanskrit. The Sanskrit language has been refined and perfected over many eons, and its impression exists in the sound and meaning of the vast literature from India.

Description

A vāsanā is more subtle than a saṃskāra. It comes from the feeling of an event rather than the event itself. Vāsanā-s can carry the energy of saṃskāra-s created during one lifetime into the next life (jāti). Any propensities we are born with are vāsanā-s.

Vāsanā-s are latent impressions of feelings arising from birth, life span, and experience (pleasure/pain), which are the consequences of karma (sensory impression, rumination, thought, word or deed, etc.). They are said to be carried along from lifetime to lifetime with their less subtle counterparts, saṃskāra-s, and can be strengthened or weakened during any lifetime. For example, a kind thought creates a kind feeling in you. The thought itself creates a memory, while the feeling of kindness produces a more subtle vāsanā. See the table below for more examples.

COMPARISON AND DISCUSSION

	SAṂSKĀRA	VĀSANĀ
DEFINITION	Impression left on the heart-mind from an event, subliminal activator	Innate predisposition or propensity, subliminal trait
BASED ON	Acquired by events experienced or actions performed in this lifetime	Saṃskāras from all previous lifetimes
HOW CREATED	Recorded each time an event takes place, then stored in the karmāśaya	Innate vāsanā is then influenced by newly acquired saṃskāra-s
WHERE STORED	Karmāśaya part of subconscious memory	Deep, subtle, subconscious memory
EXAMPLES	Color	Hue
	Good deed	Goodness
	Helping someone	Caring
	Killing	Violence

SUMMARY OF TERMS

karma	An internal or external event experienced: sensory input, internal rumination, or action performed
citta	Heart-mind field of consciousness; substratum conditioned by karma
smṛti	Memory of all karma
saṃskāra	Habitual tendency caused by intense or repeated karmic impressions. Stored in the karmāśaya part of deep memory
vāsanā	Inborn propensity influenced by the feeling experienced during a karma. Is a subtle saṃskāra
karmāśaya	Accumulation of saṃskāra-s and vāsanā-s imprinted in deep memory. Carried from birth to birth, and determines birth, life span, and experience
vṛtti	Activity (thoughts and feelings) in the heart-mind based on the content of the karmāśaya

METAPHOR

Saṃskāra-s are pieces of playdough.

Karmāśaya is a container for the playdough pieces.

Vāsana-s are the hole-shapes through which the playdough is squeezed.

When an external stimulus causes a response:

A round piece of playdough (saṃskāra) is squeezed through a star-shaped hole (vāsana), which changes the form of the original saṃskāra, influencing the resulting action.

Ultimately it is the guṇa-s that are performing action (karma). Our body, mind, and sensory organs carry out the action. A karma creates a memory. Repetition of the same karma, or a very intense karma (like a trauma) creates a new saṃskāra or strengthens an existing saṃskāra.

All karma is influenced by the karmāśaya. When an event triggers a response, here is what happens:

- The initial stimulus causes a habitual tendency (saṃskāra) to arise.
- This tendency (saṃskāra) flows through a more subtle propensity (vāsanā), which alters its effect on the action.
- If the tendency (saṃskāra) is negative, based on an affliction (kleśa), negative thoughts and feelings (kliṣṭa-vṛtti-s) occur in the heart-mind. If the tendency is positive, positive thoughts and feelings (akliṣṭa-vṛtti-s) occur in the heart-mind.

Habitual tendencies (saṃskāra-s) can be ended by discovering what caused them (pratiprasava).

Complete Translation

4.7 karmāśuklākṛṣṇaṃ yoginastrividhamitareṣām

karma-aśukla-akṛṣṇaṃ yoginaḥ trividham itareṣām

karma	action
aśukla	not white
akṛṣṇa	not black
yogin	one who practices yoga as defined in 1.2
trividha	threefold
itara	other

1. The actions of a yogin are neither white nor black. (The actions) of others are threefold.
2. Actions of non-yogins are threefold: white (positive/good/right), black (negative/bad/wrong), or gray (neutral). The actions of a yogin transcend good or bad, right or wrong.

Derivation of Terms

SAṂSKĀRA

Prefix	sam, "completely, together"
Original Root	kṛ (see above for karma)
Prefixed Root	samskṛ, "to adorn; refine, polish; consecrate by repeating mantras; purify (a person); cultivate, educate, train; prepare"
Literal Meaning	"complete training"
Dictionary	"making perfect, refining, polishing; education, cultivation, training; preparation; cooking; impression, form, mold, influence; faculty of recollection, impression on the memory"
Translation Here	"subconscious impression created from an action"
Other Translations	"habitual movement of the mind; habit; conditioning; subliminal impressions"

VĀSANĀ

Root	vās, "to scent; steep, infuse; spice, season (related to vas, "dwell, inhabit, live, stay; to exist, be found in")
Literal Meaning	"a scent, infusion"

Dictionary	"knowledge derived from memory; the impression unconsciously left on the mind by past good and bad actions, producing pleasure or pain; imagination; false idea; inclination"
Translation Here	"innate predisposition; a deep, subtle influence on actions"
Other Translations	"subliminal/subconscious trait; latent tendency; subliminal trait"

KARMA

Root	kṛ, "to do; to make; to create; to produce; act, perform"
Dictionary	karman, "action, work; performance of action; business"

Related Sūtra-s

4.8–11, 4.24

Contemplations

What patterns do I possess, and how does each influence or drive my behavior?

If any saṃskāra causes negativity to arise, how can I transform that into something positive?

What harmful habitual patterns am I reinforcing on a regular basis?

Can I reduce negative sensory impressions coming my way? How?

What new, helpful habits do I wish to cultivate?

PARIṆĀMA
Change

परिणामैकत्वाद्वस्तुतत्त्वम् ॥ ४.१४ ॥

4.14 pariṇāmaikatvādvastutattvam
Every object is a unique combination of guṇa-s at a particular moment in space-time due to the continuous changes occuring in matter.

Commentary
Everything in nature is changing from moment to moment. Even our DNA mutates ever so slowly in the background. Dense or gross objects consisting of predominantly earth and water change more slowly than subtler objects made up of air or gas. The heart-mind can change instantly on the outside, but deeply held opinions and longstanding habits are much less mutable. Deliberate change to purify the body and heart-mind in order to truly connect with our inner awareness requires sincere effort and perseverance. (See abhyāsa.)

HOW CHANGE HAPPENS

Dharmī is the substratum (3.14), the underlying substance that does not fundamentally change but simply appears differently over time. The substrata in the physical realm are the fundamental elements of nature, like hydrogen, tin, copper, gold, etc., found in the periodic table of elements. Transformation has three components to it, which apply to the citta (3.9–12) as well as to the gross elements and sensory organs (3.13):

1. Dharma: Characteristic/external form—what it looks like on the outside
2. Lakṣaṇa: Potential change over time—past, present, or future
3. Avasthā: State—for example, dirty, clean, tarnished, scratched, etc.

For example, if the substratum is gold:

Gold begins in the form of ore in the present. When the gold changes into molten form, then the ore form is past and the molten form is present. When the gold becomes a ring, then the molten form is past and the ring form is present. The ring may stay in this form for many years, during which time its condition changes from new to dirty to scratched to clean and so on. The gold remains gold through all the changes.

For another example, if the substratum is the citta (heart-mind):

1. The citta begins, scattered by vṛtti-s, and contains the potential to become one-pointed.
2. When one-pointedness occurs, then the scattered state is past/old, the one-pointed state is present/new, and the absorbed state has potential.
3. When the absorbed state (samādhi) occurs, the one-pointed state is past and the stilled state is future.
4. Finally, when the citta has reached the stilled state (niruddha; see yoga as nirodha), the absorbed state is past and only oneness (kaivalya) remains to be experienced.

CITTA	PAST FORM	PRESENT FORM	FUTURE (POTENTIAL) FORM
1. Scattered by vṛtti-s		Scattered	One-pointed
2. One-pointed	Scattered	One-pointed	Absorbed
3. Absorbed	One-pointed	Absorbed	Stilled
4. Stilled	Absorbed	Stilled	Oneness

Each change will determine the next set of potential changes (3.15). Using the example of gold above, if the molten gold became a gold coin instead of a ring, its new form would assume a different shape and go through potentially different conditions. By practicing saṃyama on these three components of change, one can understand the progression of changes and figure out the past and likely future forms (3.16). One can apply this line of reasoning to the heart-mind as well. By understanding our longstanding habitual patterns and genetic traits, we can get a glimpse into what might have happened in the past to create them and predict how these might play out in the future. For example, you meet someone who is overly cautious driving a car. By getting to know them closely (saṃyama) you might realize, even without them telling you, that they were in a car accident in the past. Another example might be someone whose posture is quite contracted—their shoulders are hunched and their heart is protected. Again, when you really focus on their posture, you might come to know how this happened and how it might affect the person's behavior now and in the future.

Another type of transformation relates to suffering (duḥkha), mentioned in 2.15. Real change is often difficult and uncomfortable. The easiest way to change is to set an intention and take small steps toward the goal. Rapid change is rarely sustainable, with the exception of change due to a trauma or a very intense and life-changing event.

The *Yoga Sūtra-s* describes several kinds of transformations, (***pariṇāma-s***), as follows:

1. Transformation into nirodha (3.9,10)
   When the saṃskāra-s supporting an active mind are weakened and those supporting a still heart-mind are strengthened (by regular practice of saṃyama), eventually the nirodha (stillness) of the heart-mind occurs more often and subjugates the lower saṃskāra, and it becomes easier to still the heart-mind than to make it active.

   This is the most important and difficult transformation because it involves replacing deep-seated habits with a pattern of clarity and stillness.
2. Transformation into samādhi (3.11)
   When scattered attention goes away and one-pointed attention arises, the state of the heart-mind changes into samādhi.
3. Transformation into ekāgratā (one-pointedness) (3.12)
   When the past thoughts are the same as the present thoughts, the state of the heart-mind becomes one-pointed.

Every object is a unique combination of the three guṇa-s: sattva, rajas, and tamas (4.14). Past memories and future potential exist in the present state of an object (4.12). Previous changes brought it to the current state, and similar changes will likely move it along to its future states. In terms of the heart-mind, its current state can be seen as the result of past habitual patterns, which, if left unchecked, will determine future actions and the future states of the heart-mind. This is how practicing saṃyama on these changes can reveal valuable information about how they arrived in their present state and what the future may look like without breaking the habitual patterns. The characteristic forms of an object may be obvious or subtle and are ultimately just the guṇa-s changing over time (4.13).

All things are created, last for a while, then transform into something else. This is due to the abundant flow of the guṇa-s (4.2). Going with nature's flow often involves ensuring there is no resistance due to obstructions. As a farmer irrigates his field by separating the earth into ditches so the water can flow by itself unobstructed, so the processes within nature (Prakṛti) are directed by removing the obstacles that block the flow from birth to birth (4.3). Removing hindrances lets nature find its way back.

When the guṇa-s stop moving, the transformations end (4.32) and the sequence of changes for an object is finally understood completely (4.33). Change is difficult to perceive while it is happening, especially when the changes occur slowly over a long period of time. Only at the end of the series of changes, when things stop changing, can we fully understand each individual step that led us to the end result. The guṇa-s are eternally changing. Puruṣa is eternally unchanging.

Complete Translation

4.14 pariṇāmaikatvādvastutattvam

pariṇāma-ekatvāt vastu-tattvam

pariṇāma	transformation, change, mutation
ekatvāt	oneness, uniqueness
vastu	object
tattva	essence, "that-ness"

1. The essence of an object is due to the uniqueness of (its) transformations.
2. Every object is a unique combination of guṇa-s at a particular moment in space-time due to the continuous changes occuring in matter.

Derivation of Terms

Prefix	pari, "around"
Original Root	nām, "to name"
Prefixed Root	pariṇam, "to bend or bow down; to be changed or transformed into, assume the form of"
Literal Meaning	same as dictionary
Dictionary	"alteration, change, transformation; digestion; result, consequence; ripening, maturity"
Translation Here	"change, transformation"

Related Sūtra-s

2.15, 3.9–16, 4.2, 3, 12, 13, 32–33

Contemplations

Do the changes I intend happen and endure? Why or why not?

How am I different than I was five years ago? Ten years ago?

Have I noticed any behavioral changes based on an event in my past?

DUḤKHA
Suffering as Opportunity

हेयं दुःखमनागतम् ॥ २.१६ ॥

2.16 heyaṃ duḥkhamanāgatam
Future suffering is avoidable.

Commentary
If we anticipate suffering, we may be able to avoid it. Sometimes we know in our gut that if we follow through with an action it will result in suffering, yet we do it anyway when our habitual patterns (saṃskāra-s) override our good intentions.

In the midst of a painful experience (***duḥkha***), the heart-mind is clouded and it is difficult to understand why it is happening. At some point we can step back and think about why. We can learn from duḥkha and use it as a tool to reveal our habitual tendencies.

We can set a deliberate intention and direction toward our own happiness and personal/spiritual evolution. If we are mindful of this long-term commitment, much suffering can be avoided by acting with discrimination. What will help us versus hinder us toward reaching our goals? Setting an intention to anticipate possible future pain and taking action to bypass it.

The cause of duḥkha is thinking that the seer (Puruṣa) and seen (Prakṛti—the manifest world) are the same (saṃyoga). Saṃyoga also implies becoming too involved in and attached to events.

We can reduce future suffering by

1. Looking closely at how our habitual patterns (saṃskāra-s) determine our actions/reactions
2. Being around wiser people/teachers, listening to them and noticing how they act
3. Using our own discrimination

The direction of yoga moves from outer (second- and thirdhand) indirect knowledge from reading, hearing, and inferring (see the pramāṇa-s āgama and anumāna under vṛtti #1: pramāṇa) toward direct experience (pratyakṣa) and inner advice. Progressing from outer to inner by means of the eight limbs, kriyā-yoga, etc., develops a solid foundation that endures. Jumping headlong into the subtle aspects of our inner self without preparing the body and heart-mind properly may not be sustainable.

There are four stages of suffering, much like the four noble truths of the Buddha:

1. Duḥkha, "suffering"—identify the symptoms of suffering
2. Duḥkha-hetu, "cause of suffering" (kleśa-s)—identify the cause
3. Duḥkha-hāna, "end of suffering" (kaivalya)—make a goal
4. Duḥkha-hāna-upāya, "the means to end suffering" (eight limbs of yoga)—the means to achieve the goal

Duḥkha is not simply physical pain, but can arise from it. Duḥkha is the suffering that occurs in the heart-mind, especially the subtle suffering of feeling disconnected from our inner light of awareness. Duḥkha can result from greed, anger, and delusion and can intensify from mild to medium to excessive (2.34) as follows:

LEVEL OF DUḤKHA	GREED	ANGER	DELUSION
Mild	Want more than we need	Annoyance	Think we know something that we do not
Medium	Take from others if necessary	Verbal spears	View what changes as permanent
Excessive	Already rich; use deceit to get more	Violence	Schizophrenia

Sūtra 2.15 mentions three kinds of duḥkha.

PARIṆĀMA-DUḤKHA	TĀPA-DUḤKHA	SAMSKĀRA-DUḤKHA
Want change, doesn't happen	Get taste, want more, can't have it	Get used to something and form an attachment to it
Don't want change, does happen	Feel deprived	Uncomfortable with something different or unavoidable
Happens too fast or too slow	Craving unsatisfied	Bad eating habits
Change	*What I want*	*What I am used to*

Pariṇāma-duḥkha is suffering caused by change. When the desired change does not happen, or an undesired change happens, it can feel uncomfortable or painful. For example, you want to change your diet but become frustrated when you cannot follow through. Or, moving from a place you have lived for a long time can make you distraught. If you want to change and it actually happens, then there is no pariṇāma-duḥkha.

Tāpa-duḥkha is suffering caused by the friction of unfulfilled desire. When we desire something and cannot have it, or when an expectation is not met, our heart-mind can be thrown off center, causing suffering. For example, you have a relative who is stingy. Every time you see them you hope they will be more generous. When they behave as stingily as usual, you might get upset again. Accepting someone's nature and not expecting anything more will avoid this kind of suffering. If you desire something and are not upset when you cannot have it, this pain is avoided. Letting go of the results of action can prevent tāpa-duḥkha.

Saṃskāra-duḥkha is suffering caused by habitual patterns. Transforming a longtime habit can feel uncomfortable. For example, an unhealthy relationship recently ended, yet you are tempted to enter into it again, knowing that you will be hurt again. If you regress into it, you are letting your old habitual patterns trump your higher thinking, thus causing more suffering. You can listen to your intuitive wisdom and choose to not go back, thus avoiding future suffering.

Complete Translation

2.16 heyaṃ duḥkhamanāgatam

heyaṃ duḥkham anāgatam

heya avoidable, endable

duḥkha suffering, pain, discomfort

anāgata "not yet come," future

1. Future suffering is avoidable.

Derivation of Terms

Prefix	duḥ, "bad, negative"
Original Root	kha, "space"
Prefixed Root	duḥkh, "to pain, afflict, distress"
Dictionary	duḥkha, "sorrow, unhappiness, pain; trouble, difficulty"
Literal Meaning:	"negative space"
Translation Here	"negativity, pain, suffering, discomfort"

Related Sūtra-s

2.17

Contemplations

Can I identify with any of these types of duḥkha?

How can I take steps to prevent future suffering?

Can I learn from my suffering?

SAṂYOGA

False Identification of Seer with Seen

स्वस्वामिशक्त्योः स्वरूपोपलब्धिहेतुः संयोगः ॥ २.२३ ॥

2.23 svasvāmiśaktyoḥ svarūpopalabdhihetuḥ saṃyogaḥ
Confusing what changes (Prakṛti) with what does not change (Puruṣa), thinking they are the same, causes suffering that leads us to inquire as to the true nature of each.

Commentary

Saṃyoga means thinking that the seer (draṣṭṛ) and the seeable (dṛśya) are the same, when they are actually distinct entities eternally mixed together. As salt and water are different until they are mixed and seem as one, so the Puruṣa invisibly pervades the manifest world. The confusion of saṃyoga partly results from applying the concepts of time and space, which are qualities of the manifest world, to something that is beyond them.

In saṃyoga we are too close to a situation. There is no space for observation and thus we lack a proper perspective. Saṃyoga causes suffering (duḥkha) (2.17). When we can distinguish between what sees and what is seen by stepping back and observing a situation, we can put what we perceive in the proper perspective. This can be called viyoga: union with discrimination, the ability to separate from things that cause suffering.

Avidyā, the shroud of ignorance covering the inner light of awareness, is the cause of saṃyoga (2.24) because it prevents our heart-mind from seeing clearly. Thus we superimpose the seer and the seen, which empowers our ego (asmitā 2.6) and keeps us trapped in the cycle of kleśa-s, karma-s, etc. Asmitā is an expression of saṃyoga when the Puruṣa and citta are taken as one and the same thing and identified as part of the individual's sense of "I."

Sūtra 2.23 reminds us of the concepts of vitarka and pratipakṣa-bhāvana, wherein a negative event triggers positive thoughts. For example, when we witness someone stealing, it reminds us that stealing is harmful, so we may try to help in some positive way. Here, the confusion itself (saṃyoga) creates suffering (2.17), which leads to stepping back and noticing that whatever changes is different from that which never changes, our divine inner awareness.

Complete Translation

2.23 svasvāmiśaktyoḥ svarūpopalabdhihetuḥ saṃyogaḥ

sva-svāmi-śaktyoḥ svarūpa-upalabdhi-hetuḥ saṃyogaḥ

sva	one's own self, what is "owned"
svāmi	master, owner
śakti	power
sva-śakti	seeable
svāmi-śakti	seer
svarūpa	one's true nature
upalabdhi	acquisition, perception attained, realization
hetu	cause, reason
saṃyoga	confusion; mistakenly identifying the seer as the seen

1. Superimposing the powers of the master (seer) and what is owned (seeable) is the reason for realizing the true nature of them both.
2. Confusing what changes (Prakṛti) with what does not change (Puruṣa), thinking they are the same, causes suffering that leads us to inquire as to the true nature of each.

Derivation of Terms

Prefix	sam, "completely, together"
Root	yuj, "unite, join, connect, yoke"
Dictionary	"join completely, associate, superimpose, involvement"
Translation Here	saṃyoga, "identification, confusion, superimposition, correlation"

Related Sūtra-s

2.17, 24–25

Contemplations

Am I aware when my perspective is biased from being too personally involved in a situation?

What can cause me to remember the distinction between the changing world and the changeless seer?

How does it feel when I remember this distinction?

VṚTTI-S

Chatter in the Citta

प्रमाणविपर्ययविकल्पनिद्रास्मृतयः ॥ १.६ ॥

1.6 pramāṇaviparyayavikalpanidrāsmṛtayaḥ
(The fluctuations of the heart-mind are) correct evaluation, misperception, imagination, sleep, and the act of memory.

Commentary

Vṛtti-s are all thoughts and emotions that keep the heart-mind preoccupied. When we are attempting to meditate or stay focused in some way, thoughts usually pop up that distract our attention. These distracting thoughts are vṛtti-s. Sūtra 1.6 lists the five vṛtti-s, then 1.7 to 1.11 define each vṛtti individually.

1.7 Vṛtti #1	Pramāṇa (valid means of perception/evaluation)
1.8 Vṛtti #2	Viparyaya (misperception)
1.9 Vṛtti #3	Vikalpa (imagination)
1.10 Vṛtti #4	Nidrā (sleep)
1.11 Vṛtti #5	Smṛti (memory)

Vṛtti-s are not necessarily bad. They can be harmful (kliṣṭa) or helpful (akliṣṭa) (1.5). The kleśa-s (mental-emotional afflictions) generate the harmful ones (kliṣṭa-vṛtti-s), which can be stilled by meditation (dhyāna) (2.11). Vṛtti-s become more sattvic as the kliṣṭa-vṛtti-s decrease from dhyāna and the kleśa-s weaken (via kriyā-yoga). It is important to be aware of the distorting and painful nature of the kliṣṭa-vṛtti-s, which are manifestations of the kleśa-s, most commonly rāga and dveṣa. Akliṣṭa-vṛtti-s do not have the afflictive quality of the kleśa-s in them, and help bring about nirodha.

The ego (ahaṅkāra) tries to define *us* as the vṛtti-s. If we let that happen, our perception and actions will be clouded by them. This is avidyā-kleśa interfering with clear perception. Slowing down and stilling the vṛtti-s requires diligent, continuous practice (abhyāsa) and a lack of desire for external objects (vairāgya) (1.12). As we cultivate these two pillars of yoga with keen discernment (viveka), eventually vairāgya occurs more and more, leading to the quelling of these activities (nirodha) and the clarification of the heart-mind (citta-prasādana).

Akliṣṭa-vṛtti-s are the manifestation of positive saṃskāra-s.

Kliṣṭa-vṛtti-s are the manifestation of negative saṃskāra-s rooted in the kleśa-s.

(See appendix F, figures 10 and 13.)

Complete Translation

1.6 pramāṇaviparyayavikalpanidrāsmṛtayaḥ

pramāṇa-viparyaya-vikalpa-nidrā-smṛtayaḥ

pramāṇa	correct way of evaluating an object (see 1.7)
viparyaya	misperception, incorrect evaluation (see 1.8)
vikalpa	imagination (see 1.9)
nidrā	sleep (see 1.10)
smṛti	the act of memory (see 1.11)

1. (The vṛtti-s are) correct evaluation, misperception, imagination, sleep, and the act of memory.
2. (The fluctuations of the heart-mind are) correct evaluation, misperception, imagination, sleep, and the act of memory.

Derivation of Terms

Root	vṛt, "to turn, revolve; engage oneself, be occupied by"
Dictionary	"action, movement, function, operation"

Related Sūtra-s

1.5, 7–12; 2.11

Contemplations

How does my perception of a situation evoke an emotion?

Is my preconceived notion clouding correct perception?

Which thoughts or emotions are not helpful to me?

PRAMĀṆA (VṚTTI #1)

Correct Evaluation

प्रत्यक्षानुमानागमाः प्रमाणानि ॥ १.७ ॥

1.7 pratyakṣānumānāgamāḥ pramāṇāni

The correct ways to evaluate what we perceive are direct experience, inference, and reliable testimony.

Commentary

Pramāṇa means correct perception, from the root "mā" and prefix "pra" taken together literally as "to measure or gauge what is in front of us." In order to perceive an object or situation accurately and completely, a broad understanding is necessary. Personal agendas, external labels, and preconceived notions can all interfere with pramāṇa.

There are three kinds of pramāṇa, all of which require viveka (discernment) to maximize the reliability of the information and decide if it is helpful or harmful. Pratyakṣa is the most important pramāṇa.

1. Pratyakṣa—direct perception, firsthand knowledge, where nothing stands between the heart-mind and the object being perceived by the senses. This is experiential knowledge, the most reliable because it is based on our actual experience. Can we know what honey tastes like if someone merely describes it to us in words?
2. Anumāna—inference, secondhand knowledge, literally "measuring after." The mind is involved here, inferring information based on what is perceived. For example, when you see smoke, the mind infers there is a fire, even though you cannot see the fire. If the smoke is due to fire, then it is correct and anumāna. If it is not smoke but something else not due to a fire, then it is misperception (viparyaya—vṛtti #2).
3. Āgama—reliable testimony, second- or thirdhand knowledge, often from reading a book or hearing it from another person. Traditionally āgama comes from texts written by people who are considered reliable; i.e., who have had direct experience of their own. This kind of perception requires our own verification from pratyakṣa (direct experience). Āgama informs and reinforces pratyakṣa.

In yoga, the progression of knowledge goes from āgama to pratyakṣa. That is, initially learning progresses from a teacher or books to inferring and extrapolating, and is finally reinforced by direct experience. Of course these three phases may overlap during our journey toward self-knowledge.

A helpful or neutral (akliṣṭa) pramāṇa is simply when we perceive something accurately and it does not disturb our heart-mind. For example, you see a flower and perceive it as such.

A harmful (kliṣṭa) pramāṇa is observing something correctly that disturbs the heart-mind. For example, watching a violent movie may cause impressions in our heart-mind that will adversely affect our future actions. If we witness an event that we simply cannot process because it is so foreign to us, our heart-mind does not know how to digest it, so the event becomes improperly recorded in memory. This undigested material has the potential to cause confusion, just as undigested food can cause physical disease.

Complete Translation

1.7 pratyakṣānumānāgamāḥ pramāṇāni

pratyakṣa-anumāna-āgamāḥ pramāṇāni

pratyakṣa	direct, firsthand perception
anumāna	inference, assumption, indirect/secondhand
āgama	testimony, knowledge from conversation or books, second- or thirdhand
pramāṇa	correct way of evaluating an object

1. The correct ways to evaluate what we perceive are direct experience, inference, and reliable testimony.

Derivation of Terms

Prefix	pra, "in front of, forward, forth"
Root	mā, "to measure, compare with"
Literal Meaning	"measuring forth, size up"
Dictionary	"a measure in general; evidence; authority; accurate; a means of arriving at correct knowledge"
Translation Here	"correct evaluation"

Contemplations

What are my primary sources of information?

Are they reliable?

How can I recognize an unreliable or biased source of information?

VIPARYAYA (VṚTTI #2)

Misperception

विपर्ययो मिथ्याज्ञानमतद्रूपप्रतिष्ठम् ॥ १.८ ॥

1.8 viparyayo mithyājñānamatadrūpapratiṣṭham
Misperception is perceiving an object incorrectly and thinking it is something else.

Commentary

Sometimes we think we understand something but we do not yet have enough information for a full picture (a "blessing in disguise," for example). A man falls off a horse and breaks his leg. This seems unfortunate until a war breaks out and all the men in the town are called upon to fight, except the man who broke his leg. His life may now be spared because the injury was a blessing in the end.

The kliṣṭa (harmful) form of ***viparyaya*** is delusion, when perception and reality do not match. If we are used to looking at things in a certain way and our expectations are not met, then our misperception is due to past conditioning (saṃskāra-s) and we suffer. Viparyaya manifests as avidyā-kleśa.

When we make assumptions based on incomplete knowledge, thinking we are right when we are actually wrong, then viparyaya is present. If it is dark and you see what looks like a snake on the ground, you may react in fear and flee—this is viparyaya. When daylight appears you see the object clearly as just a rope—this is pratyakṣa.

A helpful (akliṣṭa) form of viparyaya is its transformation into pratyakṣa by admitting we are wrong, asking questions to verify our perception, and adjusting our knowledge to fit reality. Listening to different perspectives helps reduce viparyaya and increase pramāṇa. Our goal is to clarify our heart-mind (citta-prasādana) and refine our sensory organs to the point where they are keen and alert and are fully under our control.

Viparyaya is the opposite of pramāṇa (correct perception).

Complete Translation

1.8 viparyayo mithyājñānamatadrūpapratiṣṭham
viparyayaḥ mithyā-jñānam atad rūpa-pratiṣṭham
viparyaya misconception
mithyā mistaken, false

jñāna	knowledge, cognition
atad	not that (a + tad)
rūpa	form (visual, auditory, subtle, etc.)
pratiṣṭha	based on

1. Misperception is false knowledge based upon a form which is not that.
2. Misperception is perceiving an object incorrectly and thinking it is something else.

Derivation of Terms

Prefix	vi, "separating, cutting, discerning"
Prefix	pari, "around"
Root	i, "to go"
Dictionary	"contrariety, reverse, inversion; nonexistence; misapprehension"
Translation Here	"misperception"

Contemplations

How often does assuming get me into trouble?

Do I see myself as others do?

Are there any particular kinds of events I remember differently than others do?

VIKALPA (VṚTTI #3)

Imagination

शब्दज्ञानानुपाती वस्तुशून्यो विकल्पः ॥ १.९ ॥

1.9 śabdajñānānupātī vastuśūnyo vikalpaḥ
Imagination is an idea that can be expressed in words yet has no real object.

Commentary

Vikalpa is an abstraction and has no basis in reality. It is based on a concept in the heart-mind that does not actually exist. Some words have no real objects, like "infinite" or "possible." Real knowledge is supported by fact (sūtra 1.48) and is antagonistic to vikalpa. Yet vikalpa serves the purpose of creating abstract thoughts, which may eventually manifest in a practical way (like mathematics) or lead to a higher level of understanding beyond our limited intellect (buddhi). Even the concept of Puruṣa as described in these *Yoga Sūtra-s* is a vikalpa, albeit a nonharmful one.

Helpful forms of vikalpa include high-level abstract thinking, such as theoretical mathematics or physics, or musical composition. A teacher or parent can inspire the student or child to try out ideas to see if they can become reality. Uplifting daydreams can be helpful vikalpa, while destructive daydreams are harmful. If we make decisions based on daydreams or fantasies or on our own unrealistic wishes, we may suffer. In this way vikalpa can contribute to misperception (viparyaya). For example, a potential mate sweeps us off our feet, infatuating our heart-mind so much as to result in a quick elopement. This rapid implementation of fantasy may end in suffering and regret. Or, we enroll in a "get rich quick" scheme, desirous of amassing wealth with little or no effort. Most of the time this unrealistic dream does not work, and we are left disappointed and no further along financially.

Complete Translation

1.9 śabdajñānānupātī vastuśūnyo vikalpaḥ
śabda-jñāna-anupātī vastu-śūnyaḥ vikalpaḥ

śabda	word, sound, language
jñāna	knowledge, cognition
anupātin	relying, chasing after

vastu	object
śūnya	devoid, without
vikalpa	conceptualization, imagination

1. Vikalpa is without an object, relying on knowledge from words or language.
2. Imagination is an idea that can be expressed in words, yet has no real object.

Derivation of Terms

Prefix	vi, "separating, cutting through, discerning"
Original Root	kḷp, "to be fit, worthy, ready; to produce, create; to imagine, believe"
Prefixed Root	vikḷp, "to be doubtful, be optional, guess"
Literal Meaning	vikalpa—same as dictionary
Dictionary	"doubt, uncertainty; suspicion; contrivance, art; an error; fancy, imagination"
Translation Here	"imagination or conceptualization"

Contemplations

Do daydreams or fantasies help me or not?

Are my decisions grounded in reality or based on unrealistic ideas?

Am I too caught up in abstract thinking, and do I need more grounding?

NIDRĀ (VṚTTI #4)

Sleep

अभावप्रत्ययालम्बना तमोवृत्तिर्निद्रा ॥ १.१० ॥

1.10 abhāvapratyayālambanā tamovṛttirnidrā

Sleep is when the mind slows down and is supported by a lack of conscious thoughts.

Commentary

Believe it or not, sleep is considered to be an activity of the mind. There are four sleep states: waking, dreaming, deep sleep, and turīya ("fourth," also known as yoga-nidrā).

	WAKING	DREAMING	DEEP/ DREAMLESS	BEYOND SLEEP
SANSKRIT	Jāgratā	Svapna	Nidrā/suṣupti	Turīya/yoga nidrā
STAGE	1	2	3	4
PLANE	Conscious	Subconscious	Unconscious	Superconscious
BODY	Gross	Subtle	Causal	Bliss
OBJECTS	External	Internal	Only itself	No Object
WHAT HAPPENS	Sensory perception, external interactions, record new impressions	Suppressed desires, fears, deep-seated impressions as well as positive insights express themselves	Nothing is happening	Borderline between waking and dreaming
SENSORY & MOTOR ORGANS	Active	Inactive	Inactive	Inactive
BUDDHI	Active	Active	Inactive	Inactive

Since upon awakening we remember that we were sleeping, sleep is considered an activity or fluctuation of the heart-mind, even though it is an inactive state. Deep sleep has the heaviness and inertia of tamas (the quality of inactivity and stagnation), and the restful quietness of sattva. Here tamas means inertia, and nidrā is described as a vṛtti that happens when tamas is present.

Deep sleep is quite different from meditation or samādhi although as the heart-mind becomes calmer over time it may require less sleep, even though the physical body may still need it. ***Nidrā*** is unconscious and involuntary, whereas samādhi is conscious and voluntary.

Sleep is helpful if we are naturally tired and get the rest that our body and mind require. However, if you are at a meeting where you are supposed to be attentive and you nod off in the middle and miss some important information, it could be harmful to you.

Nidrā can also be an object of focus for clarifying the heart-mind (1.38), since it represents a quiet and peaceful state of mind.

Complete Translation

1.10 abhāvapratyayālambanā tamovṛttirnidrā

abhāva-pratyaya-ālambanā tamas-vṛttiḥ nidrā

abhāva	absence
pratyaya	presented thought; current vṛtti directed toward an object
ālambanā	supporting
tamas	inertia
vṛtti	fluctuation or activity in the heart-mind
nidrā	sleep

1. Sleep is a tamasic mental activity supported by the absence of presented thoughts.
2. Sleep is when the mind slows down, supported by a lack of conscious thoughts.

Derivation of Terms

Root	nidrā, "to fall asleep, sleep"
Dictionary	"sleep, sleepiness"

Contemplations

How can I prevent myself from dozing off at inappropriate times?

Do I sleep more because of sluggishness or fatigue?

How can I remain alert and not succumb to boredom and mental fatigue?

SMṚTI (VṚTTI #5)
The Act of Memory

अनुभूतविषयासंप्रमोषः स्मृतिः ॥ १.११ ॥

1.11 anubhūtaviṣayāsaṃpramoṣaḥ smṛtiḥ
The act of memory is to store a sensory experience in our memory.

Commentary

Everything we experience is recorded in our memory. Even though no object is present, we maintain an image or impression of it in our heart-mind (citta) that may last much longer than the object itself. Memories of loved ones who died long ago, of songs we have heard, of joy we have experienced, are all retained in our ***smṛti***.

All events, whether witnessed or participated in, when very intense or repeated many times become habitual tendencies (saṃskāra-s) and are stored in the section of memory called the karmāśaya. Memory can influence the saṃskāra-s and vice versa. (See appendix F, figure 3.)

The clarity of our citta determines how accurately the experience is stored. For example, A casually smiles at B. B interprets the smile negatively as if A were making fun of B. Instead of a positive, friendly impression, B is left with negative residue in his or her heart-mind. In this way smṛti has an affinity with saṃskāra-s (4.9), both influencing each other.

An uplifting movie might become a helpful (akliṣṭa) memory if it is positive and contributes to our happiness. A film with violence or horror may cause nightmares or violent imitative actions that can lead to future suffering. Another example is the phantom-limb phenomenon. When a person loses an arm or leg, often her mind thinks it is still there and she can actually feel her nonexistent hand or foot. This type of memory could be a vāsanā, a subtle saṃskāra of the feeling experienced from an event.

Memory is necessary for reminding the heart-mind to stay on its point of focus (1.20). When the memory is completely purified, then nirvitarka-samāpatti (heart-mind state beyond thought—see samādhi) is attained (1.43). The deeper purpose of smṛti is to remember our true nature.

The smṛti is part of the heart-mind complex (citta). The phrase "learn by heart" means to learn something repeatedly until it establishes a strong saṃskāra and goes "into our bones." This complete mastery of the object at hand is called saṃprajñāta-samādhi (1.17).

Complete Translation

1.11 anubhūtaviṣayāsaṃpramoṣaḥ smṛtiḥ

anubhūta-viṣaya-asaṃpramoṣaḥ smṛtiḥ

anubhūta	experienced before
viṣaya	object of sensory perception
asaṃpramoṣa	retention, "not carrying off" (a + sam + pra + moṣa)
smṛti	the act of memory

1. The act of memory is the retention of an experienced object.
2. The act of memory is to store a sensory experience in our memory.

Derivation of Terms

Root	smṛ, "to remember, keep in mind, recollect"
Dictionary	"remembrance, recollection, memory; thinking of, calling to mind"
Translation Here	"recollection"

Related Sūtra-s

1.20, 43

Contemplations

Can I train my memory to serve my growth and happiness?

Can I deliberately experience and thus remember more sattva and less rajas and tamas?

Can memorizing a meaningful phrase redirect my attention inward?

ANTARĀYA-S
Obstacles That Distract

व्याधिस्त्यानसंशयप्रमादालस्याविरतिभ्रान्तिदर्शनालब्धभूमिकत्वानवस्थितत्वानि

चित्तविक्षेपास्ते ऽन्तरायाः ॥ १.३० ॥

1.30 vyādhistyānasaṃśayapramādālasyāviratibhrāntidarśanālabdhabhūmikatvān avasthitatvāni cittavikṣepāste 'ntarāyāḥ
The obstacles to practice are disease, apathy, doubt, carelessness, lethargy, temptation, erroneous views, ungroundedness, and regression.

Commentary

An ***antarāya*** is an obstacle that distracts our attention away from a point of focus. All nine obstacles are disruptions to the heart-mind field of consciousness and can be debilitating to a practice. Vṛitti-s arise when antarāya-s are present. Antarāya-s are also shown in appendix F, Figure 9.

Vyādhi, disease or illness, is obviously a major distraction that may be extremely difficult to remove. This is the only antarāya that does not necessarily come from a kleśa. Maintaining a quiet, focused heart-mind while sniffling, sneezing, or feeling physical pain after surgery is quite a challenge. Yet a fully focused heart-mind can actually cut off the pain signals to the brain.

Styāna is an attitude of not caring about our progress or practice. It may arise from doubt (see saṃśaya below) or from our perceived lack of progress. Patience and perseverance are key to avoid falling into this apathetic state. From this dullness we are unable to convert thoughts into actions. Stimulation of our heart-mind by means of vigorous āsana, active prāṇāyāma practice, or some other nonyogic exercise can wake us out of this tamasic state.

Saṃśaya means self-doubt or lack of confidence. This obstacle is particularly arresting, since it can cause us to stop practice for a while. Like fire, it consumes everything in its path. With it comes indecision, the inability to decide between two things. This kind of paralysis can be even worse than making a bad decision, because we are stuck in a stagnant, tamasic state of limbo. A leap of faith (śraddhā) is one way to overcome this.

Pramāda means intoxication or drunkenness, a state of not thinking clearly and an inability to focus our attention. If we act carelessly, without paying proper attention, we will likely cause ourselves and others potentially disastrous pain and suffering, with unknown future consequences.

Ālasya is simply being fatigued or tired, which makes it difficult to muster up the energy to concentrate. When the body or mind is too exhausted to practice, sitting quietly for just a few minutes will still serve to maintain the helpful habit of daily practice.

Avirati consists of sensory and sexual temptations and preoccupations. The word is built from the prefixes "a" meaning "not" and "vi" meaning "away from" and the word "rati" meaning "sensual attraction." A literal translation might be "not able to stay away from sensual attractions." This powerful energy originating in the second cakra can divert our attention in an unhealthy and potentially obsessive direction. Sexual and sensual indulgence, often driven by the ego's quest for gratification, can be difficult to control.

Bhrānti-darśana means "erroneous seeing" and implies a distorted view of the world. This is similar to the vṛtti called viparyaya (misperception). Delusion, not seeing reality as it is, clouds and twists sensory information coming into the heart-mind and stores it inaccurately so as to bias future thoughts and actions. A rigid or extreme philosophical stance, such as being too self-righteous, literal, or fundamentalist, is prone to error, since there are many paths to the same spiritual goal. The practice of yoga requires the ability to let go of our opinions and consider other viewpoints as valid.

Alabdhabhūmikatva is made up of "a," meaning "not," "labdha," meaning "obtaining," and "bhūmikatva," meaning "groundedness." A literal translation then is "not obtaining groundedness." It implies that not being fully established at one level of development prevents us from progressing further. For all but a few rare beings, yoga as a process occurs in stages. If we try to move on without being firmly grounded in the previous stages, we cannot progress fully. We are in a sense off balance, teetering between moving forward or backward.

Anavasthitatva is composed of "an," meaning "not" and "avasthitatva," meaning "stability." It is related to the previous antarāya, ungroundedness. Anavasthitatva is when we have indeed progressed but we cannot maintain that level of focus and fall back into a previous stage. Of course there will be times of upward progress and growth and plateau times when we feel like nothing is moving. During these times of apparent stagnation, patience and perseverance are crucial. The state of samādhi, especially when we acquire extraordinary powers (see saṃyama), is difficult to maintain.

The accompanying disruptions are pain (physical or mental), negativity/dejection, trembling, and disturbed breathing (1.31). These can be considered symptoms or effects of the antarāya-s. One may lead to another, in the order mentioned. Inner suffering negatively affects the heart-mind, leading to upset or frustration. This can cause nervousness and twitching of the limbs, which affects inhalation and exhalation patterns.

Repeating praṇava (most commonly the sound Om) evokes the essence of Īśvara (the universal light of knowledge) and causes these obstacles to disappear (1.28-29). (See Īśvara.) Practice (abhyāsa) on a single tattva prevents them (1.32). The word "tattva" can mean any of the twenty-five components described in the Sāṅkhya philosophy. (See appendix F, figure 1.) It could very well mean our inner awareness itself, the Puruṣa. (See appendix F, figure 9.)

Complete Translation

1.30 vyādhistyānasaṃśayapramādālasyāviratibhrāntidarśanālabdhabhūmikatvānavasthitatvāni cittavikṣepāste 'ntarāyāḥ

vyādhi-styāna-saṃśaya-pramāda-ālasya-avirati-bhrāntidarśana-alabdhabhūmikatva-anavasthitatvāni citta-vikṣepāḥ te antarāyāḥ

vyādhi	disease
styāna	apathy, dullness
saṃśaya	doubt, indecision
pramāda	carelessness, intoxication
ālasya	lethargy, laziness
avirati	temptation, sexual preoccupation
bhrānti-darśana	erroneous seeing
alabdhabhūmikatva	inability to become grounded
anavasthitatva	regression
citta	heart-mind field of consciousness
vikṣepa	disruption
te	those
antarāya	obstacle

The obstacles to practice are disease, apathy, doubt, carelessness, lethargy, temptation, erroneous views, ungroundedness, and regression.

Derivation of Terms

Prefix	antar, "in the middle, between"
Prefix	ā—reverses direction of movement
Original Root	i, "go"
Dictionary	antarāya, "impediment, hindrance, obstacle, what stands in the way"
Translation Here	"that which comes between, gets in the way"

Related Sūtra-s

1.29, 31–32

Contemplations

Am I aware of any obstacles in my life?
How do they affect me?
How do they affect my practice?

KLEŚA-S

Causes of Suffering

अविद्यास्मितारागद्वेषाभिनिवेशाः क्लेशाः ॥ २.३ ॥

2.3 avidyāsmitārāgadveṣābhiniveśāḥ kleśāḥ
The mental-emotional causes of suffering are unawareness, egotism, clinging to past pleasure, clinging to past pain, and the fear of death.

Commentary
The ***kleśa-s*** are arguably the most challenging aspects of ourselves to confront, yet the most liberating after they are weakened and eventually removed. They are emotions or instincts that arise when "our buttons are pushed." Kleśa-s cause us to suffer by tormenting our heart-mind as negative thoughts and emotions (kliṣṭa-vṛtti-s). (See vṛtti-s.) Each kleśa is described in detail in its own section.

SŪTRA	KLEŚA	MEANING
2.4–5	Avidyā	Lack of awareness
2.6	Asmitā	Egotism ("I am"-ness)
2.7	Rāga	Desire for previously experienced pleasure
2.8	Dveṣa	Aversion from previously experienced pain
2.9	Abhiniveśa	Fear of death, will to live, instinct to survive

(See appendix F, figures 10 and 13.)

Avidyā (lack of awareness), defined as a "field for the others" (2.4), is distinguished from the other four kleśa-s that only exist as long as avidyā is present. Avidyā is the shroud of ignorance, a simple lack of knowledge that prevents us from understanding something. It is the sound chamber in which the kleśa-s are heard. The other four kleśa-s can be in one of four states (2.4):

	STATE OF KLEŚA	EFFECT ON OUR ACTIONS	VOLUME CONTROL
prasupta	Dormant, potential exists	Not affecting our actions now, but can in the proper situation	On but quiet
tanu	Weakly active, weakened by kriyā-yoga	Currently affecting our actions, but weakly	Low
vicchinna	Intermittent, rises up again and again	Comes and goes	Variable
udāra	Strongly active	Currently affecting our actions in full force	Loud

All kleśa-s are fear-based. Avidyā is the fear borne of ignorance and feeds the other kleśa-s. Asmitā is the fear the ego has of losing control of decision-making power. Rāga erupts when one is afraid he will not experience a certain pleasure again, while dveṣa manifests from being afraid he will endure a painful event again. Abhiniveśa is the deepest fear of death.

In any situation, especially interpersonal relations, we have the capability to act consciously or react unconsciously. Every action we perform creates a subtle impression (saṃskāra) that is stored in our individual karmāśaya, a karmic reservoir within our consciousness. Every action we perform can also be influenced by these stored saṃskāra-s. The repetition of an action adds to the previously created saṃskāra and thus strengthens it. The stronger the impression, the more it can affect our action or reaction. Over time these become habitual patterns that are strong enough to overpower our conscious mind's intention to act differently. Our mental-emotional "baggage" (karmāśaya) predetermines our actions and often causes a kleśa to appear (2.12), resulting in some reaction that reinforces a saṃskāra and activates the kliṣṭa-vṛtti-s that continue the cycle of suffering.

The saṃskāra-s in our karmāśaya drive our future actions and ultimately determine the conditions in which we will be reborn, our life span, and our life experiences (2.13). If our past actions were virtuous/helpful/positive, joy will result. If our past actions were nonvirtuous/harmful/negative, sorrow will result (2.14). This of course is a very black-and-white generalization. The bottom line is the golden rule: whatever effects our actions have, those effects will come back to us at some point in the future.

Reincarnation is assumed to be true here, as in most other belief systems originating in India. The karmāśaya stays with us from birth to birth and contributes to our standing in the next lifetime.

When we exercise pure discrimination and understand how the guṇa-s operate, changing all the time, we realize that everything in the manifest world inherently involves some degree of discomfort (duḥkha) (2.15). Nature (Prakṛti) constantly changes as the guṇa-s change, just as the cells in our bodies are continuously transforming themselves and being recycled into other substances.

Over time the kleśa-s weaken and become more subtle through the practice of kriyā-yoga (2.1). Gradually the kleśa-s in their subtle form can be eliminated by understanding where they came from and how they were produced (pratiprasava—2.10). The related kliṣṭa-vṛtti-s can then be overcome by meditation (dhyāna) (2.11). Once the kleśa is rendered inert, unable to activate, it is as if the sound device is turned off and the volume control becomes useless. After this, any related saṃskāra-s will not affect future actions, and no new saṃskāra-s or kliṣṭa-vṛtti-s related to that particular kleśa are created. This is a prerequisite to kaivalya (3.50). (See appendix F, figure 13.)

Complete Translation

2.3 avidyāsmitārāgadveṣābhiniveśāḥ kleśāḥ

avidyā-asmitā-rāga-dveṣa-abhiniveśāḥ kleśāḥ

avidyā	lack of awareness, ignorance
asmitā	identification with our individual being
rāga	attachment to previous pleasure
dveṣa	attachment to previous suffering; dislike, aversion because of past suffering
abhiniveśa	survival instinct, will to live, fear of dying
kleśa	deep emotional affliction

1. The kleśa-s are avidyā, asmitā, rāga, dveṣa, and abhiniveśa.
2. The mental-emotional afflictions are unawareness, egotism, clinging to past pleasure, clinging to past pain, and the fear of death.

Derivation of Terms

Root	kliś, "to be tormented, afflicted; to suffer, feel pain"
Dictionary	kleśa, "pain, anguish, distress, trouble; sin"
Meaning Here	"mental-emotional affliction"

Related Sūtra-s

2.2, 4–15; 3.50

Contemplations

Do any of my actions stem from the kleśa-s?

Are the kleśa-s I am aware of weak or strong?

Which habitual patterns strengthen or weaken these kleśa-s?

AVIDYĀ (KLEŚA #1)
Lack of Awareness

अनित्याशुचिदुःखानात्मसु नित्यशुचिसुखात्मख्यातिरविद्या ॥ २.५ ॥

2.5 anityāśuciduḥkhānātmasu nityaśucisukhātmakhyātiravidyā
Lack of awareness causes one to think the ever-changing manifest world is the same as the unchanging, inner light of awareness.

Commentary

Avidyā is a lack of awareness, or being "in the dark," so to speak. Too much commotion and busyness in the heart-mind distracts our attention and neglects the pure light of awareness that rests inside of our heart-mind. As ignorance breeds fear, so avidyā feeds egoism (asmitā-kleśa) and the other kleśa-s.

Avidyā is the very first kleśa (deep affliction) (2.3), and as such carries the most importance. The other four kleśa-s exist in the *field* of avidyā (2.4), meaning they need avidyā to exist. Avidyā is like fertile soil in which the seeds of the other kleśa-s can grow and thrive.

Avidyā is the root cause of saṃyoga (2.24), falsely associating the changeable world (Prakṛti) with the changeless witness (Puruṣa). Saṃyoga is the cause of suffering (duḥkha) (2.17). Clearing the cloud of avidyā thus ends suffering and leads to the cascade of events toward kaivalya.

Avidyā can be cleared away by diligent practice (abhyāsa) and keen discernment (viveka), which lead to a state of noninvolvement (vairāgya). A sincere effort to purify the body, breath, and heart-mind will gradually clear out impurities. As this happens, our knowledge and awareness open up, illuminating the heart-mind. As darkness cannot exist in the presence of light, so ignorance disappears in the presence of knowledge.

Vidyā is the inner light of knowledge. As darkness is simply a lack of light, so avidyā is a lack of vidyā or awareness. The heart-mind has a certain amount of each at any given time. By increasing awareness/light/sattva, the ignorance/darkness/tamas-rajas are then decreased. The word "guru" means that which removes (ru) the darkness (gu) of avidyā by shedding the light of knowledge on our consciousness.

Avidyā can be a simple lack of understanding. This "being in the dark" about something can be transformed by adding the light of knowledge in the form of accurate information based on correct perception (pramāṇa). Avidyā is the dark veil that cloaks our citta, causing us to act out of blind ignorance. Practicing yoga involves the sincere and earnest pursuit of truth. Mahātma Gandhi coined his movement "Satyagraha," meaning "grasping for truth." Being open-minded contributes to learning the truth and clearing the film of avidyā off the lens of our citta.

By working to weaken and nullify the kleśa-s using kriyā-yoga (2.1), then eliminating them with pratiprasava (2.10), we render them unable to sprout and cause an unconscious reaction. When our "baggage" no longer drives our actions, our citta is clear, avidyā is gone, and our attention moves on toward kaivalya.

Complete Translation

2.5 anityāśuciduḥkhānātmasu nityaśucisukhātmakhyātiravidyā

anitya-aśuci-duḥkha-anātmasu nitya-śuci-sukha-ātma-khyātiḥ avidyā

anitya	impermanent
aśuci	impure
duḥkha	suffering, pain, discomfort
anātma	nonself
nitya	permanent
śuci	pure
sukha	happiness
ātma	self
khyāti	awareness, realization, understanding, identification
avidyā	lack of awareness, ignorance

1. Avidyā is (falsely) identifying the impermanent, impure, suffering nonself (which comprises Prakṛti) as the permanent, pure, happy Self (which describes Puruṣa).
2. Lack of awareness causes one to think the ever-changing manifest world is the same as the unchanging, inner light of awareness.

Derivation of Terms

Prefix	a, "not, without"
Root	vid, "know, understand, find"
Dictionary	avidyā, "ignorance, want of learning; illusion"
Literal Meaning	"not knowing, not seeing"
Translation Here	"lack of awareness, knowledge, or understanding; ignorance"

Related Sūtra-s

2.4, 24

Contemplations

What around me is interfering with my growth and purification?

Am I open-minded enough to accept new yet surprising information?

In what areas of my life am I unclear or confused?

Item: 31183167428124
Title: Real happiness at work : meditations for accomplishment, achievement, and peace
Call no.: 158.1 S
Due: 06/25/2022

Item: 31183197590158
Title: Heal : discover your unlimited potential and awaken the powerful healer within
Call no.: 613 N
Due: 06/25/2022

Item: 31183206593003
Title: Karmic management : what goes around come s around in your business and your life
Call no.: 658 R
Due: 06/25/2022

Total items: 6

You just saved $110.93 by using your library today.

Free to Be All In
Late fees no longer assessed for overdue items
Ask for details or visit bcpl.info

ASMITĀ (KLEŚA #2)

Distorted Sense of Self

दृग्दर्शनशक्त्योरेकात्मतेवास्मिता ॥ २.६ ॥

2.6 dṛgdarśanaśaktyorekātmatevāsmitā
The sense of "I am" makes us think that our decision-making power is the same as the unchanging witness consciousness.

Commentary

Asmitā is a mental-emotional affliction because it makes us think that we are our body and we are our mind, and therefore we are our thoughts and emotions (vṛtti-s). It causes us to believe our being is limited by things like our name, occupation, likes and dislikes, etc. Asmitā can be translated as "ego," but as a kleśa it is "egotism" or "insecurity." If our actions are self-centered and we think of ourselves as better than others, then asmitā is active. The ego (ahaṅkāra) likes to be in control, and when that control is threatened, asmitā arises to defend it. The ego will go to any lengths in order to "save face." An insecure ego is terrified of relinquishing control. Ignorance breeds fear, and thus avidyā sustains the other kleśa-s.

Asmitā can appear in various forms. It can be a distorted image of ourselves that does not match reality. We may feel puffed up, believing we are somehow more than we really are, or feel insecure and think we are less than we actually are. In the former, asmitā appears as conceit and pompousness, while the latter presents as self-doubt.

Asmitā usually strengthens into conceit when excess śakti from flattery or fame or lots of attention come our way. (See "The Power of Attention" in part 1.) The ego likes to feel powerful and in control, so it welcomes this energy. Unfortunately, once we begin to think we have power over or are in any way better than other people, the heart-mind moves away from yoga and deteriorates toward avidyā. In Indian lore, paying attention to the head represents serving the interests of the ego and wanting something from a person, while honoring the feet symbolizes humility, respect, and surrender.

Once we perceive that the buddhi (aspect of the heart-mind) is distinct from the inner light of awareness, and the ego (ahaṅkāra) becomes subservient to the buddhi, then asmitā will not cause us suffering (2.6). Our actions are now governed by our higher, inner intelligence instead of the ego, whose agenda is to make us think that we are the body and that our personality is defined by the vṛtti-s.

Through practicing kriyā-yoga (2.1), asmitā-kleśa can be weakened. To prevent pompousness, observe when your ego receives more attention using the tool of self-observation (svādhyāya), strive to not feel puffed up by means of tapas, and pass the attentive energy on up to your teacher or Īśvara, the universal teachings, by practicing īśvara-praṇidhāna. To prevent insecurity, first reflect on why you feel that way (svādhyāya), then make an effort to transform that into something positive (tapas), and finally have faith that deep in the center of your impermanent, changing body glows the eternal light of awareness (īśvara-praṇidhāna).

As asmitā weakens we will realize that in fact we are better off treating others as we would like to be treated and that we are no more or less important than anybody else. Once we allow ourselves to listen to our inner, divine voice, then our ego (ahaṅkāra) becomes a servant instead of the master, and asmitā-kleśa is destroyed.

It is important to have a healthy ego in order to function in society. A weakened asmitā means most of the time we neither think of ourselves as better than others nor less than others, and we welcome suggestions for self-improvement, even if they are difficult to hear. We are no longer embarrassed by verbal criticism, and we do not need to "save face" because our inner sense of self can withstand what it knows to be only external perceptions.

There is a story about the Buddha being invited to a house to take alms. The host proceeded to insult him, calling him "swine" and "ox" and making many other derogatory remarks. The Buddha was not the slightest bit fazed and did not respond to the insults. He calmly asked his host, "What do you do when guests enter your house?" The host replied "I prepare a feast for them." The Buddha then said. "What would you do if the guests did not partake in the feast you prepared?" The host answered, "In that case we ourselves would eat the food." The Buddha said finally, "Well my friend, you have invited me to your house for alms. You have entertained me with all manner of verbal abuse. I do not accept it. Please take it back."

This story illustrates how a healthy heart-mind does not let the ego hold on to negative stimuli. As the saying goes, "Sticks and stones may break my bones but names will never hurt me." If we let what is harmful to us pass through, and only register what is helpful to us, we will not become offended when verbal abuse comes our way. We can remain poised and unruffled like the Buddha. This may require quite a bit of tapas, especially if there is societal pressure to "save face."

Please note that asmitā is mentioned in 1.17, 3.47, and 4.4 not as an affliction (kleśa) but as the individual sense of "I-ness" that is necessary to stay alive. Refer to citta, ahaṅkāra aspect.

Complete Translation

2.6 dṛgdarśanaśaktyorekātmatevāsmitā

dṛk-darśana-śaktyoḥ eka-ātmata iva asmitā

dṛk	seer, Puruṣa
darśana	seeing
śakti	power
eka	one, single
ātmatā	identity
iva	like, as if
asmitā	sense of "I am," egoism

1. Asmitā is as if the seer (Puruṣa) and the instrument of seeing (buddhi) are the same.
2. The sense of "I am" makes us think that our decision-making power is the same as the unchanging witness consciousness.

Derivation of Terms

Verb	asmi, "I am"
Suffix	tā, "ness"
Literal Meaning	"I am-ness"
Dictionary	"egotism"
Translation Here	"as an affliction, when our ego is filled with conceit, it is egotism; when filled with self-doubt, it is insecurity"

Related Sūtra-s

2.1

Contemplations

Are there situations in which I act as if I am better than those around me?

Can I learn as much from my students as they can learn from me?

How are my relationships affected by moments of conceit or self-doubt?

RĀGA (KLEŚA #3)

Clinging to Past Pleasure

सुखानुशयी रागः ॥ २.७ ॥

2.7 sukhānuśayī rāgaḥ
Rāga is holding on to past pleasure.

Commentary

Rāga is the third kleśa and is somewhat parallel to dveṣa (see next kleśa). Both are emotional triggers based on clinging to a past experience.

When we experience pleasure, a memory is created that colors our heart-mind by making us desire that experience again. The memory becomes a saṃskāra (habitual impression) stored in the karmāśaya. The more intense the pleasure, the stronger the saṃskāra. This "pleasure-stain" remains and influences future action.

If we cannot reenact this pleasurable experience, and this upsets us, rāga has been activated. Desire is like a fire: it is always consuming, as the satisfaction of desires consumes our consciousness.

Rāga is the opposite of vairāgya (detached awareness).

Rāga is a product of asmitā (egoism).

Vairāgya removes asmitā and thus rāga.

The word rāga has several different yet related meanings and applications. Red is the color of heat or passion. Coloring indicates that our perception is tainted from a previous experience. This may affect how we act. Wearing "rose-colored glasses" means we perceive everything in an idealistic manner. A musical rāga is designed to evoke emotions upon listening to it.

For example, you just "ended" a long, passionate but unfulfilling and unhealthy relationship in which you experienced both intense pleasure and pain. It is hard to let go of that experience and move on with your life. Because the relationship lasted so long, the saṃskāra-s had time to develop deep patterns in your consciousness, which can pull you back into the relationship despite your mind telling you it is not a good idea. It is much more difficult to resist rāga and stay away from the person than to submit to rāga and return to the intense pleasure.

We can apply kriyā-yoga in this situation for its ability to weaken rāga. Tapas is the heat from the friction of resistance that we feel when we find the strength to listen to our inner voice telling us not to return to the past and to move ahead with our life. Svādhyāya allows us to observe our emotions from a distance and listen to the advice of friends and family. Īśvara-praṇidhāna is the letting go of this unhealthy relationship and having faith that life will be okay without it.

Complete Translation

2.7 sukhānuśayī rāgaḥ

sukha-anuśayī rāgaḥ

sukha	pleasure, joy
anuśayin	holding onto, dwelling on
rāga	passion, emotional attachment

1. Rāga is holding on to past pleasure.

Derivation of Terms

Root	rañj, "to color or taint; redden; to be attached to; to be enamoured by"
Dictionary	rāga, "coloring; red dye; love, passion; emotion; joy, pleasure"
Translation Here	"attachment to past pleasure"

Contemplations

What do I crave?

Why do I crave it?

How is my behavior affected by what I cling to?

DVEṢA (KLEŚA #4)

Clinging to Past Suffering

दुःखानुशयी द्वेषः ॥ २.८ ॥

2.8 duḥkhānuśayī dveṣaḥ
Aversion (to something) comes from a previous painful experience of it.

Commentary

Dveṣa is the fourth kleśa and is somewhat parallel to rāga (see previous kleśa). Both are emotional triggers based on clinging to a past experience.

When we experience pain or discomfort (duḥkha), it is natural to want to avoid that experience again. If this aversion changes our behavior in a way that is not helpful to us, then dveṣa is present. This often involves repressed emotions.

Dveṣa can arise from resistance, resentment, vengefulness, or anger toward the painful event.

A painful trauma often strengthens dveṣa. The traumatic experience creates a deep imprint in memory and an automatic aversion to some or all aspects of the event. This imprint (saṃskāra) will likely affect how you act in the future, especially when a situation arises that contains an aspect of the trauma. Your heart-mind has been programmed to avoid at all costs anything that might recreate the suffering you went through during the trauma.

Yoga provides tools to reprogram the heart-mind and root out these emotional afflictions, allowing you to act consciously and positively instead of negatively.

For example, you are walking down the street alone and someone accosts you, steals your money, throws you to the ground, and runs away. This traumatic experience may cause you to never walk down a street alone again. If the mugging causes you to become fearful every time you meet a stranger on the street, it is harming you more than helping you. Of course, there are healthy ways to try to prevent such an event from happening again, like walking with friends. Allowing the trauma to inform better, safer habits and then fade as the new habits strengthen permits the past event to take its proper place in the present.

Complete Translation

2.8 duḥkhānuśayī dveṣaḥ

duḥkha-anuśayī dveṣaḥ

duḥkha	suffering, pain, discomfort, trauma
anuśayin	holding onto, dwelling on
dveṣa	aversion, repulsion

1. Dveṣa is holding on to past pain.
2. Aversion (to something) comes from a previous painful experience of it.

Derivation of Terms

Root	dviṣ, "to hate, dislike, be hostile"
Dictionary	dveṣa, "hate, dislike, abhorence; enmity, hostility"
Translation Here	"aversion, dislike"

Contemplations

How does past suffering affect my present actions?

Is it time to let go of any aversion or grudge because it causes me to behave in a negative manner?

Am I ready to view suffering as a means to learn more about myself?

ABHINIVEŚA (KLEŚA #5)

Fear of Death

स्वरसवाही विदुषो ऽपि समारूढो ऽभिनिवेशः ॥ २.९ ॥

2.9 svarasavāhī viduṣo 'pi samārūḍho 'bhiniveśaḥ*
The fear of death is strong in everyone, as our essence of experience is carried along from lifetime to lifetime.

Commentary
The fear of death or pain exists deep in our subconscious. When we sense that our life is in danger, we either fight, flee, or freeze. This primal instinct is embedded "even in the wise," implying it is very, very difficult to overcome. Every species is hardwired to survive and avoid extinction. This genetic imprint (vāsanā) flows from one generation to another. It is natural to want to stay alive, yet it also indicates an attachment to the body.

What is wrong with death? It is a fact of life. Our ego is afraid to let go of our body, mind, habits, possessions, reputation, friends, family, etc. Once we stop clinging to the fetters of our physical existence, we become liberated while alive (jīva-mukti) and death is merely a transition from one life to the next. The soul inside (ātman) never dies and is in fact our true essence. This is the primary message of the *Bhagavad-Gītā*.

Abhiniveśa is a deep-seated involvement in the process of dualities, being caught up in joy and sorrow, good and bad, beauty and ugliness, etc. It is also an addiction to the game of the kleśa-s. Fear is based on attachments such as rāga and dveṣa. Being caught in the wheel of dualities, we identify with them and see ourselves as a conglomeration of our thoughts (vṛtti-s), possessions, preferences, family, etc. Our egotism (asmitā) keeps us bound to who it thinks we are.

Our state of mind at the time of death contributes to our state of mind in the next life. If the heart-mind imbibes the qualities of sattva at the time of death, then the next life will be more sattvic. It is one thing to cultivate an attitude of healing and perseverance in order to survive a life-threatening condition. It is another thing to cling to life, or another's life, when it is not a real life anymore. Accepting death when it is imminent conquers abhiniveśa and allows one to move on. The Hindu god of death is named "Yama," the same word as the first limb of yoga (regulations, restraints), because he restrains life itself. (See yama-s.)

For example, say you are traveling on an airplane when all of a sudden the ride becomes rough. You can feel the plane dipping and rising abruptly. How do you feel? What can you do? At that point you have no control of your fate. The fear of death can only make you worrisome and unhappy. Stepping back and realizing that you have no control (svādhyāya) and then surrendering to whatever is going to happen (īśvara-praṇidhāna) brings your consciousness back to its center. Mental and emotional calmness ensue in the midst of your chaotic surroundings. Thus abhiniveśa, fear of death, is weakened.

Complete Translation

2.9 svarasavāhī viduṣo 'pi samārūḍho 'bhiniveśaḥ*

svarasa-vāhī viduṣaḥ api samārūḍhaḥ abhiniveśaḥ

svarasa	own essence
vāhin	carried along, flowing
viduṣa	a wise person
api	even, also
samārūḍha	grown or developed completely
abhiniveśa	fear of death, will to live, survival instinct

1. Abhiniveśa is fully developed even in a wise person, carried along by its own essence.
2. The fear of death is strong in everyone, as our essence of experience is carried along from lifetime to lifetime.

* Other versions substitute "tathā" for "samā" without causing significant difference in meaning.

Derivation of Terms

Prefix	abhi, "toward, in the direction of"
Prefix	ni, "down, under, below"; "into," so "deep into"
Original Root	viś, "enter into; penetrate"
Stem Word	veśa, "entrance; access; a dwelling"
Prefixed Root	abhiniviś, "to occupy, take possession of, be attached to"
Literal Meaning	"that which has taken possession of us"
Dictionary	abhiniveśa, "instinctive clinging to worldly life and bodily enjoyments and the fear that one might be cut off from all of them"
Translation Here	"entered into from every direction," so "penetrates deep into every living creature"

Contemplations

Why am I afraid to die?
Am I attached to my body?
Is the fear of death helping me or harming me?

AṢṬĀṄGA

Eight Limbs of Yoga

यमनियमासनप्राणायामप्रत्याहारधारणाध्यानसमाधयो ऽष्टावङ्गानि ॥ २.२९ ॥

2.29 yamaniyamāsanaprāṇāyāmapratyāhāradhāraṇādhyānasamādhayo 'ṣṭāvaṅgāni

The eight parts of yoga are social ethics, personal self-care, refinement of the body, breath regulation, focusing attention away from external objects, choosing what to focus on, maintaining the focus, and assimilation of the object of focus.

Commentary

The eight limbs of yoga are a set of practices that develop our civility in society as well as our journey inward to discover our true nature. The deliberate order from external to internal is consistent with the common textual theme of moving our consciousness from a gross state to subtler and subtler states. The practice of each limb can occur simultaneously, much as the limbs of a baby grow at the same time. Implementing all eight parts into our life virtually guarantees we will develop into a well-rounded human being whose inner core understands who he or she is and acts harmoniously with other people.

The eight limbs are the easiest place to begin our journey into yoga. Of all the avenues provided in the sūtras, they are the simplest to pursue. Practicing these purifies the body and heart-mind and leads to viveka-khyāti (discriminating perception) (2.28). Each limb is explained in its own section.

The first five limbs are treated as individual outer limbs as compared to the final three limbs, which are called "antaraṅga," meaning "inner limb" (3.7), and are grouped together in a trio called "saṃyama," meaning "complete control" (3.4). Pratyāhāra is more of a side effect of its surrounding limbs and serves as a threshold point from outer to inner.

Each part of yoga stabilizes and refines a different aspect of our being:

PART/LIMB	STABILIZES AND REFINES	OUTER OR INNER
Yama-s	Social interactions	Outer
Niyama-s	Personal care	Outer
Āsana	Physical body	Outer
Prāṇāyāma	Breath	Outer
Pratyāhāra	Senses	Outer/inner
Dhāraṇā	Heart-mind, by choosing an object	Inner
Dhyāna	Heart-mind, by continuous focus on the object	Inner
Samādhi	Heart-mind, by assimilating the object	Inner

(See appendix F, figures 11 and 12.)

Complete Translation

2.29 yamaniyamāsanaprāṇāyāmapratyāhāradhāraṇādhyānasamādhayo 'ṣṭāvaṅgāni

yama-niyama-āsana-prāṇāyāma-pratyāhāra-dhāraṇā-dhyāna-samādhayaḥ aṣṭau aṅgāni

yama	social ethics, interactions, "control, restraint"
niyama	personal behavior, "internal yama"
āsana	sitting, posture, physical exercises to purify the body
prāṇāyāma	regulation of breath, breathing exercises to calm the mind
pratyāhāra	a side effect: sensory inputs no longer distract
dhāraṇā	choosing a focus and directing our attention there
dhyāna	focused and uninterrupted attention on a single place
samādhi	complete absorption of the heart-mind in the focus
aṣṭau	eight
aṅga	limb, part

1. The eight limbs are yama, niyama, āsana, prāṇāyāma, pratyāhāra, dhāraṇā, dhyāna, and samādhi.
2. The eight parts of yoga are social ethics, personal self-care, physical exercises, breath regulation, focusing attention away from external objects, choosing what to focus on, maintaining the focus, and assimilation of the object of focus.

Related Sūtra-s

2.28

Contemplations

Which parts of yoga are not being attended to?

Am I spending most of my time in āsana, and very little on the other limbs?

How can I find time to practice all eight parts of yoga as a system?

Asato Mā

May we move toward our own truth
and inner light of awareness.

असतो मा सद्गमय	asato mā sad gamaya.
तमसो मा ज्योतिर्गमय	tamaso mā jyotir gamaya.
मृत्योर्मा अमृतं गमय	mṛtyor mā amṛtaṃ gamaya.
ॐ शान्तिः । शान्तिः । शान्तिः ।	Om śāntiḥ śāntiḥ śāntiḥ.

Lead me from untruth to truth.
Lead me from darkness to light.
Lead me from death to immortality.
Om. Peace. Peace. Peace.

YAMA-S (LIMB #1)
Ethical Practices

अहिंसासत्यास्तेयब्रह्मचर्यापरिग्रहा यमाः ॥ २.३० ॥

2.30 ahiṃsāsatyāsteyabrahmacaryāparigrahā yamāḥ
The social ethics are nonviolence, truthfulness, nonstealing, conservation of vital energy, and nonpossessiveness.

Commentary

The ***yama-s*** define a list of ethical guidelines for getting along with other people. The ability to interact with others is arguably the most important of the eight limbs of yoga. Its place at the very beginning of the limbs suggests this. Social interaction is the best environment in which to ascertain how effective our practices are. The way we treat other living creatures is a testament to our inner state. Clarity in our heart-mind manifests as kindness, compassion, selflessness, keen judgment, etc. Cloudiness reveals itself as malice, selfishness, poor judgment, etc.

Yama #1 *Ahiṃsā* (nonviolence)
Yama #2 *Satya* (truthfulness)
Yama #3 *Asteya* (not taking from others)
Yama #4 *Brahmacarya* (conservation of vital energy)
Yama #5 *Aparigraha* (nonhoarding, nonpossessiveness)

The first and foremost yama is nonviolence toward other creatures. Truthfulness is next, which, when practiced alongside nonviolence, creates a powerful force for goodness in the world.

The yama-s are listed in sūtra 2.30. Each is considered a "great vow," universal ethics not limited by social class, place, time, or circumstance (2.31). This can be taken in several ways. One extreme is to practice all the yama-s strictly all the time. Another interpretation may say that observing the yama-s depends on the situation, and to use our discrimination to determine whether or not observing a yama is appropriate. For example, if you are a soldier defending your people, it seems appropriate to incapacitate the invaders, which may mean killing some of them. If you are married, you cannot be expected to practice celibacy. Many cultures perform animal sacrifices during ritual, but a person advanced in yoga has no need for such rituals.

Complete Translation

2.30 ahiṃsāsatyāsteyabrahmacaryāparigrahā yamāḥ

ahiṃsā-satya-asteya-brahmacarya-aparigrahāḥ yamāḥ

ahiṃsā	nonviolence
satya	truthfulness
asteya	nonstealing
brahmacarya	conservation of vital energy; chaste studentship
aparigraha	nonpossessiveness
yama	social ethics, interactions, "control, restraint"

1. The yama-s are ahiṃsā, satya, asteya, brahmacarya, and aparigraha.
2. The social ethics are nonviolence, truthfulness, nonstealing, chastity, and nonpossessiveness.

Derivation of Terms

Root	yam, "restrain, control"
Dictionary	"a restraint, a check"

Related Sūtra-s

2.31

Contemplations

Do I consider myself an ethical person?

Why or why not?

How can I integrate good conduct into my practice of yoga?

AHIṂSĀ (YAMA #1)

Nonviolence and Compassion

अहिंसाप्रतिष्ठायां तत्संनिधौ वैरत्यागः ॥ २.३५ ॥

2.35 ahiṃsāpratiṣṭhāyāṃ tatsaṃnidhau vairatyāgaḥ
In the presence of one practicing nonviolence,
hostility cannot exist.

> Man and his deed are two distinct things. "Hate the sin and not the sinner" is a precept rarely practised. Ahiṃsā is the basis of the search for Truth. I am realizing every day that the search is in vain unless it is founded on ahiṃsā as the basis. It is quite proper to resist and attack a *system*, but to resist and attack its author is tantamount to resisting and attacking oneself. To slight a single human being is to slight the divine powers within us, and thus harm not only that being but with him the whole world.
>
> —MAHATMA GANDHI *Autobiography*

Commentary

Ahiṃsā is the yama (social observance) of nonhurtfulness toward others and ourselves. It involves abstaining from intentionally inflicting pain or killing other creatures in thought, word, or deed. A nonjudgmental and forgiving attitude is essential to practicing this, the first and most important social observance. Ahiṃsā also implies an attitude that strives to reduce harm. All other yama-s are supposed to be practiced alongside ahiṃsā. The second yama, truthfulness (satya), is particularly powerful when observed with nonviolence.

This yama can be applied toward yourself as well. For example, if you do something wrong, do not beat yourself up about it or regret it for a long time. Be compassionate and kind to yourself, and learn from the experience.

There are three kinds of hiṃsā (violence) and therefore ahiṃsā (nonviolence):

Kāyaka: physical (deed)
Vācaka: verbal (word)
Mānasika: mental (thought)

We are responsible for our thoughts, words, and deeds. Sūtra 2.34 states that violence (a vitarka: an opposite of a yama) results in endless suffering and ignorance, whether done, authorized, or consented to. If we had our hand in any part of a violent event, by the law of action-reaction, that energy will come back to us in some fashion. Greed, anger, and delusion cause these vitarka-s. Think of how many innocent people are harmed because of someone who will do anything to acquire or maintain power.

The antidote according to sūtra 2.33 is understanding the other side of the story (pratipakṣa-bhāvana). If violence is directed toward you, use discrimination to determine your response.

Our state of mind can affect others nearby, and vice versa. If our mind is quiet, we can calm down others around us. Conversely, if we are agitated, those near us will feel that as well. The mind-state of those around us can influence us in the same way. When there is no trace of negativity around us, ahiṃsā is present. Being considerate by performing an act of kindness stimulates friendship and good will among people.

Thoughts: Whenever we direct thoughts toward another person, she receives that energy. For example, if we look at someone and think to ourselves "she is ugly," she receives that energy. Some men will look at a woman with lust in their eyes and mind and make her uncomfortable. On the other hand, thoughts of unconditional love and support will serve to uplift another person.

Words: What do we do if someone calls us insulting names? Words have a way of inciting violence. Let the words pass through you, understanding that the person is unhappy with herself and is directing frustration toward you. This may be difficult, given that the ego may try to identify and hold on to its interpretation of the words, causing asmitā-kleśa to arise and throw you into the cyclical whirlpool of negativity. The practice of nonviolence helps one to rise above this petty game of name-calling and can be cultivated more easily when the ego is under the control of the higher intelligence (buddhi).

Deeds: Who suffers when an act of violence takes place? Who benefits from an act of nonviolence? Both parties, in both cases. For example, when a bully hits an innocent student, it might feel good to him on the outside and make him feel dominant and in control, but inside he may feel guilty for accosting someone who did nothing to deserve his wrath. Giving is receiving, whether it is positive or negative. That same bully, encountering a person just injured from a car accident, may do what he can to save that person's life, and thus receive a large dose of inner joy.

Complete Translation

2.35 ahiṃsāpratiṣṭhāyāṃ tatsaṃnidhau vairatyāgaḥ

ahiṃsā-pratiṣṭhāyāṃ tad saṃnidhau vaira-tyāgaḥ

ahiṃsā	nonviolence, nonhurtfulness, kindness, compassion
pratiṣṭhā	being established in
tad	(of) that, its
saṃnidhi	vicinity, presence
vaira	hostility
tyāga	relinquishing, abandoning

1. When established in ahiṃsā, hostility is abandoned in its vicinity.
2. In the presence of one practicing nonviolence, hostility cannot exist.

Derivation of Terms

Prefix	a "not, non-, without"
Root	hiṃs, "to strike; to hurt, injure, harm; to torment; to kill"
Dictionary	"harmlessness, abstaining from killing or giving pain to others in thought, word or deed"
Translation Here	"nonviolence, nonharming"

Contemplations

What do I *do* when I witness violence and become afraid? Can I use keen discernment (viveka), judge each situation differently, and decide for myself if and to what extent I should be involved?

The next time someone insults or unduly criticizes me, how do I feel and why do I allow those words to affect me? Can I ignore them, or investigate why they are being said?

Whenever I think negative thoughts about someone, I will take time to notice why I am thinking this way, always striving to understand that the person behaves the way she does because of her previous life experience.

SATYA (YAMA #2)
Truthfulness and Sincerity

सत्यप्रतिष्ठायां क्रियाफलाश्रयत्वम् ॥ २.३६ ॥

2.36 satyapratiṣṭhāyāṃ kriyāphalāśrayatvam
Truthfulness secures confidence in the results of an action.

> Truth is like a vast tree which yields more and more fruit the more you nurture it. The deeper the search in the mine of truth the richer the discovery of the gems buried there, in the shape of openings for an ever greater variety of service.
>
> —MAHATMA GANDHI, *Autobiography*

Commentary

Satya is the yama (social observance) that occurs when our thoughts, words, and actions are consistent with one another. This mental-verbal-actual alignment is strong enough to virtually guarantee that the results we expect will happen. It is said that a yogī who has mastered satya can make something happen by willpower alone, and can effect a saṃskāra in the listener's mind that will bear fruit.

Satya has been defined as "yathā tathā," which literally means "as, so." This can be extrapolated to mean "as perceived (by means of pramāṇa-s), so words and thoughts." Speech and mind agree and conform to reality.

It is important to distinguish three Sanskrit words within the context of satya as a yama:

ṛta: fact, what actually exists
sat: truth, what we think is fact
satya: truthfulness, the truth that we communicate

We can use pramāṇa, viparyaya, and vikalpa (as helpful vṛtti-s) to ascertain sat. When our truth aligns with actual facts, whatever we communicate will be reliable.

As a yama, satya is second only to ahiṃsā (nonviolence). When satya is practiced *with* nonviolence, the remaining yama-s and niyama-s become much easier. Otherwise, if our thoughts, words, and deeds are all harmful, then although we are practicing satya, we are not engaging in yoga. This is why nonviolence is first among the yama-s. Mahatma Gandhi called his nonviolent movement "Satyagraha," meaning "grasping for truthfulness." Satya and ahiṃsā are meant to go hand in hand.

Satya with ahiṃsā means clear, honest, appropriate, helpful communication that considers the short- and long-term consequences. Sensitivity toward others and an unselfish intention for the greater good will likely produce the most positive results.

For example, say you ask a friend to pick up some bread at the store. If you say, "Pick up some bread," he will have to guess what kind you want. If you are very specific and say, "I want seven-grain bread made by ____," your communication is clear enough to produce the desired result: the loaf of bread bought will be what you expected.

Satya also involves a high degree of responsibility and follow-through. If we give our word that we will do something, then it becomes our responsibility to finish it. Following through on commitments develops confidence in ourselves and others that we will do what we say. If we think one thing and say another, or say one thing and do another, the energy becomes diffracted and much less potent. When all three energies are the same, they are focused like a laser beam and the intention is much more likely to come true.

For example, you think *I need to lose weight* and say to yourself and others, "I will lose weight by changing my diet and exercising more." If you follow through with your intention, you are practicing satya and the results are likely to be what you expect; i.e., you will lose weight. On the other hand, if you do not significantly change your diet or lifestyle, your actions are not consistent with your thoughts and words and the desired result of weight loss will probably not happen.

Complete Translation

2.36 satyapratiṣṭhāyāṃ kriyāphalāśrayatvam

satya-pratiṣṭhāyāṃ kriyā-phala-āśrayatvam

satya truthfulness

pratiṣṭhā being established in

kriyā action

phala results

āśrayatva confidence, surity

1. When established in truthfulness, one can be sure of the results of action.
2. Truthfulness secures confidence in the results of an action.

Derivation of Terms

Root as, "to be, exist; to become; to take place"

Word sat, "being, existing; true; virtuous"

Literal Meaning	"being truthful"
Dictionary	satya, "truth, sincerity, virtue"
Translation Here	"truthfulness, sincerity"

Contemplations

How do I feel when I think one thing and say something different?
How does a lie affect my conscience?
How may lying lead to further lies?

ASTEYA (YAMA #3)

Not Taking from Others

अस्तेयप्रतिष्ठायां सर्वरत्नोपस्थानम् ॥ २.३७ ॥

2.37 asteyapratiṣṭhāyāṃ sarvaratnopasthānam
Prosperity comes to one who does not steal.

Commentary

Asteya is the yama (social observance) of not taking from others and only accepting what is earned or freely given. If we do not covet another's property, more prosperity will come to us. When our actions show that we can be trusted, others will share everything with us. Asteya shares the principle of honesty with satya, the previous yama.

By giving, we receive much more, if only on a subtle level. Being generous toward others without expecting anything in return nurtures our heart-mind and promotes lovingkindness. Giving with an expectation of a future favor is tainted with tamasic residue and does not nourish our heart-mind.

A vitarka is the opposite: stealing. When we covet something belonging to another person, they will not trust us and therefore will not share.

For example, say you become a housesitter for a few months. Inside the house are many valuable works of art, electronic equipment, etc. If you steal out of greed or envy, you will reap the negative energy described in 2.34. If you refrain and take care of the house as expected, the owners will trust you and probably have you housesit for them again.

If we interrupt someone during a conversation, we are stealing his or her attention. Plagarizing or taking undue credit for someone else's ideas are also forms of stealing.

Complete Translation

2.37 asteyapratiṣṭhāyāṃ sarvaratnopasthānam
asteya-pratiṣṭhāyāṃ sarva-ratna-upasthānam

asteya	nonstealing, not taking
pratiṣṭhā	being established in
sarva	all
ratna	jewels, wealth
upasthāna	close proximity

1. Established in nonstealing, all jewels come close.
2. Prosperity comes to one who does not steal.

Derivation of Terms

Prefix	a, "not, without"
Root	sten, "to steal, rob; to be dishonest in speech"
Dictionary	"not stealing"
Translation Here	"not taking from others"

Contemplations

How can I become more of a giver than a taker?
If I am a giver, can I allow myself to receive as well?
How do I feel when I am interrupted?

BRAHMACARYA (YAMA #4)

Conservation of Vital Energy

ब्रह्मचर्यप्रतिष्ठायां वीर्यलाभः ॥ २.३८ ॥

2.38 brahmacaryapratiṣṭhāyāṃ vīryalābhaḥ
Vitality is gained when sexual energy is conserved and directed inward.

Commentary

Brahmacarya is the yama (social observance) of conserving vital energy, especially sexual impulses, in order to channel it in more productive directions. Moving (carya) toward supreme truth (Brahma) directs the heart-mind away from sensual indulgence, reduces the libido, and thus conserves the sexual fluids that contribute to overall health and vitality. According to Āyurveda, the ultimate product of digestion is the most refined tissue in the body, called śukra ("pure, radiant"), the reproductive fluids. This fuels ojas, the subtle force behind the immune system.

Sexual desire is a powerful force. Regular physical exercise can divert some of this energy. Moderation combined with responsible and appropriate sexual behavior is the key to brahmacarya. A vitarka is its opposite: promiscuity.

Many translate this yama as "celibacy." In India, traditionally one goes through four stages of life (see table below). Brahmacarya is practiced as celibacy throughout puberty in order to direct all that hormonal energy into one's studies. Once one is married, brahmacarya is practiced as fidelity, sexual monogamy. If the final two stages are pursued, brahmacarya means celibacy again.

The Four Stages of Life (āśrama-s) are chronological:

LIFE STAGE	ROLE	AGE (APPROXIMATE)
Brahmacarya	Celibate student	Five to twenty-five
Gārhasthya	Householder	Twenty-five to fifty
Vānaprastha	Forest dweller, hermit	Fifty to seventy-five
Saṃnyāsa	Renunciate, monk, swāmī	Seventy five and up

These stages are distinct from the Four Aims of Life (puruṣārtha-s), which are not chronological:

AIM	MEANING	DESCRIPTION
Dharma	Virtue	Being a good person
Artha	Means	Work, earn money
Kāma	Desire	Marry, have children
Mokṣa	Liberation	Experience the inner light within

Complete Translation

2.38 brahmacaryapratiṣṭhāyāṃ vīryalābhaḥ

brahmacarya-pratiṣṭhāyām vīrya-lābhaḥ

brahmacarya	moving as Brahma, celibacy, conservation of sexual energy
pratiṣṭhā	being established in
vīrya	vitality
lābha	obtainment

1. When established in brahmacarya, vitality is obtained.
2. Vitality is gained when sexual energy is conserved and directed inward.

Derivation of Terms

Word	brahma, "supreme divinity; creative energy of the universe"
Root	car, "walk, move, roam; to do, act; to practice; to conduct oneself"
Word	carya, "going about; behavior, conduct"
Literal Meaning	"behaving honorably; acting from our inner divinity"
Dictionary	brahmacarya, "religious studentship; celibacy practiced during a boy's learning stage of life"
Translation Here	"conservation of vital energy"

Contemplations

In what other productive and helpful directions can I divert any excess sexual energy?

Am I able to practice moderation of my sensory organs and not indulge them so much?

Can physical exercise, like āsana, replace other ways of channelling excess energy?

APARIGRAHA (YAMA #5)
Non-Hoarding

अपरिग्रहस्थैर्ये जन्मकथंतासंबोधः ॥ २.३९ ॥

2.39 aparigrahasthairye janmakathaṃtāsaṃbodhaḥ
When no longer grasping for things,
we discover why we were born.

Commentary

Aparigraha is the yama (social observance) of not being possessive. This applies to material objects, our body, and our thoughts. Rejecting the concept of "mine" will be difficult for the ego but is indeed necessary to progress in yoga. Once this is achieved, the sūtra states that we will understand how we came to be born into this particular life situation. Our current life is a culmination of many births and deaths, all molded by past actions and their impressions (saṃskāra-s).

Nonpossessiveness of the heart-mind means not holding on to rigid opinions and not regarding ideas as our own. Whenever we come up with something that appears to be new and original, it is important to realize that we are just tapping into knowledge that already exists, represented by Īśvara. Our ego (ahaṅkāra—see citta) loves to hold on to things and call them its own. Everything changes. An inflexible heart-mind is not easy to interact with.

Nonhoarding also involves not controlling other people when there is a power differential, as a boss might try to control his or her employees, threatening them if they speak up or rock the boat. Money can be used as leverage to control the actions of others as well.

The vitarka (opposing, negative form of aparigraha) would be "parigraha," grasping things (graha) all around us (pari). As we accumulate "stuff," more of our time is spent maintaining it, leaving less time for our own internal development. The "shop 'til you drop" attitude feeds our bottomless desire to acquire. We are bombarded with advertisements pushing us to buy "stuff" that we often do not need.

Applied to a conversation, aparigraha means allowing others to speak and share their point of view. The vitarka here would be dominating the conversation and barely allowing anyone else to chime in.

Complete Translation

2.39 aparigrahasthairye janmakathaṃtāsaṃbodhaḥ

aparigraha-sthairye janma-kathaṃtā-saṃbodhaḥ

aparigraha	nonpossessiveness, not being greedy
sthairya	being firm in
janma	birth
kathaṃtā	"how-ness," the reason for, what sort of manner
saṃbodha	complete knowledge

1. When firm in aparigraha, complete knowledge of the reason we were born.
2. When no longer grasping for things, we discover why we were born.

Derivation of Terms

Prefix	a, "not, without"
Prefix	pari, "around"
Original Root	gṛh, "to accept, take, seize"
Prefixed Root	parigṛh, "to clasp around, hug; to surround; to take; to accept"
Literal Meaning	"not taking from all around"
Dictionary	"nonacceptance; rejection; renunciation"
Translation Here	"not hoarding, not accepting inappropriately"

Contemplations

Do I actually use all the things I own?

If not, can someone else use them?

How can I reduce my material footprint and use of resources?

PRATIPAKṢA-BHĀVANA

Cultivating the Opposite

वितर्कबाधने प्रतिपक्षभावनम् ॥ २.३३ ॥

2.33 vitarkabādhane pratipakṣabhāvanam

When disturbed by an event opposed to the yama-s,
one should cultivate an attitude that counteracts that
(and acts according to the yama-s).

Commentary

Vitarka means "opposing beliefs" and is equated with any behavior that opposes social ethics (yama-s) (2.34). It can be expanded to mean all negative and disturbing actions. These can be mild, moderate, or excessive, and they are based on greed, anger, and delusion. Whether they are done, approved of, or consented to, they inevitably result in pain (duḥkha) and ignorance (ajñāna, same as avidyā).

When we witness vitarka-s, i.e., events that are contrary to the yama-s, they may very well disturb us. Automatically we are reminded of opposite, virtuous qualities like the yama-s, and strive to cultivate those instead. Negative thoughts can be used as opportunities to create positive thoughts. In this way ***pratipakṣa-bhāvana*** supports the yama-s.

For example, assume you see someone shoplifting and become a little uncomfortable. You know in your heart-mind that stealing is wrong; therefore nonstealing is right. Whether or not to act is up to your discretion. In traditional Indian medicine (Āyurveda), when we eat foods that create imbalance, the treatment is to eat foods that have qualities opposed to the imbalances. Even when practicing āsana, we often do a pose, then a counterpose, to maintain a balanced body. Opposing action brings stability, focus, and endurance.

Pratipakṣa-bhāvana can also mean understanding another's point of view, putting ourselves in another's shoes. Most people act according to their habitual patterns based on their past. What would the world look like if we all attempted to understand the other side of every story? For example, when a relationship involving a friend of yours ends, you probably only hear your friend's side of the story, which may make the other person look like the "bad guy." Only when you hear the other person's version of the breakup can you truly understand it yourself.

This concept can also help avoid future suffering (duḥkha). By listening to both sides of a story in a nonjudgmental way, you can maintain a decent relationship with both parties and do not run the risk of spreading false information based on one person's opinion.

In any interaction, remember that you may be entering the situation influenced by your own assumptions based on past experience. A kleśa may arise. Before actually doing anything, immediately distance yourself from the resulting emotion that is about to cause a reaction. Then visualize the other side and ask yourself, "How will the other person be affected?" "How much is my own perception of the situation causing this emotion?" At this point there is an opportunity to see what is going on from a more objective vantage point. By acting consciously and compassionately instead of reacting negatively based on your own issues, you build a new, helpful, positive saṃskāra.

Complete Translation

2.33 vitarkabādhane pratipakṣabhāvanam

vitarka-bādhane pratipakṣa-bhāvanam

vitarka	anti-yama, adverse to logic, negative thought or action
bādhana	troubling, disturbing, binding
pratipakṣa	"other wing," other side, opposite side
bhāvana	cultivating, attitude, manifestation

1. When disturbed by negative thoughts or events, cultivation of opposite thoughts or events.
2. When disturbed by an event opposed to the yama-s, one should cultivate an attitude that counteracts that (acting according to the yama-s).

Derivation of Terms

PRATIPAKṢA

Prefix	prati, "against, opposed to"
Root	pakṣ, "take, seize, accept, side with"
Literal Meaning	pratipakṣa, "opposite side"
Dictionary	pakṣa, "wing, side, faction, half of"
Translation Here	"opposite side"

BHĀVANA

Root	bhū, "to be, exist, become, be produced, happen"
Dictionary	"creating, manifesting; promoting any of our interests; conception, imagination, idea; feeling of devotion, faith; meditation, contemplation; observing, investigating, determining; infusing; scenting"
Translation Here	"cultivation, intention, attitude, feeling"

VITARKA

Prefix	vi, "separating, discerning"
Original Root	tark, "to suppose, guess; to reason, speculate about; to ascertain"
Prefixed Root	vitark, "to guess, think, suppose, believe, reflect, reason, expect, anticipate"
Dictionary	"argument, reasoning, inference; guess, supposition, belief; fancy, thought; purpose, intention"
Translation Here	"an attitude contrary to the yama-s"

Related Sūtra-s

2.34

Contemplations

How can I understand someone I do not like, but have to be around?

How can I transform a negative experience into a positive one?

Can I listen to both sides of a story fairly, even when I am closer to one person than the other?

NIYAMA-S (LIMB #2)

Personal Practices

शौचसंतोषतपःस्वाध्यायेश्वरप्रणिधानानि नियमाः ॥ २.३२ ॥

2.32 śaucasantoṣatapaḥsvādhyāyeśvarapraṇidhānāni niyamāḥ
Personal practices are cleanliness, contentment, practice causing change, self-study, and letting go.

Commentary

Niyama means "internal control or restraint" and defines practices to use for taking care of ourselves on a personal level. Each is discussed in its own section.

The most external niyama is cleanliness: keeping the body, mind, and surroundings free of clutter and impurities. Next is being content with and grateful for who we are and what we have. The final three niyama-s constitute kriyā-yoga and are discussed in that section.

Niyama #1: *Śauca* (cleanliness of body, heart-mind, and surroundings)
Niyama #2: *Santoṣa* (contentment)
Niyama #3: *Tapas* (practice causing positive change)
Niyama #4: *Svādhyāya* (study by and of oneself)
Niyama #5: *Īśvara-praṇidhāna* (humility and faith)

Complete Translation

2.32 śaucasantoṣatapaḥsvādhyāyeśvarapraṇidhānāni niyamāḥ
śauca-santoṣa-tapas-svādhyāya-īśvarapraṇidhānāni niyamāḥ

śauca	cleanliness, purity, personal hygiene
santoṣa	contentment
tapas	practice causing change
svādhyāya	self-study, self-observation, reciting our mantra
īśvara-praṇidhāna	honoring the divine inner teacher, letting go
niyama	personal practice or observance

1. Niyama-s are śauca, santoṣa, tapas, svādhyāya, and īśvara-praṇidhāna.
2. Personal practices are cleanliness, contentment, practice causing change, self-study, and letting go.

Derivation of Terms

Prefix	ni, "down, into"
Root	yam, "restrain, control"
Literal Meaning	"internal yama"
Dictionary	"restraint, check; a rule; self-imposed religious observance"

Related Sūtra-s

2.40–45

Contemplations

How much emphasis do I put on outer and inner cleanliness?

Do I take the time to care for myself?

Am I ignoring any of these niyama-s?

ŚAUCA (NIYAMA #1)
Cleanliness

शौचात्स्वाङ्गजुगुप्सा परैरसंसर्गः ॥ २.४० ॥

2.40 śaucātsvāṅgajugupsā parairasaṃsargaḥ
From cleanliness, a disfavor of our own body and of contact with other (bodies).

Commentary
Śauca is the niyama (personal behavior) of maintaining a clean body and clear heart-mind. The body is purified through tapas (2.43) and āsana, while the heart-mind can be cleansed from those and the other limbs of yoga. The process of yoga is a gradual purification of all layers of our individual self. The body is never completely sanitary and requires regular care to keep functioning. Because of this, the physical body itself can never be pure. When our goal is to become clear, and we realize that the body is inherently dirty, an aversion develops toward our body and other bodies.

Good personal hygiene, uncluttered surroundings, and the process of yoga all contribute to a clear heart-mind. Śauca leads to a heart-mind that is sattvic, happy, focused, not distracted by sensory perceptions, and ready for experiencing the divine light (2.41). A vegetarian diet aligns with śauca, since it supports nonviolence (ahiṃsā) and promotes the quality of sattva.

Cleanliness can be taken to an extreme when we become uptight because our surroundings are not spic-and-span all the time. This may be the ego's way of controlling its environment or making up for a deep sense of insecurity from perceived internal impurity. Sometimes if we feel unclean on the inside, often from a past painful experience, it can manifest as obsessive cleaning on the outside.

Keeping the body clean can remind us of its impermanence, since it is always changing, which in turn can make us realize what does not change and requires no maintenance (the light within). All the stuff we spend time cleaning can also reveal what we are attached to.

"Coming clean" by admitting something we have been holding in because of potential embarassment is another form of śauca. Expressing deep emotion in a nonviolent way purges the heart-mind of pent-up feelings. Mourning the death or suffering of a loved one cleanses our heart-mind as well. Apologizing is extremely cathartic for the heart-mind, and weakens the kleśa asmitā (egotism).

Complete Translation

2.40 śaucātsvāṅgajugupsā parairasaṃsargaḥ

śaucāt svāṅga-jugupsā paraiḥ asaṃsargaḥ

śauca	cleanliness, purity of body, mind, and surroundings
svāṅga	our own limbs/body
jugupsā	disgust
para	another
asaṃsarga	nonassociation, noncontact

1. From cleanliness, aversion to our own body (and) nonassociation with others.
2. From cleanliness, a disfavor of our own body and of contact with other (bodies).

Derivation of Terms

Root	śuc, "to mourn; to regret; to be sorry; to be wet; to shine; to be pure or clean"
Dictionary	"purity, clearness; cleansing; uprightness, honesty; purification from personal defilement caused by the death of a relative"
Translation Here	"cleanliness, purity, personal hygeine, neatness"

Related Sūtra-s

2.41

Contemplations

How is the clutter on my desk affecting the clarity of my heart-mind?

Am I too clean?

If so, why?

SANTOṢA (NIYAMA #2)

Contentment and Gratitude

सन्तोषादनुत्तमः सुखलाभः ॥ २.४२ ॥

2.42 santoṣādanuttamaḥ sukhalābhaḥ

When we are content with who we are, we become happy.

Commentary

Santoṣa is the niyama (personal behavior) of being grateful for what we have and content with who we are and where we are in life. Contentment is related to being unattached to the results of our actions. If the result is less than we expected, we accept what happens, learn from it, and move on. If we have unreasonable expectations, we may be setting ourselves up for disappointment.

If we cultivate gratitude even when we are content, we strengthen that saṃskāra in the heart-mind, like amending its soil, and make it easier to access when needed. Gratefulness is like eating food; it nourishes our heart-mind and creates a sense of fulfillment. Slowing down, stepping back, and appreciating the little things in life create inner happiness.

The opposite (vitarka) of santoṣa is discontent or dissatisfaction, a form of duḥkha. Noticing this feeling is the first step toward converting it. By applying the principle of pratipakṣa-bhāvana, we must be grateful for what we have and where we are instead of focusing on what we do not have or why we are not where we want to be. As long as we are *doing* something in a positive direction, time and patience will lead us to the desired result. Contentment is not stagnant because of the changeable nature of our life and the world around us. We are aware that we are moving forward and satisfied with our progress.

So often we judge our progress based on comparison to others. Granted, those who have practiced for many years can show us what we may be capable of, but it usually takes time and effort to reach that level. As long as we are moving in a positive direction, it doesn't matter. Our culture is used to immediate gratification. Yet a delicious soup results from a slow simmer over time, not a quick and furious boil.

How we look can be another source of dissatisfaction. If we attend a yoga lecture and feel uncomfortable sitting on the floor for hours on end, why not just sit in a chair? Even for meditation it is better to be relaxed and upright in a chair than tense, in pain, and slouched sitting on the floor. When we conform to what we think others expect of us in order to "save face" and be accepted by others, we are not content with ourselves.

Āsana progress is falsely judged by our level of flexibility. If someone can perform all of the "difficult" postures, are they really good at āsana? If so, then a ballet dancer or gymnast could walk into a class and be judged the most advanced student. Obviously, this is misperception (viparyaya). In fact, even someone who is inflexible can be an expert in āsana if they exert sincere effort and understand their body and its limitations.

Complete Translation

2.42 santoṣādanuttamaḥ sukhalābhaḥ

santoṣāt anuttamaḥ sukha-lābhaḥ

santoṣa	contentment
anuttama	unexcelled
sukha	happiness
lābha	obtainment, attainment

1. From santoṣa, (one) obtains unexcelled happiness.
2. When we are content with who we are, we become happy.

Derivation of Terms

Prefix	sam, "completely, together"
Root	tuṣ, "to be pleased, satisfied, content with anything"
Dictionary	santoṣa, "satisfaction, contentment; delight, joy"

Contemplations

When am I happiest? Why?

What makes me feel content and satisfied? How might that change?

How can I become a happier person?

KRIYĀ-YOGA

Practice in Action

तपःस्वाध्यायेश्वरप्रणिधानानि क्रियायोगः ॥ २.१ ॥

2.1 tapaḥsvādhyāyeśvarapraṇidhānāni kriyāyogaḥ
The yoga of active practice consists of practice causing change, self-observation, and honoring the divine inner teacher.

Commentary

Kriyā-yoga is a synergistic set of tools that bring about real change. It consists of the last three niyama-s—tapas, svādhyāya, and īśvara-praṇidhāna—each of which has its own separate commentary. Tapas, practice causing change, involves conscious and deliberate action. Svādhyāya, observation by and of ourselves, allows us to see what about ourselves needs improvement. Īśvara-praṇidhāna keeps us humble and respectful by acknowledging and honoring knowledge itself.

When this triad is practiced in collaboration, it becomes a powerful mechanism for learning and growth. Kriyā-yoga is one of the easiest systems to understand but is quite difficult to implement since it involves real on-the-ground change to our personality. It is a simple, straightforward formula on the path of yoga if practiced with great tenacity and purpose. Since each component informs the others, change is more profound and noticeable when they are practiced together.

Kriyā-yoga is the seed for the eight limbs of yoga (aṣṭāṅga-yoga). The threefold set of tools is to be integrated into the other practices. Inner growth involves changing the way we look at things, the way we operate, our attitudes, and our expectations. Some questions you might ask yourself are:

Tapas: How can you implement changes?

- Set an intention to commit to positive changes in your life.
- Formulate specific actions to take, or ways you wish to respond when certain buttons are pushed.

Svādhyāya: How do you discover who you really are?

- Observe how you act in uncomfortable situations (duḥkha management, monitoring our levels of reactivity).
- Notice any tendencies you have.

- Reflect on how much of your action is controlled by your past (rāga, dveṣa).
- See how your actions and reactions affect outcomes.

Īśvara-praṇidhāna: How can you let go of your attachments and expectations?

- Understand that all things change.
- When your heart-mind is still, listen to your inner teacher.
- Remember that unreasonable or unrealistic expectations will likely lead to disappointment and unhappiness.

The purpose of kriyā-yoga is twofold: to cultivate an intention toward samādhi and to cause a weakening of the kleśa-s (2.2). Note that kriyā-yoga does not eliminate the kleśa-s; it only serves to weaken them. Continuous meditation (dhyāna) ends the outer, gross form of the kleśa-s known as kliṣṭa-vṛtti-s. Pratiprasava ends the kleśa-s in their subtle form, as saṃskāra-s (2.10).

NIYAMA	YOGA	REALM
Tapas	Karma	Physical
Svādhyāya	Jñāna	Mental
Īśvara-praṇidhāna	Bhakti	Emotional/spiritual

Complete Translation

2.1 tapaḥsvādhyāyeśvarapraṇidhānāni kriyāyogaḥ
tapaḥ-svādhyāya-īśvarapraṇidhānāni kriyā-yogaḥ

tapas	practice causing positive change
svādhyāya	self-study, self-observation
īśvara-praṇidhāna	honoring the divine inner teacher
kriyā-yoga	the yoga of active practice or work

1. Kriyā-yoga consists of tapas, svādhyāya, and īśvara-praṇidhāna.
2. The yoga of active practice consists of practice causing change, self-observation, and honoring the divine inner teacher.

Derivation of Terms

Root	kṛ, "to do, act, make"
Literal Meaning	kriyā, "action, work"
Dictionary	"doing, execution; action, business, undertaking; practice"
Translation Here	"active practice"

Related Sūtra-s

2.2

Contemplations

Am I willing to do the work necessary for lasting inner transformation?

How can I apply kriyā-yoga in my life?

Is there anything I cannot apply this to?

TAPAS (NIYAMA #3)

Practice Causing Positive Change

कायेन्द्रियसिद्धिरशुद्धिक्षयात्तपसः ॥ २.४३ ॥

2.43 kāyendriyasiddhiraśuddhikṣayāttapasaḥ
Perfection of the body and sensory organs is from the destruction of impurities due to tapas.

Commentary

Tapas, along with svādhyāya and īśvara-praṇidhāna, make up kriyā-yoga, a powerful triad of tools for weakening the kleśa-s and realizing samādhi (2.1-2).

Tapas is the niyama (personal behavior) of deliberately acting in a way that causes positive change in ourselves. The word is derived from the root "tap" meaning "to heat." The heat generated by practicing tapas will incinerate physical, mental, and emotional impurities and refine the body, sensory organs, and heart-mind. A vigorous āsana sequence with enough effort to create heat and change in the body is one of the most common forms of tapas. The heat of tapas comes from the friction generated by resistance to a new and different action.

Habitual behavior causes stagnation. When we consciously change a habit, discomfort (duḥkha) arises and creates heat in the body. This is the priceless heat of real change. If we are aware that the discomfort is good for us, it becomes a desirable effect and may encourage our continued practice. Because we are consciously challenging long-standing patterns of behavior, tapas burns up those deep saṃskāra-s. The heat generated by tapas results in spiritual and physiological transformation.

For example, think of a strong habit, some action that you have done the same way for many years. Let's say it's the way you brush your teeth. Try to brush them using the opposite hand, or moving through your mouth in a different order. This will feel uncomfortable at first, but with enough repetition a new saṃskāra will form and it will become easier. Next, try choosing a habit that you know is obstructing some aspect of your life. Set an intention and make a commitment to change the habit. An attitude of satya will help you follow through with your plan.

In Indian tradition, heat is also called agni and is responsible for change, just as heat added or removed is required to change solid to liquid or liquid to gas and vice versa. Fire is central to ritual and ceremony; it transforms what is offered into its most basic elements.

A traditional, orthodox view sees tapas as an austere practice of enduring physical pain in order to become detached from the mortal body. One such practice is called "pañcāgni," meaning "five fires," in which a person sits in the hot sun (fire #1) surrounded by four fires and tries to meditate. The idea is to become impervious to the "pairs of opposites" like heat/cold, wet/dry, etc. that assail the sensory organs and draw the attention outward toward external objects. The manifest world (Prakṛti) is the realm of duality. Our heart-mind is constantly bombarded with external stimuli we try to make sense of. Distinguishing one thing from another allows us to function in society. By deliberately enduring various extremes like heat or cold, an ascetic was said to become immune to their effect on the heart-mind. This kind of ascetic practice may have merit in a different culture, time, or place, but in contemporary society it may not be appropriate. Tapas should never be harmful to ourselves or others.

Tapas requires discipline and effort. In Indian lore, sages practice tapas and celibacy for thousands of years to accumulate lots of power. When the gods notice that their power may be threatened, they send a beautiful nymph down who tries to distract the sage from his meditation. If she succeeds in seducing him, he loses his seed and thus his power. (See brahmacarya.)

Complete Translation

2.43 kāyendriyasiddhiraśuddhikṣayāttapasaḥ
kāya-indriya-siddhiḥ aśuddhi-kṣayāt tapasaḥ

kāya	body
indriya	sensory organ
siddhi	perfection, power
aśuddhi	impurity
kṣaya	destruction
tapas	practice causing positive change

1. Perfection of the body and sensory organs is from the destruction of impurities due to tapas.

Derivation of Terms

Root	tap, "to shine, blaze; to heat up; to suffer pain; to undergo penance"
Literal Meaning	same as dictionary
Dictionary	"warmth, heat, fire, light; pain, suffering; religious austerity"
Translation Here	"practice causing change"

Related Sūtra-s

2.1–2

Contemplations

What habits do I want to change?

How can I actually implement real changes in the way I act?

Am I willing to endure some discomfort or suffering if it serves to create positive changes in myself?

SVĀDHYĀYA (NIYAMA #4)

Study by and of Oneself

स्वाध्यायादिष्टदेवतासंप्रयोगः ॥ २.४४ ॥

2.44 svādhyāyādiṣṭadevatāsaṃprayogaḥ

By observing ourself in action, we can connect with our higher truth.

Commentary

Svādhyāya is the niyama (personal behavior, 2.32) of learning about and developing the heart-mind (citta). Through reading and listening that promote self-reflection, recitation of mantra, or insightful observation of ourselves in action, we bring awareness to our strengths and shortcomings. Once we understand where we are, we can set an intention toward letting go of our negative qualities and reinforcing those that have a positive effect. Svādhyāya includes understanding our physical body (in terms of Āyurvedic doṣa-s), mental body (in terms of guṇa-s), and how we act (karma-s).

Studying ancient scriptures is helpful if they are meaningful to us. In our society, it may be more applicable to study books that cause us to ponder ourselves and our surroundings, or books/CDs that help us refine our yoga practice. Keeping a daily diary of actions we were not proud of is extremely beneficial, since it brings awareness to parts of ourselves that can improve and may involve vṛtti-s, kleśa-s, and saṃskāra-s.

Traditionally svādhyāya means learning and repeating a mantra (japa) chosen by our teacher for us and studying sacred texts that guide us inward, like the *Veda-s, Upaniṣad-s,* or *Bhagavad-Gītā.* The mantra Om is the most common mantra, whose repetition connects us with Īśvara (1.27–28). If we have chosen a deity to relate to, then a mantra to that deity activates the energetic link between us and it. For example, Gaṇeśa represents the energy of abundance and clearing away obstacles. Chanting a mantra specifically to Gaṇeśa will connect us to that energy and help bring it into our life.

Tapas, practice causing change, naturally leads to svādhyāya as we observe the changes happening and adjust our practice to maintain our desired direction. It may be easier to wait until the heat diminishes, and then, in a quieter space, reflect back on our tapas experience.

Svādhyāya, along with tapas and īśvara-praṇidhāna, constitute kriyā-yoga, a powerful triad of tools for weakening the kleśa-s and realizing samādhi (2.1–2).

Through svādhyāya it is possible to understand anything.

Complete Translation

2.44 svādhyāyādiṣṭadevatāsaṃprayogaḥ

svādhyāyāt iṣṭa-devatā-saṃprayogaḥ

svādhyāya	self-study, self-observation
iṣṭa-devatā	desired deity, something to look up to, strive for
saṃprayoga	communion

1. From svādhyāya, communion with our desired deity.
2. By observing ourself in action, we can connect with our higher truth.

Derivation of Terms

Prefix	sva, meaning "own/self"
Root	adhī, meaning "to study, learn by heart, read; to notice, observe, understand"
Literal Meaning	"self-study, self-observation"
Dictionary	"self-recitation, study of sacred books"
Translation Here	"study by and of oneself"

Contemplations

Am I aware of my actions as they are happening?

Do I reflect on them later?

Is it easy or difficult to observe myself deeply or see myself as others do?

ĪŚVARA-PRAṆIDHĀNA (NIYAMA #5)
Humility and Faith

समाधिसिद्धिरीश्वरप्रणिधानात् ॥ २.४५ ॥

2.45 samādhisiddhirīśvarapraṇidhānāt
Samādhi is experienced from surrendering the results of action to and deeply respecting the inner, universal light of knowledge.

Commentary

Īśvara-praṇidhāna, along with tapas and svādhyāya, make up kriyā-yoga, a powerful triad of tools for weakening the kleśa-s and realizing samādhi (2.1-2).

Īśvara-praṇidhāna is the niyama (personal behavior) of deep respect, admiration, and faith in a higher, inner knowledge. The results of, and credit for, all actions are offered to Īśvara. A clear and receptive heart-mind promotes insight into this infinite reservoir of knowledge. Serving others is serving Īśvara, since it is subtly present in the heart of all beings.

According to this sūtra, the practice of Īśvara-praṇidhāna leads to the attainment of samādhi. As long as the self-identity (ahaṅkāra) secures our "self" as a distinct entity, we will always be separate from external objects. Samādhi occurs when the ego relinquishes control, allowing the heart-mind to reflect the object like a mirror and causing the subject (mirrorlike heart-mind) to look exactly like the object. Īśvara-praṇidhāna is one way toward this state. In fact, īśvara-praṇidhāna can be a direct path to samādhi bypassing the usual stages of practice (1.23).

Īśvara can mean lord, personal God, or an omniscient entity. Praṇidhāna implies a state of humility in the presence of something higher. We all have limitations, yet we share the uniquely human ability to self-reflect and the capacity to experience something beyond our conditioned heart-mind. The words "namaḥ te" combine to form "namaste," a common greeting in India that literally means "salutations to you" and implies "salutations to the divine within you." Cultivating a heart-mind that sees the divine energy inside each person is the practical culmination of this niyama. There is then no perceived difference between us and others, which cuts through unawareness (avidyā), demotes egotism (asmitā), and is a form of samādhi.

Focus on the action and accept the results without hesitation. Act out of inspiration. Humility means the asmitā-kleśa is not active and anything the ego thinks it owns can be passed through us to our teacher or to the universe. For example, if you think that what you teach or purport belongs to you, asmitā-kleśa has reared its possessive head. Any teaching that you think is uniquely your own is the result of an integration and extrapolation of past learning and experience. Let the accolades coming toward you pass right through by honoring, respecting, and giving credit to the past teachers and teachings that have contributed to your unique way of transmitting useful information.

Īśvara-praṇidhāna cannot happen if doubt (see antarāya-s) is present. This is especially true if this is practiced as devotion or bhakti-yoga, where one bypasses the heart-mind and connects directly with the object of devotion. To be successful, there can be nothing in the way.

Complete Translation

2.45 samādhisiddhirīśvarapraṇidhānāt

samādhi-siddhiḥ īśvara-praṇidhānāt

samādhi	complete absorption of the heart-mind in the focus
siddhi	power
īśvara-praṇidhāna	honoring the divine inner teacher

1. The power of samādhi is due to Īśvara-praṇidhāna.
2. Samādhi is experienced from surrendering the results of action to, and deeply respecting, the inner, universal light of knowledge.

Derivation of Terms

Prefix	pra, "front"
Prefix	ni, "in, beneath"
Root	dhā, "to place, lay"
Literal Meaning	"placing (ourself) beneath and in front of"
Dictionary	"applying, employing; application, use; great effort; profound religious meditation; entrance, access; respectful behavior toward; renunciation of the fruit of actions"
Translation Here	"deeply respecting and honoring, having faith in, letting go"

Related Sūtra-s

1.23; 2.1–2

Contemplations

Am I able to let go of my ego and intellect and make room for another kind of experience?

Am I too afraid to take any risk, even when it is safe and there is nothing to lose?

Can I be thankful for compliments and pass any flattery or accolades through me so they do not stick and inflate my ego?

ĀSANA (LIMB #3)

Refinement of the Body

स्थिरसुखमासनम् ॥ २.४६ ॥

2.46 sthirasukhamāsanam
Correct posture has a balance of firmness and pliability.

Commentary

Āsana means sitting or seat, and implies sitting in meditation. This third limb of yoga involves stretching and exercising the physical body. The body needs to be strong and pliable to ground the prāṇa coursing through the nervous system. The aim of āsana is to reduce any hyperactivity in the nervous system (rajas guṇa) and prepare for prāṇāyāma. If one cannot sit still comfortably with the spine erect, the prāṇa cannot flow unobstructed. On the other hand, prāṇāyāma is important during the practice of āsana, so they work hand in hand.

In the West, the connotation of "yoga" is āsana. If I say I practice yoga, everyone thinks I mean working with the physical postures. Āsana is that small fraction of yoga meant for refining the physical body so the prāṇa can move without obstruction. Patañjali does not emphasize āsana and devotes only three sūtra-s to it. There are other Sanskrit texts that go into detail about āsana, mentioning hundreds of postures that focus more on physical purification than the *Yoga Sūtra-s.* (See part 1 for a list of these texts.)

Āsana acheives stability and comfort when accompanied by relaxed effort and samāpatti (2.47). (See samādhi.) In this kind of āsana we are no longer affected by our surroundings—heat and cold, pleasure and pain, etc. (2.48). When we can sit effortlessly still and relaxed, with our heart-mind focused on the infinite within, then the prāṇa is stable and pratyāhāra occurs, leaving one invulnerable to sensory stimuli (the pairs of opposites).

Āsana can also imply our posture during interactions with others. If we are too rigid with our opinions, closed-minded, and not open to a different way of looking at something, then there is too much sthira (rigidity) and not enough sukha (openness). On the other hand, if we have no opinion about anything and go along with whatever anyone says, then we are like a spineless worm, with too much sukha (looseness) and not enough sthira (firmness).

Complete Translation

2.46 sthirasukhamāsanam

sthira-sukham āsanam

sthira	stable, steady, firm, alert
sukha	comfortable, adaptable, relaxed
āsana	sitting, seat, posture

1. Āsana (sitting) is (should be) stable and comfortable.

Related Sūtra-s

2.47–48

Derivation of Terms

Root	ās, "sit, rest"
Literal Meaning	"sitting, seat, resting"
Dictionary	"sitting down; seat, place, stool; posture; encamping; dwelling"
Translation Here	"postural development, physical exercises"

Contemplations

Do I emphasize the form of a posture more than the function?

What specific āsana-s can I do to be able to sit comfortably and relaxed for meditation?

How can I apply the principles of āsana to my social interactions?

PRĀṆĀYĀMA (LIMB #4)

Regulation of Prāṇa

तस्मिन्सति श्वासप्रश्वासयोर्गतिविच्छेदः प्राणायामः ॥ २.४९ ॥

2.49 tasminsati śvāsapraśvāsayorgativicchedaḥ prāṇāyāmaḥ
Once (the sitting posture) is (stable and comfortable), then the regulation of breath is cutting off the movements of inhalation and exhalation (so the breath is still).

Commentary

Breath is a physical manifestation of prāṇa, the life-force, that connects all aspects of perception. (See appendix F, figures 4 and 5.) Prāṇa is one of the most important aspects of yoga and the Vedic philosophy from which yoga developed. (See prāṇa in part 1.)

Prāṇāyāma comprises both the practices involving the breath and the resulting breath regulation and control. Breathing exercises manipulate the prāṇa and directly affect the body and the mind (see appendix F, figure 2) through the nervous system, and thus have the potential to be very helpful or very harmful. It is safest to learn from an experienced teacher who takes into consideration our Āyurvedic constitution, breath capacity, etc. The overall goal of prāṇāyāma is to calm the nervous system, quell the activity in the heart-mind (nirodha), and quietly focus inward.

When the life-force is obstructed, the breath becomes irregular. For example, when we are frightened our prāṇa is shocked, causing us to gasp. The antarāya-s can cause irregular breathing (1.31), which when corrected can help clarify the citta (1.34).

According to 2.50, the practice of prāṇāyāma consists of three breathing activities:

1. Exhalation, externally directed, relaxing, also known as recaka, "emptying"
2. Inhalation, internally directed, stimulating, also known as pūraka, "filling"
3. Retention, no direction, space between breath, known as kumbhaka, "holding"

Each of these three can be done

1. With our attention on a certain location in the body
2. For a certain duration
3. A certain number of times

The result of prāṇāyāma is breathing that is protracted and subtle (2.50), smooth as silk with no blips.

The fourth activity of prāṇāyāma (2.51) is inactivity: stillness of the breath, as if the air in the lungs is passively mixing with the air outside. This illustrates another example, like the guṇa-s, of a trinity (exhalation, inhalation, retention) representing the manifest world, then a fourth state going beyond that. In the fourth prāṇāyāma, which is really a state more than a process, the shroud of ignorance (avidyā) disappears (2.52) and the outer mind is now ready for the inner limbs (antaraṅga/saṃyama), beginning with dhāraṇā (2.53). Why don't the sūtra-s say "ready for pratyāhāra," which is the next limb? Because pratyāhāra is a side effect of prāṇāyāma and the last three limbs. Prāṇāyāma stabilizes the heart-mind, allowing the attention to focus on a single object in preparation for saṃyama.

Complete Translation

2.49 tasminsati śvāsapraśvāsayorgativicchedaḥ prāṇāyāmaḥ

tasmin sati śvāsa-praśvāsayoḥ gati-vicchedaḥ prāṇāyāmaḥ

tasmin	upon that (āsana)
sat	being present, existing
śvāsa	inhalation
praśvāsa	exhalation
gati	movement, gait
viccheda	separation, cutting off
prāṇāyāma	regulation of breath

1. When that (āsana) is present, prāṇāyāma is breaking the (irregular) movements of inhalation and exhalation.
2. Once the sitting posture is (stable and comfortable), then the regulation of breath is cutting off the movements of inhalation and exhalation (so the breath is still).

Derivation of Terms

Prefix	pra, "front, lead"
Root	an, "breathe"
Literal Meaning	prāṇa, "lead breath"
Translation Here	prāṇa, "breath; life force"

Prefix	ā, "enhance"
Root	yam, "to restrain, control, regulate"
Suffix	āyāma, "enhanced control, regulation"
Literal Meaning	prāṇāyāma, "enhanced regulation of the prāṇa"
Dictionary	"restraining or suspending the breath"
Translation Here	"regulation of prāṇa/breath via breathing exercises"

Related Sūtra-s

2.50–53

Contemplations

How is my breath obstructed or irregular?

Do I realize how my breath can cause me to become anxious or tired?

Am I consciously aware of my breath while practicing āsana?

PRATYĀHĀRA (LIMB #5)

Tuning Out Sensory Input

स्वविषयासंप्रयोगे चित्तस्य स्वरूपानुकार इवेन्द्रियाणां प्रत्याहारः ॥ २.५४ ॥

2.54 svaviṣayāsaṃprayoge cittasya svarūpānukāra
ivendriyāṇāṃ pratyāhāraḥ
Turning off sensory inputs is directing the attention inward following the true nature of the heart-mind, thus disconnecting with external objects.

Commentary

Pratyāhāra is the last of the outer limbs and the pivotal juncture between outer and inner. It is considered an outer, external limb (3.7) because it involves the sensory organs.

Pratyāhāra is not a practice, but a side effect of prāṇāyāma (breath regulation) and saṃyama (focusing on a single object by practicing the last three limbs of yoga). Prāṇāyāma serves to slow and smooth out the breath, a prerequisite to being able to focus the attention. When our attention is inwardly concentrated (saṃyama), we do not register other sights and sounds around us, and we are no longer distracted by external objects. Therefore, our senses are essentially turned off. The sensory organs now follow the heart-mind (2.55) instead of the heart-mind catering to external sensory distractions. Sensory perceptions, food for the outer mind (manas), are not ingested and therefore do not cause any reaction or disturbance in the heart-mind.

In terms of perception and action, manas is the instrument and buddhi is the agent. A traditional example, mentioned in the *Kaṭha Upaniṣad* (3.3–4), is riding a chariot. The road represents sense objects, the horses are the sensory organs, the reins are the dual-natured mind, the chariot driver is the buddhi, and the chariot master is the ātman/Puruṣa. If the driver lets the horses run wild, chaos results. When a discerning intellect (driver) listens to the higher self (master), it can guide the outer mind (reins) in the desired direction, with the sensory organs (horses) following the reins.

In the *Bhagavad-Gītā*, in a conversation between Arjuna (representing a human) and Kṛṣṇa (representing his inner, higher self), Arjuna experiences the universal struggle between spiritual development and sensory indulgence. His inner voice attempts to help him understand that true happiness is detaching from sensory experience and going inward to connect with the light of awareness. To reach that state he must actively battle the parts of himself that are drawing him outward.

Complete Translation

2.54 svaviṣayāsaṃprayoge cittasya svarūpānukāra ivendriyāṇām pratyāhāraḥ
sva-viṣaya-asaṃprayoge cittasya svarūpa-anukāraḥ iva indriyāṇām pratyāhāraḥ

sva	own
viṣaya	sensory object
asaṃprayoga	not connecting
citta	heart-mind field of consciousness
svarūpa	true nature
anukāra	following, imitating
iva	as if
indriya	sensory organ (see Sāṅkhya)
pratyāhāra	exclusion, turning off

1. Pratyāhāra is when the sensory organs no longer connect with their own objects, as if following the true nature of citta.
2. Turning off sensory inputs is directing the attention inward following the true nature of the heart-mind, thus disconnecting with external objects.

Derivation of Terms

Prefix	prati, "against, opposed to"
Prefix	ā, "up to, near to"
Root	hṛ, "carry away, remove, lead away"
Word	āhāra, "bringing near, procuring, ingesting food"
Literal Meaning	pratyāhāra, "reversing ingestion, against procuring" and so "not taking in"
Dictionary	"retreat; withholding; restraining the organs of sense"
Translation Here	"tuning out sensory perceptions"

Related Sūtra-s

2.55

Contemplations

Am I able to concentrate amid the hustle and bustle around me?
Which senses are the most difficult for me to reign in?
How can I improve that?

CITTA-PRASĀDANA
Clarifying the Heart-Mind

मैत्रीकरुणामुदितोपेक्षाणां सुखदुःखपुण्यापुण्यविषयाणां

भावनातश्चित्तप्रसादनम् ॥ १.३३ ॥

1.33 maitrīkaruṇāmuditopekṣāṇāṃ sukhaduḥkhapuṇyāpuṇyaviṣayāṇāṃ bhāvanātaścittaprasādanam

Purification of our field of consciousness occurs from an attitude of friendship when encountering happiness, compassion when encountering suffering, gladness when encountering virtue, and neutrality when encountering vice.

Commentary

When another person is happy, be friendly toward her. Many people who are deeply unhappy in their own lives become hateful and envious toward those who are successful or happy. Do not envy one who is happy. Cultivate santoṣa (contentment) by being grateful for what you have. For example, a colleague was promoted instead of you. If you congratulate the person and sincerely wish her well, this will purify your heart-mind. If you envy and become upset with her, your heart-mind will suffer.

When another person is suffering, being compassionate toward her sends positive, loving energy her way and helps her in her healing process. Do not avoid one who is suffering. Love thine enemy. For example, Nelson Mandela, who suffered himself for many years in prison, understands that those who made him suffer must be suffering themselves. Instead of punishing people, his Truth and Reconciliation Commission allowed the criminals to face their victims and admit what they had done and apologize to them. Not only did Mandela show compassion for apartheid's worst leaders, he provided an opportunity for them to dig deep down and express compassion toward those whose suffering they caused.

Witnessing a virtuous act fosters a feeling of reciprocal gladness and allows us to appreciate another person. For example, when a whistleblower at work speaks out about unfair or illegal activities, he risks losing his job. This action is very courageous as the employee is risking his neck for the benefit of himself and others. Appreciating virtuous acts will encourage others to do likewise in the future.

When we encounter a person who is mean, negative, or performing illegal or unjust actions, we must step back and ask these questions: "Should I get involved?" "What is my role here?" Each individual situation will determine our level of involvement: gentle caution, restraint sharing our opinions, or complete avoidance for self-protection. For example, say you see a thief in the act of shoplifting. What should you do? Failing to act at all allows him to get away with the crime, yet protects you. Talking to a store employee is a safe, indirect way to let the perpetratee go after the perpetrator. Approaching the thief directly could cause you and others to be hurt.

The heart-mind can also be purified (see appendix F, figure 6):

- Through breathing exercises, especially exhaling (which relaxes the body and heart-mind) and retention (1.34).
- By developing finer sensory perceptions (1.35). This can occur through the practice of saṃyama, the inner limbs of yoga consisting of dhāraṇā, dhyāna, and samādhi.
- If perception is imbued with sattva—sorrowless and luminous (1.36).
- When the heart-mind is focused on an object that does not arouse rāga-kleśa, the affliction of attachment to past pleasure (1.37).
- When the heart-mind's focus draws from a sattvic dream or inactive sleep state (1.38). Dreams and deep sleep shut out external events. Either will contribute to calming the heart-mind.
- By meditation (dhyāna) as desired (1.39). The object of focus should be something you like but are not attached to in any way and that does not cause a disturbance in your heart-mind.

Psychological healing, arousing positive emotions as an antidote to negative emotions (pratipakṣa-bhāvana), also purifies the heart-mind.

Complete Translation

1.33 maitrīkaruṇāmuditopekṣāṇāṃ sukhaduḥkhapuṇyāpuṇyaviṣayāṇāṃ bhāvanātaścittaprasādanam

maitrī-karuṇā-mudita-upekṣāṇāṃ sukha-duḥkha-puṇya-apuṇya-viṣayāṇāṃ bhāvanātaḥ citta-prasādanam

maitrī	friendliness
karuṇā	compassion
mudita	joyfulness
upekṣāṇa	neutrality
sukha	happiness
duḥkha	suffering, pain, discomfort

puṇya	virtue
apuṇya	nonvirtue, vice
viṣaya	sensory object
bhāvana	attitude, disposition
citta	heart-mind field of consciousness
prasādana	purification, clarification

1. Purification of our field of consciousness occurs from an attitude of friendship when encountering happiness, compassion when encountering suffering, gladness when encountering virtue, and neutrality when encountering vice.
2. Purification of our heart-mind is the result of cultivating a mindset that is usually positive, never negative or critical, and sometimes cautious (neutrality).

Derivation of Terms

Prefix	pra, "in front, forward, forth"
Original Root	sad, "to sit, settle; rest"
Prefixed Root	prasad, "to be gracious; to be a soother; to be pure or clear"
Dictionary	prasādana, "purifying, clarifying; soothing, calming; composing"
Translation Here	"clarification, purification"

Related Sūtra-s

1.34–39

Contemplations

Can I be happy with another person's success, even if it could have been mine?

How can I best be compassionate toward someone in pain?

Does seeing a courageously kind act affect my future actions?

Am I able to maintain composure in the face of vice?

DHĀRAṆĀ (LIMB #6)
Choosing a Focus

देशबन्धश्चित्तस्य धारणा ॥ ३.१ ॥

3.1 deśabandhaścittasya dhāraṇā
Dhāraṇā is choosing a focus and directing our attention there.

Commentary
Dhāraṇā is the sixth limb of aṣṭāṅga-yoga and the first of three inner limbs collectively called saṃyama (3.4). Dhāraṇā as defined in this sūtra means keeping the attention in a single place. Viveka (keen discernment) and vairāgya (detached awareness) must be present for dhāraṇā to take place.

At this stage, one proactively chooses an object to focus on, either external, internal, or abstract. It does not have to be a physical object, but should be something that has the quality of sattva and does not bring up rāga or dveṣa. Examples include a flame, cakra, or mantra, the breath, an idea, or even Īśvara. We should like the object but not be attached to it in any way. If there is any resistance to it, or if it brings up negative or distracting thoughts, we choose something else.

A traditional, common place of focus is the heart cakra, regarded as the center of our being. It is said in the *Kaṭha Upaniṣad* that a flame the size of a thumb burns continuously in the heart, like a pilot light of life. This glow represents our inner light, the Puruṣa, the warm splendor of pure awareness. The name of this energy sphere in the heart area is "anāhata," meaning "unstruck." External sounds begin when something is struck or physical objects collide. The innermost pulsation of life is a subtle sound that has no beginning and no end, and so is called unstruck. Sound and light are the fundamental waves of the manifest world.

Dhāraṇā alone can be intermittent: attention drifting away, then back again. When it becomes continuous, then it is dhyāna. In dhāraṇā, we are aware of our surroundings but they do not distract our focus very much. In dhyāna, peripheral commotion does not cause any distraction. Prāṇāyāma prepares the heart-mind for dhāraṇā (2.53). Pratyāhāra is a side effect of dhāraṇā, dhyāna, and samādhi. (See appendix F, figure 12.)

What is the difference between dhāraṇā and dhyāna?

Dhāraṇā: There is a location where the focus is
Periphery still distracts
Water dripping

Dhyāna: Peripheral distractions go away
Continuous, uninterrupted
Honey flowing

Examples:

PLACE OF FOCUS	DHĀRAṆĀ	DHYĀNA
External: flower	Stare at it but can still see everything around it	Stare at it but do not see anything else
Internal: heart cakra	Direct attention there, but it may wander at times	Attention stays there

Complete Translation

3.1 deśabandhaścittasya dhāraṇā

deśa-bandhaḥ cittasya dhāraṇā

deśa place, point, location

bandha bound, fixed

citta heart-mind field of consciousness

dhāraṇā establishing a locus

1. Dhāraṇā is the focus of citta at a locus.
2. Dhāraṇā is choosing a focus and directing our attention there.

Derivation of Terms

Root dhṛ, "to hold, support"

Literal Meaning "concentration, holding, locking, binding, streaming, focusing"

Dictionary dhāraṇā, "holding, supporting, preserving, keeping the mind collected"

Translation Here "confining our attention to a chosen place"

Contemplations

What object can I choose to focus my attention on?

Does that object have the quality of sattva?

What distractions are throwing off my ability to concentrate?

DHYĀNA (LIMB #7)

Continuous Meditation

तत्र प्रत्ययैकतानता ध्यानम् ॥ ३.२ ॥

3.2 tatra pratyayaikatānatā dhyānam
Once dhāraṇā is in place, then, when the heart-mind's focus on one object is uninterrupted, dhyāna occurs.

Commentary

Dhyāna is the seventh limb of aṣṭāṅga-yoga, and the middle of the "inner limbs" comprising saṃyama. Dhyāna is continuous dhāraṇā, so focused that peripheral noise does not interfere with our concentration. Dhāraṇā is focusing on a single place, but thoughts about the object vary. Dhyāna is the same, but only one thought (pratyaya) exists toward the object. Just as water drips intermittently on a single spot (dhāraṇā), honey flows continuously when poured (dhyāna).

Dhyāna can overcome the kliṣṭa-vṛtti-s (2.11), those afflicting activities in the heart-mind that are responsible for troubling thoughts. During dhyāna there is room for only one vṛtti in the heart-mind, the current and continuous thought (pratyaya) directed toward the focal point. Dhyāna does not remove the deeper kleśa-s, but will block the afflicting activities from strengthening the kleśa-s further.

The clarification and stabilization of the heart-mind (citta-prasādana) can result from dhyāna as well (1.39). The more attention is focused, the fewer distractions occur, and the heart-mind becomes more serene and composed.

The powers described in chapter 3 of the sūtra-s can be accomplished in many ways (4.1), one of which is samādhi, a product of dhyāna. Heart-minds that achieve these powers will keep depositing residue (saṃskāra-s) into the subconscious memory, whereas a heart-mind trained over time through the practice of dhyāna will not (4.6).

Complete Translation

3.2 tatra pratyayaikatānatā dhyānam
tatra pratyaya-eka-tānatā dhyānam

tatra	there
pratyaya	presented thought; current vṛtti directed toward an object
eka	one, single, uniform

tānatā continuous flow, extension

dhyāna focused and uninterrupted attention on a single place

1. There (in dhāraṇā), dhyāna is the continuous flow (of attention) on a single pratyaya.
2. Once dhāraṇā is in place, then when the heart-mind's focus on one object is uninterrupted, dhyāna occurs.

Derivation of Terms

Root	dhi, "disregard, propitiate, hold, contain, fulfill"
Root	dhyai, "meditate upon, ponder over, contemplate"
Dictionary	dhyāna, "meditation, reflection, thought, contemplation"
Translation Here	dhyāna, "continuously focused meditation"

Related Sūtra-s

1.39; 2.11; 4.6

Contemplations

What can I do to maintain my focus?

What external stimuli are distracting my attention?

How can I resolve them?

SAMĀDHI (LIMB #8)

Complete Attention

तदेवार्थमात्रनिर्भासं स्वरूपशून्यमिव समाधिः ॥ ३.३ ॥

3.3 tadevārthamātranirbhāsaṃ svarūpaśūnyamiva samādhiḥ
Meditation becomes complete absorption when the object alone is reflected in the heart-mind and subject and object seem the same.

Commentary

Samādhi is the eighth and final limb of aṣṭāṅga-yoga and is functionally identical to yoga as citta-vṛtti-nirodhaḥ (1.2). At this stage, there is no perception of a subject separate from its object. Both seem as one entity, uniting in the heart-mind's eye, even though in physical reality the practitioner is still different from the object. Yoga is often defined as "union" in this sense. Specifically, the stages of samādhi transform the buddhi aspect of the heart-mind into a pure state of sattva, a transparent quality that is the buddhi's natural state. In samādhi the ego (ahaṅkāra) takes a vacation; it is removed from the equation since it can only function when the object can be distinguished from the subject.

Samādhi can be applied in everyday life. For example, anytime we get lost in something and our consciousness is completely absorbed in it, we are experiencing a type of samādhi. A hypnotic trance is another example. Intoxication and addiction can be considered tamasic samādhi-s. Full participation in an activity, when we are so in it that nothing else exists except what we are focused on, can be samādhi. The samādhi defined by Patañjali as the final third of saṃyama is conscious and has the qualities of sattva.

There are several kinds of samādhi mentioned in the text:

- Sabīja, "with seed"
- Nirbīja, "without seed"
- Saṃprajñāta, "full insight or mastery"
- Asaṃprajñāta, "beyond mastery" (this is implied in the text but not specifically mentioned)

Sabīja-samādhi relies on an object, even if it seems to be merged with the subject. The heart-mind needs an object to provoke it toward nirodha. For example, in sabīja-samādhi, our citta reflects the object perfectly and we seem to become the object. Nirbīja-samādhi has no object associated with it. Our citta does not even reflect the object; it becomes transparent. The samādhi that is the eighth limb of yoga, which is also the third and final part of saṃyama, is sabīja-samādhi, since in 3.8 it states that saṃyama is an external limb relative to nirbīja-samādhi.

Complete Translation

3.3 tadevārthamātranirbhāsaṃ svarūpaśūnyamiva samādhiḥ
tat eva artha-mātra-nirbhāsaṃ svarūpa-śūnyam iva samādhiḥ

tat	that
va	indeed
artha	purpose
mātra	alone
nirbhāsa	shining forth, apparent
svarūpa	own form
śūnya	void, empty
iva	like, as
samādhi	complete absorption of the heart-mind in the focus

1. That (dhyāna) is samādhi (when) the object alone shines forth (in the citta) as if devoid of its own form.
2. Meditation becomes complete absorption when the object alone is reflected in the heart-mind and subject and object seem the same.

Derivation of Terms

Prefix	sam, "complete, full, together"
Prefix	ā, "enhance, up to"
Root	dhā, "put, place"
Word	dhi, "putting, placing"—this can also represent the buddhi
Literal Meaning	samādhi "putting completely together"
Dictionary	samādhi "collecting, composing, concentrating; perfect absorption of thought into the one object of meditation"
Translation Here	"assimilation, complete absorption"

Related Sūtra-s

1.17–23, 40–51

SAṂPRAJÑĀTA-SAMĀDHI: MASTERING AN OBJECT (1.17)

Saṃprajñāta is a type of samādhi encompassing four levels of comprehension. The goal is to utterly and completely understand something so it becomes part of our being. Once this happens, then we let go of even that understanding, called asaṃprajñāta-samādhi. There are four stages of saṃprajñāta-samādhi, progressing from a superficial to a deep level of understanding.

1. Vitarka: gross/superficial attempt of mind to understand an object
   - Understanding through reasoning, logic, inference, conjecture
   - Every word has an object, and each word may be interpreted differently among people
   - Intellectual, hotly debatible, influenced by the kleśa-s
2. Vicāra: subtler/deeper attempt of mind to understand an object
   - Understanding through more careful examination and reflection
   - Involves discernment, more pramāṇa, and less vikalpa
   - More refined, pure, accurate, truthful
   - Cooler, no more arguing, not influenced by the kleśa-s, includes irrational ideas that stun the mind, like a zen koan
3. Ānanda: the joy and satisfaction of fully understanding something
4. Asmitā-rūpa: "form of I-ness"—knowledge becomes completely internalized
   - Freedom to experiment with new, unknown ideas
   - Union of subject and object

Another samādhi referred to by some as asaṃprajñāta-samādhi, is due to practicing paravairāgya (1.16, 3.50), a subtler form of vairāgya, and is characterized by the stoppage of all pratyaya-s (thoughts currently in the forefront of our mind), but it still contains residual saṃskāra-s (1.18). (See appendix F, figure 7.)

According to 1.20, most practitioners begin with faith in their own ability to move ahead and inward (śraddhā). This creates vitality (vīrya) for determination, enthusiasm, and energy that supports a clear memory (smṛti), which leads first to (saṃprajñāta-) samādhi. This precedes deep insight (1.48), which then leads to asaṃprajñāta-samādhi. When our practice is enthusiastic, it creates intense momentum that accelerates our progress (1.21). The level of practice, whether mild, medium, or ardent (1.22), also makes a difference to our progress. This is all powered by abhyāsa leading to vairāgya, then paravairāgya.

Patañjali offers another option to achieve this other samādhi. Īśvara-praṇidhāna by itself can bring one to asaṃprajñāta-samādhi (1.23). In contrast to what has been mentioned in the previous few sūtra-s, one who has enough faith in the divine, or who truly sees the divine light inside all beings, can reach this samādhi. This is discussed further in the sections on Īśvara and īśvara-praṇidhāna.

STAGES OF SAṂPRAJÑĀTA-SAMĀDHI

	1	2	3	4
Stage	Vitarka	Vicāra	Ānanda	Asmitā
Description of stage	Superficial attempt of mind to grasp an object, argument, reasoning, inference, guess, conjecture, supposition	Subtle attempt . . . Reflection, deliberation, examination, judgment, discernment	Joy, satisfaction—become part of experience	"I know it completely"
What we do	Read, hear, see the obvious	Observe more closely	Do on our own	Master; can now teach others
Level of perception	Partial, superficial perception	More accurate perception	Temporarily becomes part of us	Becomes part of our identity
Example: learning how to drive a car	Read the manual, talk about how to drive with a driver, learn the basics (starting, steering, braking, etc.), observe as a passenger	Watch as a passenger	Just after driver's education	After driving for a year or more
Example: learning a musical instrument	Play notes from the written sheet, basic chord progressions, key changes, tempo, etc.	How tempo and volume affect the feeling of the music	Joy when we can play it by heart	Play a piece perfectly without having to think about it, with awareness of our surroundings

Derivation of Terms

Prefix	sam, "complete, together"
Prefix	pra, "forth, in front of"
Original Root	jñā, "know, understand"
Word Here	saṃprajñāta, "complete understanding, mastery"

Dictionary	saṃprajñāta, "a kind of samādhi in which the object of meditation remains distinct even though the mind is absorbed in its contemplation—as opposed to the next stage, asaṃprajñāta, in which the distinction between knowledge and its object is completely obliterated."

SAMĀPATTI-SAMĀDHI: SATURATION OF THE HEART-MIND (1.41–51)

Samāpatti is the concentration attained in a habitually one-pointed mind. Its four stages, all involving an object of focus, comprise sabīja-samādhi (1.46: see table). In the first stage (1.42), savitarka-samāpatti, perception of an object is affected by our knowledge of it or of the words used to describe it. In the second stage of nirvitarka (1.43), the object is perceived clearly without any preconceived notions. The distinction between subject, object, and act of perceiving is dissolved in the heart-mind, which reflects the object perfectly, as a transparent crystal appears to be whatever object it reflects. This is the highest knowledge to be obtained for a gross object.

The third and fourth stages, savicāra and nirvicāra-samāpatti, are similar to the first two stages except we now apply reasoning and reflection toward a subtle object (1.44). Concentrating on subtle objects leads one all the way back to unmanifest matter (original Prakṛti—see appendix F, figure 1) (1.45).

The fourth stage of nirvicāra-samāpatti occurs when the buddhi is clear and sattva predominates (1.47). The insight thus experienced reveals the actual truth (ṛta) of an object (1.48). This particular insight is considered pratyakṣa (see pramāṇa-vṛtti) because it allows one to distinguish objects. The other pramāṇa-s (inference and testimony) are secondhand and cannot provide a complete picture of an object (1.49). This final stage of samāpatti, called nirvicāra, is also the last stage of sabīja-samādhi. Here, although an object is still present, the saṃskāra of the truth-bearing insight (prajñā) will inhibit and ultimately supersede other, harmful saṃskāra-s that involve the afflictions (kleśa-s). Strengthening the sattvic saṃskāra-s digs new and improved grooves in the heart-mind toward a closer connection to our inner self. Ultimately even those saṃskāra-s disintegrate, leading to nirbīja-samādhi or kaivalya (1.51).

Saṃprajñāta refers to the level of knowledge acquired in samāpatti.

Derivation of Terms

Prefix	sam, "complete, together"
Prefix	ā, "enhance, up to"
Original Root	pad, "go, move, approach, attain"
Prefixed Root	samāpad, "to get, obtain, attain to, happen"

Word Here	samāpatti, "to get completely"
Dictionary	samāpatti, "meeting, encountering; accident, chance, accidental encounter; assuming an original form; completion, conclusion"
Other Translations	"cognitive blending, coalescence, saturation, pervasion, perfusion, meeting face-to-face"

STAGES OF SAMĀDHI (1.41–51)

	STAGES OF SAMĀPATTI THAT COMPRISE SABĪJA-SAMĀDHI (1.46)				NIRBĪJA-SAMĀDHI
STAGE	Savitarka	Nirvitarka	Savicāra	Nirvicāra	
MEANING	With superficial thought	Beyond superficial thought	With reasoning or reflection	Beyond reasoning or reflection	"Without seed"
SŪTRA-S	1.42, mixed with words, meaning, and conceptual knowledge	1.43, object reflects true meaning (without distortion from words), or conceptual knowledge	1.44, subtler, see 1.17	1.47, purity of the higher self	1.51, after the nirodha of all saṃskāra-s
OBJECT	Gross	Gross	Subtle	Subtle	None
LEVEL	Most superficial knowledge	Highest knowledge of gross objects	Superficial knowledge of subtle object	Deepest inner reflection on object	
NOTES	Attempt to make things logical; understand what it represents intellectually, can analyze it	Object is clear and perception is accurate		All gross and subtle qualities of object appear =state of yoga	
BASED ON	Labels, culture, personal opinions	Labels, etc., are no longer present			

Contemplations

Have I ever felt the state of total absorption in one particular activity?

Is my ego afraid of becoming transparent and losing control of my being?

How might the ability to achieve samādhi affect my future actions?

SAṂYAMA
Focusing Inward

त्रयमेकत्र संयमः ॥ ३.४ ॥

3.4 trayamekatra saṃyamaḥ
Complete control (of attention) is dhāraṇā, dhyāna, and samādhi directed toward the same place or object.

Commentary

Saṃyama is the practice of the final three "inner" limbs of yoga all focused on a single place or object. At this point the breath should be stable and without obstruction or irregularity so the attention can be directed inward. As our heart-mind progresses from dhāraṇā to dhyāna to samādhi, pratyāhāra occurs naturally and completely. (See appendix F, figure 12.)

Dhāraṇā, dhyāna, and samādhi are more internal compared to the previous five limbs (3.7) yet are external in relation to nirbīja-samādhi (3.8). In other words, saṃyama is the final stage of sabīja-samādhi (absorption involving an object of focus) and the harbinger of nirbīja-samādhi, objectless absorption, also known as kaivalya.

Saṃyama is interiorizing the object of focus, ultimately making it appear as if it *is* the citta. The inner limbs are compared below. Each is discussed separately on pages 148–157.

DHĀRAṆĀ	DHYĀNA	SAMĀDHI
Holding attention but interrupted	Holding attention continuously	Notion of subject as different from object disappears
Dripping water on the same spot	Stream of honey poured in same place	Appears as the water or honey itself
Citta focused on one object but aware of periphery	Citta 100 percent focused on object; peripheral activity is closed off	Subject perceives object as itself; object appears empty of independent existence

From mastery of saṃyama comes the light of deep insight, called prajñā (3.5). Understanding of the object of focus is complete from the inside out, and on all levels (gross to subtle). From that penetrating insight arise unusual powers, called vibhūti-s or siddhi-s. (See appendix D.) These extraordinary abilities are side effects that are to be only noticed, never abused or demonstrated, and are obstacles to nirbīja-samādhi (3.37).

The application of saṃyama is in stages (3.6) as follows:

- dhāraṇā: choosing and attempting to focus on an object/place
- dhyāna: continuously maintaining that focus
- samādhi: stages of samāpatti and/or samprajñāta

Most practitioners need to progress step by step, gradually refining their heart-mind from outer, coarser thoughts toward inner, subtler thoughts. Some commentators add that it may be possible to skip over these stages via īśvara-praṇidhāna (1.23).

These siddhi-s and other unlisted powers can also be developed in other ways (4.1). Some people are born with supernormal powers such as clairvoyance or ESP. The external and/or internal application of concentrated medicinal concoctions is said to achieve siddhi-s as well. The same is true for chanting mantra-s or practicing intense tapas. Samādhi is considered the best way to develop these abilities, because they are side effects of a sattvic discipline, not a deliberate attempt to gain power.

Complete Translation

3.4 trayamekatra saṃyamaḥ

trayam ekatra saṃyamaḥ

traya	triad
ekatra	a single place
saṃyama	turning the attention inward toward a focus

1. Saṃyama is the (previous) three (focused in) one place.
2. Complete control (of attention) is dhāraṇā, dhyāna, and samādhi directed toward the same place or object.

Derivation of Terms

Prefix	sam, "completely, together"
Original Root	yam, "check, curb, restrain, control, subdue; offer, give; sustain; raise up; extend"
Prefixed Root	saṃyam, "restrain, control, subdue; confine, gather; shut, close; hold together"
Dictionary	saṃyama, "restraint, check, control; concentration of mind; religious devotion; feeling of compassion"
Literal Meaning	"control completely, confine (attention) completely"
Translation Here	"the process of focusing inward"

Related Sūtra-s

3.5–8, 16–48, 52–53; 4.1

Contemplations

What distractions are throwing off my focus?

Am I too interested in seeking extraordinary powers?

How can I avoid wanting to achieve those powers?

PRATIPRASAVA
Returning to the Source

ते प्रतिप्रसवहेयाः सूक्ष्माः ॥ २.१० ॥

2.10 te pratiprasavaheyāḥ sūkṣmāḥ
When we notice subtle signs of a kleśa erupting,
we nip it in the bud before it becomes full-blown.

Commentary
Yoga is partly about getting to know who we are inside and why we act the way we do. Whenever we react automatically to a stimulus, instead of stepping back and acting consciously, we allow our deep triggers (kleśa-s), habitual patterns (saṃskāra-s), and mental commotion (vṛtti-s) to determine our action. In order to prevent this, we can learn from the suffering these cause (duḥkha), trace our reaction back, and discover where it came from. What happened in my past that made me act this way? How can I improve myself so that I act in a way I am proud of and feel good about?

Just as the only way to truly eliminate disease is by removing its cause, the way to get rid of negative and harmful reactions is to destroy a kleśa or saṃskāra. Kleśa-s are weakened by practicing kriyā-yoga (2.2). A saṃskāra is rendered ineffective when another saṃskāra becomes strong enough to supersede it.

If we notice when a kleśa is manifesting in a subtle form and view it as a warning sign or symptom of something deeper, we can nip it in the bud before it controls our actions. In fact, reflecting on our kleśa-s and saṃskāra-s even when they are not active allows us to prepare ourselves for their inevitable arousal.

For example, let's say you composed a song that became a big hit. All of a sudden you are famous and many people are throwing their attention your way. If you notice yourself (svādhyāya) beginning to feel better than others (asmitā-kleśa), and understand where it came from, there is an opportunity to pass the credit through your heart-mind to Īśvara by practicing Īśvara-praṇidhāna. This prevents asmitā-kleśa from fully activating by turning it around and sending it back into dormancy (***pratiprasava***). If you are vigilant enough, you can save yourself from conceit. Otherwise, once the ego accepts and holds on to all that attention, asmitā-kleśa grows inside your heart-mind like a noxious weed and will be much more difficult to remove.

Pratiprasava is a powerful exercise, and is necessary to

- End the kleśa-s when in their subtle form (2.10)
- End any remaining saṃskāra-s (4.28)
- Understand the guṇa-s deeply, the final step before kaivalya (4.34)

Complete Translation

2.10 te pratiprasavaheyāḥ sūkṣmāḥ

te pratiprasava-heyāḥ sūkṣmāḥ

te	those
pratiprasava	returning back to the origin
heya	endable
sūkṣma	subtle

1. Those (kleśa-s) when subtle are to be removed by pratiprasava (the reverse of how they were produced).
2. When we notice subtle signs of a kleśa erupting, we nip it in the bud before it becomes full-blown.

Derivation of Terms

Prefix	prati, "opposed to, against"
Prefix	pra, "in front, forward, forth"
Root	sū, "to bring forth, beget, produce; to impel"
Literal Meaning	"impel backward, reverse propagation, against manifestation"
Dictionary	pratiprasava, "a counterexception, exception to an exception; a contrary effect"
Translation Here	"turning back to the cause"

Related Sūtra-s

4.28, 34

Contemplations

Can I cultivate a watchful attitude to be able to catch myself before acting unconsciously?

How can deep self-reflection help me trace my reactions back to their source?

Once I understand what caused a reaction, how can I prevent that same reaction from happening again?

KAIVALYA
Permanent Oneness

सत्त्वपुरुषयोः शुद्धिसाम्ये कैवल्यम् ॥ ३.५५ ॥

3.55 sattvapuruṣayoḥ śuddhisāmye kaivalyam
When the heart-mind is transparent,
still and pure as the inner Self, then kaivalya is experienced.

Commentary
Kaivalya literally means "aloneness" and is the final state of emancipation, where we are not affected by any conditioning in our heart-mind whatsoever. The inner light of awareness shines right through our consciousness to illuminate the world around us, turning any action into a selfless, compassionate offering to that awareness. Kaivalya cannot be understood with words; it requires direct experience. Practicing yoga is a process of self-refinement. As our heart-mind becomes clarified, glimpses of our inner light of awareness occur more and more often.

Kaivalya can be interpreted in many different ways, using many different words, none of which can do justice to the actual experience. Some English words that may reflect some characteristics of kaivalya are permanent oneness, quiet simplicity, conscious isolation, emancipation, freedom, and liberation.

After all the preliminary practices and stages, when turning inward (saṃyama) is being practiced, one finally distinguishes between sattva and Puruṣa (3.49), then detaches from even that idea to end up in kaivalya (3.50). Patañjali next advises against being tempted by other energies lest they cause our attention to slip back into undesirable states (3.51).

Chapter 4 of the *Yoga Sūtra-s* contains a veritable cascade of events leading up to kaivalya. Once the distinction is made between the sattvic buddhi and the Puruṣa, the final steps are assured.

4.25 Sense of self ceases
4.26 Citta, oriented toward viveka, moves closer to kaivalya
4.27 Between moments of viveka, thoughts that occur are due to previous saṃskāra-s
4.28 The pratiprasava process ends these saṃskāra-s

4.29	Once continuous, unbroken viveka-khyāti is present, one is fully content and not interested in moving forward anymore. Trying and seeking come to an end, and full relaxation of the heart-mind ensues, causing one to become completely soaked in the virtue field called dharma-megha-samādhi.
4.30	Karma-s and kleśa-s end (cease to affect our attention)
4.31	Clear, untainted access to Īśvara (all knowledge) results
4.32	Perception of time stops as the guṇa-s stop their sequential changes
4.33	When the sequential changes end, knowledge of them arises
4.34	The guṇa-s return to their original state of equilibrium. Prakṛti is in stillness with Puruṣa.

Kaivalya is the ultimate end of yoga, and is defined at the end of chapters 3 and 4:

3.55	When the buddhi is 100 percent pure, just like the Puruṣa
4.34	The pratiprasava of the guṇa-s, or When the power of pure awareness rests in its own nature

Complete Translation

3.55 sattvapuruṣayoḥ śuddhisāmye kaivalyam

sattva-puruṣayoḥ śuddhi-sāmye kaivalyam

sattva	guṇa of light, intelligence, purity, goodness, etc.
puruṣa	the inner light of Awareness, the observer
śuddhi	purity
sāmya	equal, same
kaivalya	final emancipation

1. Upon the equal purity of Puruṣa and sattva (buddhi), kaivalya.
2. When the heart-mind is transparent, still, and pure as the inner Self, then kaivalya is experienced.

Derivation of Terms

Root	kev, "serve, attend to; enjoy"
Original Word	kevala, "exclusive; alone, sole; whole, absolute; bare; simple"
Literal Meaning	"having the nature of exclusivity, wholeness, perfection, simplicity"
Dictionary	"perfect isolation, soleness, exclusiveness; individuality; detachment of the soul from matter; final emancipation"
Translation Here	"permanent oneness, absolute wholeness"

Related Sūtra-s

3.49–51, 4.25–34

Contemplations

Can I do my practice without seeking any goal?

How would it feel if I stopped seeking and instead rested my attention inward, experiencing that simple glow of inner awareness in my heart?

part 3

The Yoga Sutras in Translation

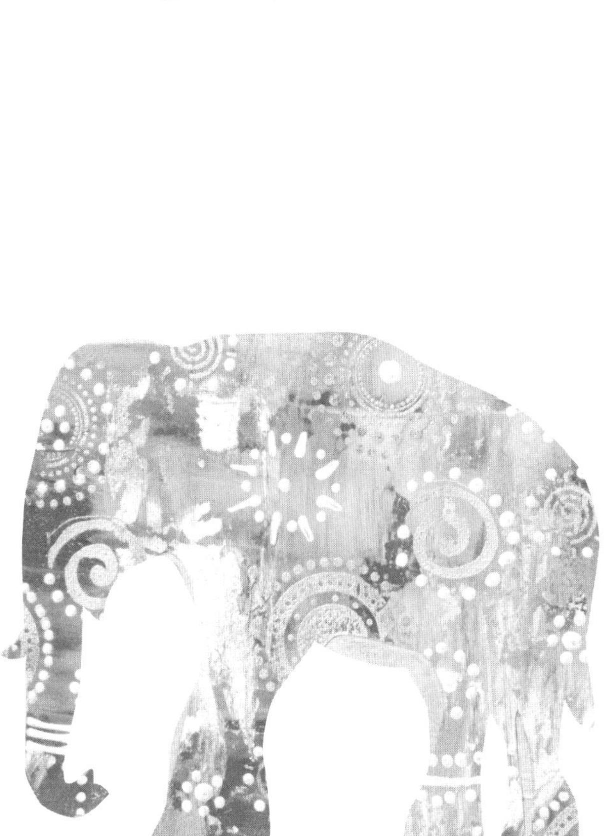

A complete translation of the *Yoga Sūtra-s* text follows. Each sūtra is presented like this:

Line 1	Sūtra in the original Sanskrit Devanāgarī script.
Line 2	Sūtra in the Romanized transliteration, representing the original exactly.
Line 3	Sūtra words before the sounds joined together via Sanskrit sound blending (sandhi). All case-endings are now visible.
Words	Individual words (in stem form) with their translation and grammar (if any) in square brackets [ ].

See appendix E for more information about Sanskrit endings and grammar.

At the end:

1. Literal translation of sūtra
2. More readable and understandable translation of sūtra

पातञ्जलयोगदर्शनम्

PĀTAÑJALA-YOGA-DARŚANAM

१. समाधिपादः

SAMĀDHIPĀDAḤ

The Chapter on Complete Attention

अथ योगानुशासनम् ॥ १.१ ॥

1.1 atha yogānuśāsanam

atha yoga-anuśāsanam

atha	now (in sequence, not at this moment)
yoga	process of calming the fluctuations in the heart-mind (defined in 1.2); topic of this text
anuśāsana	the following teaching, a teaching that follows [am subj sg n-a]

1. Now, the teaching of yoga.
2. Here begins the instruction of yoga.

योगश्चित्तवृत्तिनिरोधः ॥ १.२ ॥

1.2 yogaścittavṛttinirodhaḥ

yogaḥ citta-vṛtti-nirodhaḥ

yoga	connection, relationship, union, application [aḥ subj sg m-a]
citta	heart-mind field of consciousness
vṛtti	fluctuation or activity in the heart-mind
nirodha	stilling, settling, calming, breaking [aḥ subj sg m-a]

1. Yoga is the stilling of fluctuations in the field of consciousness.
2. Yoga occurs when one focuses completely on a single object so that thought waves do not distract one's heart-mind field of consciousness.

तदा द्रष्टुः स्वरूपे ऽवस्थानम् ॥ १.३ ॥

1.3 tadā draṣṭuḥ svarūpe 'vasthānam

tadā draṣṭuḥ svarūpe avasthānam

tadā	then
draṣṭṛ	the seer, the individual's witness state, Puruṣa [uḥ "of" sg m-ṛ]
svarūpa	its own form [e "in/on/at" sg n-a]
avasthāna	resting, dwelling [am subj sg n-a]

1. Then (in the state of yoga) the radiant seer (is seen clearly) resting in its own form.
2. When the citta-vṛtti-s no longer cloud perception, then pure awareness (Puruṣa) shines through and is experienced within ourself.

वृत्तिसारूप्यमितरत्र ॥ १.४ ॥

1.4 vṛttisārūpyamitaratra

vṛtti-sārūpyam itaratra

vṛtti	fluctuation or activity in the heart-mind
sārūpya	conformity, identification [am subj sg n-a]
itaratra	otherwise

1. Otherwise (not in yoga) we are identified with the vṛtti-s.
2. Otherwise yoga/nirodha is not present and mental activity is distracting the attention and blocking access to the inner light of pure awareness.

वृत्तयः पञ्चतय्यः क्लिष्टाक्लिष्टाः ॥ १.५ ॥

1.5 vṛttayaḥ pañcatayyaḥ kliṣṭākliṣṭāḥ

vṛttayaḥ pañcatayyaḥ kliṣṭa-akliṣṭāḥ

vṛtti	fluctuation or activity in the heart-mind [ayaḥ subj pl f-i]
pañcatayī	fivefold [yaḥ subj pl f-i]
kliṣṭa	harmful, afflicting, originating from a kleśa
akliṣṭa	not harmful, nonafflicting, not originating from a kleśa, so helpful or neutral [āḥ subj pl f-a]

1. Vṛtti-s are fivefold, (and can be) afflicting or nonafflicting.
2. There are five different fluctuations of the heart-mind, and each can be harmful or helpful.

प्रमाणविपर्ययविकल्पनिद्रास्मृतयः ॥ १.६ ॥

1.6 pramāṇaviparyayavikalpanidrāsmṛtayaḥ

pramāṇa-viparyaya-vikalpa-nidrā-smṛtayaḥ

pramāṇa	correct way of evaluating an object (see 1.7)
viparyaya	misperception, incorrect evaluation (see 1.8)

vikalpa imagination (see 1.9)
nidrā sleep (see 1.10)
smṛti the act of memory (see 1.11) [ayaḥ subj pl f-i]

1. (The vṛtti-s are) correct evaluation, misperception, imagination, sleep, and the act of memory.
2. (The fluctuations of the heart-mind are) correct evaluation, misperception, imagination, sleep, and the act of memory.

प्रत्यक्षानुमानागमाः प्रमाणानि ॥ १.७ ॥

1.7 pratyakṣānumānāgamāḥ pramāṇāni

pratyakṣa-anumāna-āgamāḥ pramāṇāni

pratyakṣa direct, firsthand perception
anumāna inference, assumption, indirect/secondhand
āgama testimony, knowledge from conversation or books, second/thirdhand [āḥ subj pl m-a]
pramāṇa correct way of evaluating an object [āni subj pl n-a]

1. The correct ways to evaluate what we perceive are direct experience, inference, and reliable testimony.

विपर्ययो मिथ्याज्ञानमतद्रूपप्रतिष्ठम् ॥ १.८ ॥

1.8 viparyayo mithyājñānamatadrūpapratiṣṭham

viparyayaḥ mithyā-jñānam atad rūpa-pratiṣṭham

viparyaya misconception [aḥ subj sg m-a]
mithyā mistaken, false
jñāna knowledge, cognition [am subj sg n-a]
atad not that (a + tad) [pronoun]
rūpa form (visual, auditory, subtle, etc.)
pratiṣṭha based on [am subj sg n-a]

1. Misperception is false knowledge based upon a form which is not that.
2. Misperception is perceiving an object incorrectly and thinking it is something else.

शब्दज्ञानानुपाती वस्तुशून्यो विकल्पः ॥ १.९ ॥

1.9 śabdajñānānupātī vastuśūnyo vikalpaḥ

śabda-jñāna-anupātī vastu-śūnyaḥ vikalpaḥ

śabda word, sound, language
jñāna knowledge, cognition
anupātin relying, chasing after [ī subj sg m-in]
vastu object

śūnya devoid, without [aḥ subj sg m-a]
vikalpa conceptualization, imagination [aḥ subj sg m-a]

1. Vikalpa is without an object, relying on knowledge from words or language.
2. Imagination is an idea that can be expressed in words, yet has no real object.

अभावप्रत्ययालम्बना तमोवृत्तिर्निद्रा ॥ १.१० ॥

1.10 abhāvapratyayālambanā tamovṛttirnidrā

abhāva-pratyaya-ālambanā tamas-vṛttiḥ nidrā

abhāva absence
pratyaya presented thought; current vṛtti directed toward an object
ālambanā supporting [ā subj sg f-ā]
tamas inertia
vṛtti fluctuation or activity in the heart-mind [iḥ subj sg f-i]
nidrā sleep [ā subj sg f-ā]

1. Sleep is a tamasic mental activity supported by the absence of presented thoughts.
2. Sleep is when the mind slows down, supported by a lack of conscious thoughts.

अनुभूतविषयासंप्रमोषः स्मृतिः ॥ १.११ ॥

1.11 anubhūtaviṣayāsaṃpramoṣaḥ smṛtiḥ

anubhūta-viṣaya-asaṃpramoṣaḥ smṛtiḥ

anubhūta experienced before
viṣaya object of sense
asaṃpramoṣa retention, "not carrying off"
(a + sam + pra + moṣa) [aḥ subj sg m-a]
smṛti the act of memory [iḥ subj sg f-i]

1. The act of memory is the retention of an experienced object.
2. The act of memory is to store a sensory experience in our memory.

अभ्यासवैराग्याभ्यां तन्निरोधः ॥ १.१२ ॥

1.12 abhyāsavairāgyābhyāṃ tannirodhaḥ

abhyāsa-vairāgyābhyāṃ tat nirodhaḥ

abhyāsa diligent, continuous practice over a period of time
vairāgya unattached awareness, noninvolvement, noninterference
[ābhyām "by/with/from/due to" du n-a]
tad (of) those [pronoun]
nirodha stilling [aḥ subj sg m-a]

1. Nirodha of those (vṛtti-s) is due to abhyāsa and vairāgya.
2. The stilling of those (vṛtti-s) is due to diligent practice and unattached awareness.

तत्र स्थितौ यत्नो ऽभ्यासः ॥ १.१३ ॥

1.13 tatra sthitau yatno 'bhyāsaḥ

tatra sthitau yatnaḥ abhyāsaḥ

tatra	there
sthiti	staying, remaining [au "in/on/upon" sg f-i]
yatna	effort [aḥ subj sg m-a]
abhyāsa	diligent, continuous practice, vigilance [aḥ subj sg m-a]

1. Abhyāsa is the effort at remaining there.
2. Diligent practice is the effort put forth to maintain a point of focus.

स तु दीर्घकालनैरन्तर्यसत्कारादरासेवितो दृढभूमिः ॥ १.१४ ॥

1.14 sa tu dīrghakālanairantaryasatkārādarāsevito dṛḍhabhūmiḥ*

sa tu dīrgha-kāla-nairantarya-satkāra-ādarā-sevitaḥ dṛḍha-bhūmiḥ

sa	that (abhyāsa) [pronoun subj sg m-p]
tu	and, moreover
dīrgha-kāla	a long time, over the long term
nairantarya	without interruption (nir + antar = nothing between, without interval)
satkāra	acting with truth, sincerity
ādara	eagerness, respect, care
sevita	pursued, practiced, followed [aḥ subj sg m-a]
dṛḍha	firm
bhūmi	ground, earth [iḥ subj sg m-i]

1. Moreover, that (abhyāsa) becomes firmly established when pursued with eagerness, sincerity, and continuity for a long time.

* The following variation occurs in other translations: sa tu dīrghakālanairant aryasatkārāsevito dṛḍhabhūmiḥ

दृष्टानुश्रविकविषयवितृष्णस्य वशीकारसंज्ञा वैराग्यम् ॥ १.१५ ॥

1.15 dṛṣṭānuśravikaviṣayavitṛṣṇasya vaśīkārasaṃjñā vairāgyam

dṛṣṭa anuśravika-viṣaya-vitṛṣṇasya vaśīkāra-saṃjñā vairāgyam

dṛṣṭa	seen
anuśravika	heard after
viṣaya	sensory object
vitṛṣṇa	nonclinging, noncraving (vi + tṛṣṇa) [asya "of" sg m-a]
vaśīkāra-saṃjñā	full knowledge of mastery [ā subj sg f-ā]
vairāgya	unattached awareness, noninvolvement, noninterference [am subj sg n-a]

1. Vairāgya is the complete mastery of nonclinging to sensory objects heard or seen.
2. Vairāgya is a state of consciousness in which the mind no longer thirsts for objects perceivable by the senses, heard about, or read.

तत्परं पुरुषख्यातेर्गुणवैतृष्ण्यम् ॥ १.१६ ॥

1.16 tatparaṃ puruṣakhyāterguṇavaitṛṣṇyam

tat-paraṃ puruṣa-khyāteḥ guṇa-vaitṛṣṇyam

tad	(than) that [pronoun stem]
para	higher [am subj sg n-a]
puruṣa	the inner light of awareness, the observer
khyāti	awareness, realization, understanding, identification [eḥ "from" sg f-i]
guṇa	quality of nature
vaitṛṣṇya	a more subtle and higher form of vitṛṣṇa (nonclinging) [am subj sg n-a]

1. The higher (and more subtle vairāgya) is the nonclinging to the guṇa-s due to the realization of one's individual Self.

वितर्कविचारानन्दास्मितारूपानुगमात्संप्रज्ञातः ॥ १.१७ ॥

1.17 vitarkavicārānandāsmitārūpānugamātsaṃprajñātaḥ

vitarka-vicāra-ānanda-asmitā-rūpa-anugamāt saṃprajñātaḥ

vitarka	logical thought on a gross level
vicāra	reflective thought on a subtler level
ānanda	joy
asmitā	identification
rūpa	form
anugama	following, comprehending [āt "from" sg m-a]
saṃprajñāta	complete understanding [aḥ subj sg m-a]

1. Saṃprajñāta-samādhi occurs from following vitarka to vicāra to ānanda to asmitā-rūpa.
2. Complete mastery of an object occurs from comprehending it on four levels: logical reasoning, subtle reflection, the joy of deeper understanding, and finally completely identifying with it (knowing it "in your bones").

विरामप्रत्ययाभ्यासपूर्वः संस्कारशेषो ऽन्यः ॥ १.१८ ॥

1.18 virāmapratyayābhyāsapūrvaḥ saṃskāraśeṣo 'nyaḥ

virāma-pratyaya-abhyāsa-pūrvaḥ saṃskāra-śeṣaḥ anyaḥ

virāma	cessation, cutting off
pratyaya	presented thought; current vṛtti directed toward an object
abhyāsa	diligent practice
pūrva	preceded [pronoun aḥ subj sg m-p]
saṃskāra	strong impression in memory causing a habitual tendency
śeṣa	leftover [aḥ subj sg m-a]
anya	other [aḥ subj sg m-p]

1. The other (i.e., asaṃprajñāta-samādhi), preceded by diligent practice on the cessation of presented thoughts, still contains residual saṃskāra-s.

भवप्रत्ययो विदेहप्रकृतिलयानाम् ॥ १.१९ ॥

1.19 bhavapratyayo videhaprakṛtilayānām

bhava-pratyayaḥ videha-prakṛtilayānām

bhava	existence, becoming
pratyaya	inclination; a presented thought, current vṛtti directed toward an object [aḥ subj sg m-a]
videha	out of body, separated from the body
prakṛtilaya	absorbed back into nature [ānām "of" plural m-a]

1. (Asaṃprajñāta-samādhi is also preceded by) one's inclination toward existing, for those who innately know yoga.
2. Those who are born with a heart-mind that is naturally undistracted by vṛtti-s act simply because they have a body, based on the residual saṃskāra-s from previous incarnations.

श्रद्धावीर्यस्मृतिसमाधिप्रज्ञापूर्वक इतरेषाम् ॥ १.२० ॥

1.20 śraddhāvīryasmṛtisamādhiprajñāpūrvaka itareṣām

śraddhā-vīrya-smṛti-samādhi-prājñā-pūrvakaḥ itareṣām

śraddhā	faith,determination
vīrya	vitality, courage, strength, energy
smṛti	memory, remembering to stay focused
samādhi	complete absorption of the heart-mind in the focus
prajñā	deep insight
pūrvaka	preceded by [aḥ subj sg m-a]
itara	another [pronoun ending eṣām "of" plural m-p]

1. For most people, (asaṃprajñāta-samādhi) is preceded by (in sequence) faith, vitality, (strong and sustained) memory, samādhi, then deep insight.

तीव्रसंवेगानामासन्नः ॥ १.२१ ॥

1.21 tīvrasaṃvegānāmāsannaḥ

tīvra-saṃvegānām āsannaḥ

tīvra	intense
saṃvega	momentum [ānām "of" plural m-a]
āsanna	closest, nearest [aḥ subj sg m-a]

1. (Asaṃprajñāta-samādhi) is closest to those with intense momentum (in their practice and faith).
2. Intense momentum of practice and faith accelerates them toward samādhi.

मृदुमध्याधिमात्रत्वात्ततो ऽपि विशेषः ॥ १.२२ ॥

1.22 mṛdumadhyādhimātratvāttato 'pi viśeṣaḥ

mṛdu-madhya-adhimātratvāt tataḥ api viśeṣaḥ

mṛdu	mild, soft
madhya	medium
adhimātratva	extraordinary [āt "from" sg n-a]
tataḥ	from that [pronoun aḥ "from" sg n-p]
api	also
viśeṣa	difference [aḥ subj sg m-a]

1. Whether their (practice or faith) is mild, medium, or extraordinary also makes a difference.

ईश्वरप्रणिधानाद्वा ॥ १.२३ ॥

1.23 īśvarapraṇidhānādvā

īśvara-praṇidhānāt vā

Īśvara	the teachings, universal teacher, eternal teacher
praṇidhāna	devotion, surrender, faith [āt "from" sg m-a]
īśvara-praṇidhāna	honoring the divine inner teacher
vā	or

1. Or because of īśvara-praṇidhāna (samādhi is attained).
2. Or due to truly seeing the same light of knowledge in all beings.

क्लेशकर्मविपाकाशयैरपरामृष्टः पुरुषविशेष ईश्वरः ॥ १.२४ ॥

1.24 kleśakarmavipākāśayairaparāmṛṣṭaḥ puruṣaviśeṣa īśvaraḥ

kleśa-karma-vipāka-āśayaiḥ aparāmṛṣṭaḥ puruṣa-viśeṣaḥ īśvaraḥ

kleśa	deep emotional affliction
karma	action
vipāka	ripening, fruition
āśaya	container, storehouse [aiḥ "by/with" pl m-a]

aparāmṛṣṭa	not connected in any way, unaffected by, untouched by [aḥ subj sg m-a]
puruṣa	the inner light of awareness, the observer
viśeṣa	special, distinct, separate [aḥ subj sg m-a]
Īśvara	the teachings, universal teacher, eternal teacher, omniscience [aḥ subj sg m-a]

1. Īśvara is a distinct (and separate) Puruṣa, in no way connected to the storehouse of ripened karma-s and kleśa-s (known as the karmāśaya, or here āśaya).
2. Īśvara is a different kind of Puruṣa, unaffected by anything that happens in the manifest world.

तत्र निरतिशयं सर्वज्ञबीजम् ॥ १.२५ ॥

1.25 tatra niratiśayaṃ sarvajñabījam*

tatra niratiśayaṃ sarvajñabījam

tatra	there
niratiśaya	beyond compare [am subj sg n-a]
sarva-jña	all-knowing
bīja	seed [am subj sg n-a]

1. There, the seed of all-knowing is beyond compare.
2. Īśvara represents all knowledge that exists, known or as yet unknown.

* The following variation occurs in other translations: tatra niratiśayaṃ sarvajñatvabījam

स एष पूर्वेषामपि गुरुः कालेनानवच्छेदात् ॥ १.२६ ॥

1.26 sa eṣa pūrveṣāmapi guruḥ kālenānavacchedāt*

saḥ eṣaḥ pūrveṣām api guruḥ kāla-ānavacchedāt

sa	that [pronoun aḥ subj sg m-p]
eṣa	this [pronoun aḥ subj sg m-p]
pūrva	before, previous [eṣām "of" pl m-p]
api	even, also
guru	teacher [uḥ subj sg m-u]
kāla	time [ena "by/with" sg m-a]
anavaccheda	not limited [āt "from" sg m-a]

1. That, this, not limited by time, is the teacher, even of those who came before.
2. Īśvara represents the eternal teachings, available to those in the past, present, and future.

* The following variation occurs in other versions: sa pūrveṣāmapi guruḥ kālenānavacchedāt

तस्य वाचकः प्रणवः ॥ १.२७ ॥

1.27 tasya vācakaḥ praṇavaḥ

tasya vācakaḥ praṇavaḥ

tasya	of that (Īśvara) [pronoun "of" sg m-p]
vācaka	spoken, speaker [aḥ subj sg m-a]
praṇava	the sound from which creation arose (Om in India) [aḥ subj sg m-a]

1. The spoken expression of Īśvara is praṇava (which in India is Om).

तज्जपस्तदर्थभावनम् ॥ १.२८ ॥

1.28 tajjapastadarthabhāvanam

tad japaḥ tad artha-bhāvanam

tad	(of) that [pronoun stem]
japa	repetition [aḥ subj sg m-a]
tad	of that, of it, its [pronoun stem]
artha	meaning
bhāvana	feeling, attitude, disposition; intention; cultivation [am subj sg n-a]

1. Repeating that (praṇava) is feeling its meaning (Īśvara).
2. The repetition of the praṇava (Om in India) leads us to understand the meaning of Īśvara.

ततः प्रत्यक्चेतनाधिगमो ऽप्यन्तरायाभावश्च ॥ १.२९ ॥

1.29 tataḥ pratyakcetanādhigamo 'pyantarāyābhāvaśca

tataḥ pratyak cetana-adhigamaḥ api antarāya-abhāvaḥ ca

tataḥ	from that
pratyak	inward
cetana	consciousness
adhigama	go toward [aḥ subj sg m-a]
api	even, also
antarāya	obstacle (see 1.30)
abhāva	disappear [aḥ subj sg m-a]
ca	and

1. From that our consciousness goes inward and the antarāya-s disappear.
2. Chanting the praṇava (Om in India) causes introspection and removes the distractions to practice.

व्याधिस्त्यानसंशयप्रमादालस्याविरतिभ्रान्तिदर्शनालब्धभूमिकत्वानवस्थितत्वानि चित्तविक्षेपास्ते ऽन्तरायाः ॥ १.३० ॥

1.30 vyādhistyānasaṃśayapramādālasyāviratibhrāntidarśanālabdhabh ūmikatvānavasthitatvāni cittavikṣepāste 'ntarāyāḥ

vyādhi-styāna-saṃśaya-pramāda-ālasya-avirati-bhrāntidarśana-alabdhabhūmikatva-anavasthitatvāni citta-vikṣepāḥ te antarāyāḥ

vyādhi	disease
styāna	apathy, dullness
saṃśaya	doubt, indecision
pramāda	carelessness, intoxication
ālasya	lethargy, laziness
avirati	temptation, sexual preoccupation
bhrānti-darśana	erroneous seeing
alabdhabhūmikatva	inability to become grounded
anavasthitatva	regression [āni subj pl n-a]
citta	heart-mind field of consciousness
vikṣepa	disruption [āḥ subj pl m-a]
te	those [pronoun e subj pl m-p]
antarāya	obstacle [āḥ subj pl m-a]

1. The obstacles to practice are disease, apathy, doubt, carelessness, lethargy, temptation, erroneous views, ungroundedness, and regression.

दुःखदौर्मनस्याङ्गमेजयत्वश्वासप्रश्वासा विक्षेपसहभुवः ॥ १.३१ ॥

1.31 duḥkhadaurmanasyāṅgamejayatvaśvāsapraśvāsā vikṣepasahabhuvaḥ

duḥkha-daurmanasya-aṅgamejayatva-śvāsa-praśvāsāḥ vikṣepa-sahabhuvaḥ

duḥkha	pain, suffering, discomfort
daurmanasya	mental pain, depression, negativity
aṅgamejayatva	agitation, nervousness
śvāsa	inhalation
praśvāsā	exhalation [āḥ subj pl m-a]
vikṣepa	disruption
sahabhuva	accompanying [aḥ subj sg m-a]

1. The accompanying disruptions are suffering, negative thinking, trembling of the body, and (disturbed) inhalation and exhalation.

तत्प्रतिषेधार्थमेकतत्त्वाभ्यासः ॥ १.३२ ॥

1.32 tatpratiṣedhārthamekatattvābhyāsaḥ

tat pratiṣedha-ārtham eka-tattva-abhyāsaḥ

tad	(of) those (antarāya;—see 1.30–31) [pronoun stem]
pratiṣedha	prevention, counteracting
artha	purpose [am subj sg m-a]
eka	one, single
tattva	thing
abhyāsa	diligent practice [aḥ subj sg m-a]

1. Abhyāsa on a single tattva is for the purpose of preventing those (anatarāya-s and their symptoms).
2. The obstacles and their effects can be prevented by diligent practice focused on one thing.

मैत्रीकरुणामुदितोपेक्षाणां सुखदुःखपुण्यापुण्यविषयाणां भावनातश्चित्तप्रसादनम् ॥ १.३३ ॥

1.33 maitrīkaruṇāmuditopekṣāṇāṃ sukhaduḥkhapuṇyāpuṇyaviṣayāṇāṃ bhāvanātaścittaprasādanam

maitrī-karuṇā-mudita-upekṣāṇāṃ sukha-duḥkha-puṇya-apuṇya-viṣayāṇāṃ bhāvanātaḥ citta-prasādanam

maitrī	friendliness
karuṇā	compassion
mudita	joyfulness
upekṣaṇa	neutrality [ānām "of" pl m-a]
sukha	happiness
duḥkha	suffering, pain, discomfort
puṇya	virtue
apuṇya	nonvirtue, vice
viṣaya	sensory object [ānām "of" pl m-a]
bhāvana	feeling, attitude, disposition; intention; cultivation [āt "from/due to" sg n-a]
citta	heart-mind field of consciousness
prasādana	purification, clarification [am subj sg n-a]

1. Purification of our field of consciousness occurs from an attitude of friendship when encountering happiness, compassion when encountering suffering, gladness when encountering virtue, and neutrality when encountering vice.
2. Purification of our heart-mind is the result of cultivating a mindset that is usually positive, never negative or critical, and sometimes cautious (neutrality).

प्रच्छर्धनविधारणाभ्यां वा प्राणस्य ॥ १.३४ ॥

1.34 pracchardhanavidhāraṇābhyāṃ vā prāṇasya

pracchardhana-vidhāṛaṇābhyāṃ vā prāṇasya

pracchardhana	exhaling
vidhāraṇa	extending, holding [ābhyām "by/with/from" du n-a]
vā	or
prāṇa	breath, life-force [asya "of" sg m-a]

1. Or (the heart-mind is clarified) by exhalation and retention of the prāṇa (through prāṇāyāma).

विषयवती वा प्रवृत्तिरुत्पन्ना मनसः स्थितिनिबन्धिनी ॥ १.३५ ॥

1.35 viṣayavatī vā pravṛttirutpannā manasaḥ sthitinibandhinī

viṣayavatī vā pravṛttiḥ utpannā manasaḥ sthiti-nibandhinī

viṣayavatī	having a sensory object [ī subj sg f-ī]
vā	or
pravṛttiḥ	finer sensory activity [iḥ subj sg f-i]
utpannā	development, arising [ā subj sg f-ā]
manas	outer mind [aḥ "of" sg n-cons]
sthiti	steadiness, calmness
nibandhinī	maintaining [ī subj sg f-in]

1. Or the development of finer sensory perceptions (results in) maintaining steadiness of mind.

विशोका वा ज्योतिष्मती ॥ १.३६ ॥

1.36 viśokā vā jyotiṣmatī

viśokā vā jyotiṣmatī

viśokā	sorrowless [ā subj sg f-ā]
vā	or
jyotiṣmatī	having light, radiant [ī subj sg f-ī]

1. Or (by perception that is) free from sorrow and filled with light (sattvic), (it is clarified).

वीतरागविषयं वा चित्तम् ॥ १.३७ ॥

1.37 vītarāgaviṣayaṃ vā cittam

vīta-rāga-viṣayaṃ vā cittam

vīta	without
rāga	attachment to pleasure (a kleśa)
vīta-rāga	without attachment to pleasure
viṣaya	object [am subj sg n-a]

vā	or
citta	heart-mind field of consciousness [am subj sg n-a]

1. Or when the heart-mind (is focused on) an object without rāga (the kleśa), (it is clarified).

स्वप्ननिद्राज्ञानालम्बनं वा ॥ १.३८ ॥

1.38 svapnanidrājñānālambanaṃ vā

svapna-nidrā-jñāna-ālambanaṃ vā

svapna	dream
nidrā	sleep
jñāna	knowledge
ālambana	support [am subj sg n-a]
vā	or

1. Or (the heart-mind is clarified when focused on an object) supported by the knowledge from dreams or deep sleep.
2. The heart-mind is clarified by focusing on a sattvic memory from a dream, or the quietness of deep sleep.

यथाभिमतध्यानाद्वा ॥ १.३९ ॥

1.39 yathābhimatadhyānādvā

yatha-abhimata-dhyānāt vā

yatha	as, whatever
abhimata	conceived, thought up
dhyāna	focused and uninterrupted attention on a single place [āt "from/due to" sg m-a]
vā	or

1. Or due to dhyāna (meditation) on whatever we like (and has the sattva quality).

परमाणुपरममहत्त्वान्तो ऽस्य वशीकारः ॥ १.४० ॥

1.40 paramāṇuparamamahattvānto 'sya vaśīkāraḥ

parama-aṇu-parama-mahattva-antaḥ asya vaśīkāraḥ

parama	great
aṇu	tiny, minuscule
parama	great
mahattva	magnitude, "largeness"
anta	end [aḥ subj sg m-a]
asya	of that [pronoun "of" sg m-p]
vaśīkāra	mastery [aḥ subj sg m-a]

1. Mastery of that (heart-mind) extends from the infinitesmally small to the infinitely large.
2. Once the heart-mind is clarified, its realm of perception spans the smallest objects to the largest.

क्षीणवृत्तेरभिजातस्येव मणेर्ग्रहीतृग्रहणग्राह्येषु तत्स्थतदञ्जनता समापत्तिः ॥ १.४१ ॥

1.41 kṣīṇavṛtterabhijātasyeva maṇergrahītṛgrahaṇagrāhyeṣu tatsthatadañjanatā samāpattiḥ

kṣīṇa-vṛtteḥ abhijātasya iva maṇeḥ grahītṛ-grahaṇa-grāhyeṣu tat-stha-tad-añjanatā samāpattiḥ

kṣīṇa	reduced
vṛtti	fluctuation or activity in the heart-mind f-i
abhijāta	perfect, flawless [asya "of" sg m-a]
iva	like
maṇi	jewel [eḥ "of" sg m-i]
grahītṛ	grasper
grahaṇa	grasping
grāhya	to be grasped [eṣu "in/on/upon" pl n-a]
tad	(on) that [pronoun stem]
stha	staying, resting, focused on
tad	(by) that [pronoun stem]
añjanatā	saturation [ā subj sg f-ā]
samāpatti	saturation of the heart-mind with the focus (see samādhi) [iḥ subj sg f-i]

1. When the (heart-mind's) vṛtti-s have been reduced, (it acts) like a flawless gemstone in terms of the perceiver, act of perceiving, and the object of perception. Samāpatti is the (gradual) saturation of that (heart-mind) due to focusing on that (object).
2. When most of the vṛtti-s in the heart-mind are cleared out, the heart-mind, like a transparent crystal, reflects the object of focus better and better, eventually saturating the heart-mind to make it seem as though the heart-mind *is* the object. The distinction between subject, object, and act of perceiving has gone away.

तत्र शब्दार्थज्ञानविकल्पैः संकीर्णा सवितर्का समापत्तिः ॥ १.४२ ॥

1.42 tatra śabdārthajñānavikalpaiḥ saṃkīrṇā savitarkā samāpattiḥ

tatra śabda-artha-jñāna-vikalpaiḥ saṃkīrṇā savitarkā samāpattiḥ

tatra	there
śabda	word, sound

artha	meaning
jñāna	knowledge
vikalpa	conceptual [aiḥ "by/with" sg m-a]
saṃkīrṇā	mixed [ā subj sg f-ā]
savitarkā	without thought [ā subj sg f-ā]
samāpatti	saturation of the heart-mind with the focus (see samādhi) [iḥ subj sg f-i]

1. There (in a heart-mind whose vṛtti-s have subsided), samāpatti is "with thought," mixed with words, meaning, and conceptual knowledge.

स्मृतिपरिशुद्धौ स्वरूपशून्येवार्थमात्रनिर्भासा निर्वितर्का ॥ १.४३ ॥

1.43 smṛtipariśuddhau svarūpaśūnyevārthamātranirbhāsā nirvitarkā

smṛti-pariśuddhau svarūpa-śūnya-iva artha-mātra-nirbhāsā nirvitarkā

smṛti	memory
pariśuddhi	purification [au "in/upon" sg f-i]
svarūpa	own form
śūnyā	empty, devoid, zero [ā subj sg f-ā]
iva	like
artha	object
mātra	alone
nirbhāsā	appearing [ā subj sg f-ā]
nirvitarkā	beyond thought [ā subj sg f-ā]

1. When the memory has been completely purified, (samāpatti is) "beyond thought" (when) the object alone appears (as a reflection in the heart-mind, which is) as if empty of its own form.
2. When the memory is purified, no more analysis takes place and the object is seen in its simplicity.

एतयैव सविचारा निर्विचारा च सूक्ष्मविषया व्याख्याता ॥ १.४४ ॥

1.44 etayaiva savicārā nirvicārā ca sūkṣmaviṣayā vyākhyātā

etayā eva savicārā nirvicārā ca sūkṣma-viṣayā vyākhyātā

etayā	by this [pronoun "by/with" sg f-p]
eva	specifically
savicārā	with reflection [ā subj sg f-ā]
nirvicārā	beyond reflection [ā subj sg f-ā]
ca	and
sūkṣma	subtle
viṣayā	object [ā subj sg f-ā]
vyākhyātā	explained [ā subj sg f-ā]

1. Specifically by this, savicārā and nirvicārā (samāpatti is explained) for subtle objects.
2. Saturation with and beyond reflection focus on subtle objects, parallel to saturation with and beyond thought, which focus on gross objects.

सूक्ष्मविषयत्वं चालिङ्गपर्यवसानम् ॥ १.४५ ॥

1.45 sūkṣmaviṣayatvaṃ cāliṅgaparyavasānam

sūkṣma-viṣayatvaṃ ca aliṅga-paryavasānam

sūkṣma	subtle
viṣayatva	objectness [am subj sg n-a]
ca	and
aliṅga-	unmanifest, "unmarked"
paryavasāna	tracing back [am subj sg n-a]

1. The subtlety of objects traces back to unmanifest matter. (See aliṅga; appendix F, figure 1.)

ता एव सबीजः समाधिः ॥ १.४६ ॥

1.46 tā eva sabījaḥ samādhiḥ

tā eva sabījaḥ samādhiḥ

tā	those [pronoun subj pl f-p]
eva	only
sabīja	"with seed" [aḥ subj sg m-a]
samādhi	complete absorption of the heart-mind in the focus [iḥ subj sg m-i]

1. Only those (aforementioned kinds of samāpatti, constitute) sabīja-samādhi (samādhi involving an object).

निर्विचारवैशारद्ये ऽध्यात्मप्रसादः ॥ १.४७ ॥

1.47 nirvicāravaiśāradye 'dhyātmaprasādaḥ

nirvicāra-vaiśāradye adhyātma-prasādaḥ

nirvicāra	beyond reflection
vaiśāradya	proficiency [e "in/upon" sg m-a]
adhyātma	inner instrument, individual self
prasāda	purity, clarity [aḥ subj sg m-a]

1. When proficient in nirvicāra-samāpatti, purity of the inner instruments of perception. Sattva predominates over rajas and tamas in the buddhi.

ऋतम्भरा तत्र प्रज्ञा ॥ १.४८ ॥

1.48 ṛtambharā tatra prajñā

ṛtam-bharā tatra prajñā

ṛtam-bharā	truth-bearing, revealing the truth [ā subj sg f-ā]
tatra	there
prajñā	insight [ā subj sg f-ā]

1. There (in nirvicāra-samāpatti) prajñā (deep insight) bears the actual truth. We see all aspects of the object clearly and accurately, without distortion because the heart-mind is clear.

श्रुतानुमानप्रज्ञाभ्यामन्यविषया विशेषार्थत्वात् ॥ १.४९ ॥

1.49 śrutānumānaprajñābhyāmanyaviṣayā viśeṣārthatvāt

śruta-anumāna-prajñābhyām anya-viṣayā viśeṣa-arthatvāt

śruta	testimony, "heard" or read from second- or thirdhand source
anumāna	inference, assumption
prajña	insight [ābhyām "by/with/to/for/from/due to/than" du f-a]
anya	other
viṣayā	object [ā subj pl f-ā]
viśeṣa	different, distinct
arthatva	purposefulness [āt "from" sg n-a]

1. Because it is different, (this higher prajñā has) an object other than the knowledge from inference or testimony. The scope of this prajñā is much broader and involves pratyakṣa, direct perception.

तज्जः संस्कारो ऽन्यसंस्कारप्रतिबन्धी ॥ १.५० ॥

1.50 tajjaḥ saṃskāro 'nyasaṃskārapratibandhī

tajjaḥ saṃskāraḥ anya-saṃskāra-pratibandhī

tad	(from) that [pronoun stem]
ja	born [aḥ subj sg m-a]
saṃskāra	strong impression in memory causing a habitual tendency [aḥ subj sg m-a]
anya	other
saṃskāra	same as above
pratibandhī	inhibition [ī subj sg m-in]

1. The saṃskāra born from that (higher prajñā) inhibits other saṃskāra-s.

तस्यापि निरोधे सर्वनिरोधान्निर्बीजः समाधिः ॥ १.५१ ॥

1.51 tasyāpi nirodhe sarvanirodhānnirbījaḥ samādhiḥ

tasya api nirodhe sarva-nirodhāt nirbījaḥ samādhiḥ

tasya of that [pronoun "of" sg m-p]
api even, also
nirodha stilling [e "on/upon" sg m-a]
sarva all
nirodha stilling [āt "from" sg m-a]
nirbīja without seed [aḥ subj sg m-a]
samādhi complete absorption of the heart-mind in the focus [iḥ subj sg m-i]

1. Seedless samādhi occurs when nirodha of even that (saṃskāra of prajñā) happens due to the nirodha of all (saṃskāra-s).

२. साधनपादः

SĀDHANAPĀDAḤ

The Chapter on Practice

तपःस्वाध्यायेश्वरप्रणिधानानि क्रियायोगः ॥ २.१ ॥

2.1 tapaḥsvādhyāyeśvarapraṇidhānāni kriyāyogaḥ

tapaḥ-svādhyāya-īśvarapraṇidhānāni kriyā-yogaḥ

tapas practice causing positive change
svādhyāya self-study, self-observation
īśvara-praṇidhāna honoring the divine inner teacher [āni subj pl n-a]
kriyā-yoga the yoga of active practice or work [aḥ subj sg m-a]

1. Kriyā-yoga consists of tapas, svādhyāya, and īśvara-praṇidhāna.
2. The yoga of active practice consists of practice causing change, self-observation, and honoring the divine inner teacher.

समाधिभावनार्थः क्लेशतनूकरणार्थश्च ॥ २.२ ॥

2.2 samādhibhāvanārthaḥ kleśatanūkaraṇārthaśca

samādhi-bhāvana-arthaḥ kleśa-tanū-karaṇa-arthaḥ ca

samādhi complete absorption of the heart-mind in the focus
bhāvana feeling, attitude, disposition; intention; cultivation

artha purpose, reason [aḥ subj sg m-a]
kleśa deep emotional affliction
tanū weakening
karaṇa cause
artha purpose, reason [aḥ subj sg m-a]
ca and

1. The purpose (of kriyā-yoga) is a bhāvana of samādhi and to cause the weakening of the kleśa-s.
2. The purpose of tapas, svādhyāya, and īśvara-praṇidhāna is to weaken the kleśa-s and experience samādhi.

अविद्यास्मितारागद्वेषाभिनिवेशाः क्लेशाः ॥ २.३ ॥

2.3 avidyāsmitārāgadveṣābhiniveśāḥ kleśāḥ

avidyā-asmitā-rāga-dveṣa-abhiniveśāḥ kleśāḥ

avidyā lack of awareness, ignorance
asmitā identification with one's individual being
rāga attachment to previous pleasure
dveṣa attachment to previous suffering; dislike, aversion because of past suffering
abhiniveśa survival instinct, will to live, fear of dying [āḥ subj pl m-a]
kleśa deep emotional affliction [āḥ subj pl m-a]

1. The kleśa-s are avidyā, asmitā, rāga, dveṣa, and abhiniveśa.
2. The mental-emotional afflictions are unawareness, egotism, clinging to past pleasure, clinging to past pain, and the fear of death.

अविद्या क्षेत्रमुत्तरेषां प्रसुप्ततनुविच्छिन्नोदाराणाम् ॥ २.४ ॥

2.4 avidyā kṣetramuttareṣāṃ prasuptatanuvicchinnodārāṇām

avidyā kṣetram-uttareṣāṃ prasupta-tanu-vicchinna-udārāṇām

avidyā lack of awareness, ignorance [ā subj sg f-ā]
kṣetram field [am subj sg n-a]
uttara other, subsequent ones [eṣāṃ "of" pl m-p]
prasupta dormant, sleeping
tanu weak
vicchinna intermittent, come and go
udāra active [āṇām "of" pl m-a]

1. Avidyā is a field for the others, which can be dormant, weakly active, intermittent, or strongly active.

अनित्याशुचिदुःखानात्मसु नित्यशुचिसुखात्मख्यातिरविद्या ॥ २.५ ॥

2.5 anityāśuciduḥkhānātmasu nityaśucisukhātmakhyātiravidyā

anitya-aśuci-duḥkha-anātmasu nitya-śuci-sukha-ātma-khyātiḥ avidyā

anitya	impermanent
aśuci	impure
duḥkha	suffering, pain, discomfort
anātma	nonself [su "in/upon" pl m-an]
nitya	permanent
śuci	pure
sukha	happiness
ātma	self
khyāti	awareness, realization, understanding, identification [iḥ subj sg f-i]
avidyā	lack of awareness, ignorance [ā subj sg f-ā]

1. Avidyā is (falsely) identifying the impermanent, impure, suffering nonself (which constitutes Prakṛti) as the permanent, pure, happy Self (which describes Puruṣa).
2. Lack of awareness causes us to think the ever-changing manifest world is the same as the unchanging, inner light of awareness.

दृग्दर्शनशक्त्योरेकात्मतेवास्मिता ॥ २.६ ॥

2.6 dṛgdarśanaśaktyorekātmatevāsmitā

dṛk-darśana-śaktyoḥ eka-ātmatā iva asmitā

dṛk	seer, Puruṣa
darśana	seeing
śakti	power [yoḥ "of/between" du f-i]
eka	one, single
ātmatā	identity, "self-ness" [ā subj sg f-ā]
iva	like, as if
asmitā	sense of "I am," egoism [ā subj sg f-ā]

1. Asmitā is as if the seer (Puruṣa) and the instrument of seeing (buddhi) are the same.
2. The sense of "I am" makes us think that our decision-making power is the same as the unchanging witness consciousness.

सुखानुशयी रागः ॥ २.७ ॥

2.7 sukhānuśayī rāgaḥ

sukha-anuśayī rāgaḥ

sukha	pleasure, joy
anuśayin	holding on to, dwelling on [ī subj sg m-in]

rāga	passion, emotional attachment [aḥ subj sg m-a]

1. Rāga is holding on to past pleasure.

दुःखानुशयी द्वेषः ॥ २.८ ॥

2.8 duḥkhānuśayī dveṣaḥ

duḥkha-anuśayī dveṣaḥ

dukha	suffering, pain, discomfort, trauma
anuśayin	holding on to, dwelling on [ī subj sg m-in]
dveṣa	aversion, repulsion [aḥ subj sg m-a]

1. Dveṣa is holding on to past pain.
2. Aversion (to something) comes from a previous painful experience of it.

स्वरसवाही विदुषो ऽपि समारूढो ऽभिनिवेशः ॥ २.९ ॥

2.9 svarasavāhī viduṣo 'pi samārūḍho 'bhiniveśaḥ*

svarasa-vāhī viduṣaḥ api samārūḍhaḥ abhiniveśaḥ

svarasa	"own essence"
vāhin	carried along, flowing [ī subj sg m-in]
viduṣa	a wise person [aḥ "of" sg m-cons]
api	even, also
samārūḍha	grown or developed completely [aḥ subj sg m-a]
abhiniveśa	fear of death, will to live, survival instinct [aḥ subj sg m-a]

1. Abhiniveśa is fully developed even in a wise person, carried along by its own essence.
2. The fear of death is strong in everyone, as our essence of experience is carried along from lifetime to lifetime.

* The following variation occurs in other translations: svarasavāhī viduṣo 'pi tathārūḍho 'bhiniveśaḥ.

ते प्रतिप्रसवहेयाः सूक्ष्माः ॥ २.१० ॥

2.10 te pratiprasavaheyāḥ sūkṣmāḥ

te pratiprasava-heyāḥ sūkṣmāḥ

te	those [pronoun subj pl m-p]
pratiprasava	returning back to the origin
heya	endable [āḥ subj pl m-a]
sūkṣma	subtle [āḥ subj pl m-a]

1. Those kleśa-s, when subtle, are to be removed by pratiprasava (the reverse of how they were produced).
2. When we notice subtle signs of a kleśa erupting, nip it in the bud before it becomes full-blown.

ध्यानहेयास्तद्वृत्तयः ॥ २.११ ॥

2.11 dhyānaheyāstadvṛttayaḥ

dhyāna-heyāḥ tad-vṛttayaḥ

dhyāna	focused and uninterrupted attention on a single place
heya	endable [āḥ subj pl f-ā]
tad	that, those
vṛtti	fluctuation or activity in the heart-mind [ayaḥ subj pl f-i]

1. The vṛtti-s of those (subtle kleśa-s) are to be overcome by dhyāna.
2. The disturbing fluctuations in the heart-mind (kliṣṭa-vṛtti-s) are endable by meditation.

क्लेशमूलः कर्माशयो दृष्टादृष्टजन्मवेदनीयः ॥ २.१२ ॥

2.12 kleśamūlaḥ karmāśayo dṛṣṭādṛṣṭajanmavedanīyaḥ

kleśa-mūlaḥ karmāśayaḥ dṛṣṭa-adṛṣṭa-janma-vedanīyaḥ

kleśa	deep emotional affliction
mūla	root [aḥ subj sg m-a]
karmāśaya	collection/reservoir of saṃskāra-s stored in the memory of the heart-mind [aḥ subj sg m-a]
dṛṣṭa	seen
adṛṣṭa	unseen
janma	birth
vedanīya	experienced, come to be known [aḥ subj sg m-a]

1. The source of the kleśa-s is the karmāśaya (collection of past impressions resulting from past actions) experienced in seen and unseen births.

सति मूले तद्विपाको जात्यायुर्भोगाः ॥ २.१३ ॥

2.13 sati mūle tadvipāko jātyāyurbhogāḥ

sati mūle tad-vipāko jāti-āyur-bhogāḥ

sat	existence [i "on/upon" sg n-cons]
mūle	root [e "on/upon" pl n-a]
tad	that, of those [pronoun stem]
vipāka	ripening [aḥ subj sg m-a]
kāti	birth class/condition/status; caste
āyur	life span
bhoga	life experience, enjoyment [āḥ subj pl m-a]

1. When the root (karmāśaya) is present, it ripens as our birth class (the familial condition or species one is born into), life span, and life experience.

ते ह्लादपरितापफलाः पुण्यापुण्यहेतुत्वात् ॥ २.१४ ॥

2.14 te hlādaparitāpaphalāḥ puṇyāpuṇyahetutvāt

te hlāda-paritāpa-phalāḥ puṇya-apuṇya-hetutvāt

te	those [pronoun e subj sg m-p]
hlāda	joy, gladness
paritāpa	sorrow
phala	result [āḥ subj pl m-a]
puṇya	virtue
apuṇya	nonvirtue
hetutva	because of [āt "from/due to" sg n-a]

1. Those (birth-class, life span, and life experience) result in joy or sorrow, depending on whether they result in actions that are virtuous (positive/helpful) or nonvirtuous (negative/harmful).

परिणामतापसंस्कारदुःखैर्गुणवृत्तिविरोधाच्च दुःखमेव सर्वं विवेकिनः ॥ २.१५ ॥

2.15 pariṇāmatāpasaṃskāraduḥkhairguṇavṛttivirodhācca duḥkhameva sarvaṃ vivekinaḥ

pariṇāma-tāpa-saṃskāra-duḥkhaiḥ guṇa-vṛtti-virodhāt ca duḥkham eva sarvaṃ vivekinaḥ

pariṇāma	transformation, change, mutation
tāpa	heat
saṃskāra	habitual tendency caused by strong or repeated impressions in memory
duḥkha	pain, suffering, discomfort [aiḥ "by/with" pl n-a]
guṇa	quality of nature
vṛtti	fluctuation or activity in the heart-mind
virodha	conflict, obstruction [āt "from" sg m-a]
ca	and
duḥkha	pain, suffering, discomfort [am subj sg n-a]
eva	just, indeed
sarva	all, everything [am subj sg n-p]
vivekin	one who has discernment [aḥ "of/in" sg m-in]

1. To a person who has discrimination, everything is only duḥkha (painful/uncomfortable) due to the naturally conflicting activities of the guṇa-s (sattva, rajas, and tamas) and through the suffering caused by (unintended) change, craving, or habitual patterns.

हेयं दुःखमनागतम् ॥ २.१६ ॥

2.16 heyaṃ duḥkhamanāgatam

heyaṃ duḥkham anāgatam

heya	avoidable, endable [am subj sg n-a]
duḥkha	suffering, pain, discomfort [am subj sg n-a]
anāgata	"not yet come," future [am subj sg n-a]

1. Future suffering is avoidable.

द्रष्टृदृश्ययोः संयोगो हेयहेतुः ॥ २.१७ ॥

2.17 draṣṭṛdṛśyayoḥ saṃyogo heyahetuḥ

draṣṭṛ-dṛśyayoḥ saṃyogaḥ heyahetuḥ

draṣṭṛ	the seer
dṛśya	the seeable [ayoḥ "of/between" du m-a]
saṃyoga	confusion; mistakenly identifying the seer as the seen [aḥ subj sg m-a]
heya	the endable (duḥkha; see 2.16)
hetu	cause [uḥ subj sg m-u]

1. The cause of what is to be ended (duḥkha) is saṃyoga between the seer and seeable.
2. The false identification of the seer as the seen causes suffering.

प्रकाशक्रियास्थितिशीलं भूतेन्द्रियात्मकं भोगापवर्गार्थं दृश्यम् ॥ २.१८ ॥

2.18 prakāśakriyāsthitiśīlaṃ bhūtendriyātmakaṃ bhogāpavargārthaṃ dṛśyam

prakāśa-kriyā-sthiti-śīlaṃ bhūta-indriya-ātmakaṃ bhoga-apavarga-arthaṃ dṛśyam

prakāśa	light, effulgence
kriyā	action
sthiti	stability, inertia
śīla	property, characteristic [am subj sg n-a]
bhūta	fundamental elements (earth, water, fire, air, space)
indriya	sensory organs
ātmaka	having the nature of, consists of [am subj sg n-a]
bhoga	experience
apavarga	end of association, completion, emancipation
artha	purpose [am subj sg n-a]
dṛśya	seeable [am subj sg n-a]

1. The seeable has the (dual) purpose of experience and emancipation, consists of the elements and sensory organs, and has the qualities of light (sattva-guṇa), activity (rajas-guṇa), and inertia (tamas-guṇa).

विशेषाविशेषलिङ्गमात्रालिङ्गानि गुणपर्वाणि ॥ २.१९ ॥

2.19 viśeṣāviśeṣaliṅgamātrāliṅgāni guṇaparvāṇi

viśeṣa-aviśeṣa-liṅgamātra-aliṅgāni guṇa-parvāṇi

viśeṣa	specific, differentiated
aviśeṣa	nonspecific, undifferentiated
liṅgamātra	primary manifestation
aliṅga	unmanifest [āni subj pl n-a]
guṇa	quality of nature
parvan	stage, phase [āṇi subj pl n-a]

1. The stages of the guṇa-s are specific (five elements, five sense organs, five action organs, and the mind), non-specific (five sense objects, ego, and buddhi), primary matter (mahat), and unmanifest (Prakṛti). (See appendix F, figure 1.)

द्रष्टा दृशिमात्रः शुद्धो ऽपि प्रत्ययानुपश्यः ॥ २.२० ॥

2.20 draṣṭā dṛśimātraḥ śuddho 'pi pratyayānupaśyaḥ

draṣṭā dṛśi-mātraḥ śuddhaḥ api pratyaya-anupaśyaḥ

draṣṭā	seer [ā subj sg m-ṛ]
dṛśi	seeing
mātra	alone [aḥ subj sg m-a]
śuddha	pure [aḥ subj sg m-a]
api	also, even
pratyaya	presented thought; current vṛtti directed toward an object
anupaśya	"watching after" [aḥ subj sg m-a]

1. The seer only sees, and remains pure even when watching thoughts in the buddhi.

तदर्थ एव दृष्यस्यात्मा ॥ २.२१ ॥

2.21 tadartha eva dṛṣyasyātmā

tad-arthaḥ eva dṛṣyasya ātmā

tad	(of) that (draṣṭṛ—the seer, observer) [pronoun stem]
artha	purpose [aḥ subj sg m-a]
eva	only
dṛṣya	the seeable, seen, observed, manifest world [asya "of" sg n-a]
ātmā	nature [ā subj sg m-an]

1. The nature of the seen exists only for the purpose of that (seer).
2. The manifest world exists only so the seer has something to perceive.

कृतार्थं प्रति नष्टमप्यनष्टं तदन्यसाधारणत्वात् ॥ २.२२ ॥

2.22 kṛtārthaṃ prati naṣṭamapyanaṣṭaṃ tadanyasādhāraṇatvāt

kṛta-arthaṃ prati naṣṭam-apyanaṣṭaṃ tad-anya-sādhāraṇatvāt

kṛta	done
artha	purpose, reason [am subj sg n-a]
prati	with regard to
naṣṭa	ended, destroyed, disappeared [am subj sg n-a]
api	also
anaṣṭa	not ended, not destroyed [am subj sg n-a]
tat	it [pronoun subj sg n-p]
anya	other(s)
sādhāraṇatva	commonness [āt "from" sg n-a]

1. For one whose purpose is done (awareness of their inner Puruṣa is present), (the seeable seems to) disappear, even though it does not actually disappear since it is common to others.

स्वस्वामिशक्त्योः स्वरूपोपलब्धिहेतुः संयोगः ॥ २.२३ ॥

2.23 svasvāmiśaktyoḥ svarūpopalabdhihetuḥ saṃyogaḥ

sva-svāmi-śaktyoḥ svarūpa-upalabdhi-hetuḥ saṃyogaḥ

sva	one's own self, what is "owned"
svāmi	master, owner
śakti	power [yoḥ "of/in" du f-i]
sva-śakti	seeable
svāmi-śakti	seer
svarūpa	one's true nature
upalabdhi	acquisition, perception attained, realization
hetu	cause, reason [uḥ subj sg m-u]
saṃyoga	confusion; mistakenly identifying the seer as the seen [aḥ subj sg m-a]

1. Superimposing the powers of the master (seer) and what is owned (seeable) is the reason for realizing the true nature of them both.
2. Confusing what changes (Prakṛti) with what does not change (Puruṣa), thinking they are the same, causes suffering that leads us to inquire as to the true nature of each.

तस्य हेतुरविद्या ॥ २.२४ ॥

2.24 tasya heturavidyā

tasya hetuḥ avidyā

tasya	of that [pronoun "of" sg m-p]
hetu	cause [uḥ subj sg m-u]
avidyā	lack of awareness, ignorance [ā subj sg f-ā]

1. Avidyā is the cause of that (saṃyoga).
2. Lack of awareness causes the erroneous belief that there is no difference between the seer and seen.

तदभावात्संयोगाभावो हानं तद्दृशेः कैवल्यम् ॥ २.२५ ॥

2.25 tadabhāvātsaṃyogābhāvo hānaṃ taddṛśeḥ kaivalyam

Tad-abhāvāt saṃyoga-abhāvaḥ hānaṃ tad dṛśeḥ kaivalyam

tad	that, of that [pronoun stem]
abhāva	absence, disappearance [āt "from/due to" sg m-a]
saṃyoga	confusion; mistakenly identifying the seer as the seen
abhāvaḥ	absence, disappearance [aḥ subj sg m-a]
hānaṃ	end [am subj sg n-a]
tad	that [pronoun subj sg n-p]
dṛśi	seeing [eḥ "of" sg m-i]
kaivalya	final emancipation [am subj sg n-a]

1. From the absence of that (avidyā), the disappearance of saṃyoga, the end. That is kaivalya (aloneness) of seeing.
2. When ignorance goes away, misunderstanding of seer and seen disappears, leading to final liberation.

विवेकख्यातिरविप्लवा हानोपायः ॥ २.२६ ॥

2.26 vivekakhyātiraviplavā hānopāyaḥ

viveka-khyātiḥ aviplavā hāna-upāyaḥ

viveka	discrimination, discernment
khyāti	awareness, realization, understanding, identification [iḥ subj sg f-i]
viveka-khyāti	identification with viveka; integration of viveka f-i
aviplavā	flowing continuously, uninterrupted [ā sg f-a]
hāna	end
upāya	way [aḥ subj sg m-a]

1. Continuous viveka-khyāti is the way to the end (kaivalya).
2. Mindful and continuous discriminating perception is the way to the goal (kaivalya).

तस्य सप्तधा प्रान्तभूमिः प्रज्ञा ॥ २.२७ ॥

2.27 tasya saptadhā prāntabhūmiḥ prajñā

tasya saptadhā prāntabhūmiḥ prajñā

tasya	of that [pronoun "of" subj sg m-p]
saptadhā	sevenfold [ā subj sg f-ā]
prānta	last, final
bhūmi	stage [iḥ subj sg f-i]
prajñā	insight [ā subj sg f-ā]

1. Prajñā (insight) of that (viveka-khyāti) is the final, sevenfold stage.

योगाङ्गानुष्ठानादशुद्धिक्षये ज्ञानदीप्तिराविवेकख्यातेः ॥ २.२८ ॥

2.28 yogāṅgānuṣṭhānādaśuddhikṣaye jñānadīptirāvivekakhyāteḥ

yoga-aṅga-anuṣṭhānāt aśuddhi-kṣaye jñāna-dīptiḥ ā-viveka-khyāteḥ

yoga	process of calming the fluctuations in the heart-mind
aṅga	limb, part
anuṣṭhāna	practicing, executing [āt "from/due to" sg n-a]
aśuddhi	impure
kṣaye	destructions [e "in/on/upon/at" sg m-a]
jñāna	knowledge
dīpti	light [iḥ subj sg f-i]
ā	leading up to
viveka	discernment
khyāti	awareness, realization, understanding, identification [eḥ "from/due to" sg f-i]
viveka-khyāti	identification with viveka; integration of viveka

1. From practicing the (eight) limbs of yoga, when impurities are eliminated, (we experience) the light of knowledge leading to viveka-khyāti.

यमनियमासनप्राणायामप्रत्याहारधारणाध्यानसमाधयो ऽष्टावङ्गानि ॥ २.२९ ॥

2.29 yamaniyamāsanaprāṇāyāmapratyāhāradhāraṇādhyānasamādhayo 'ṣṭāvaṅgāni

yama-niyama-āsana-prāṇāyāma-pratyāhāra-dhāraṇā-dhyāna-samādhayaḥ aṣṭau aṅgāni

yama	social ethics, interactions, "control, restraint"
niyama	personal behavior, "internal yama"
āsana	sitting, posture, physical exercises to purify the body
prāṇāyāma	regulation of breath, breathing exercises to calm the mind
pratyāhāra	a side effect, sensory inputs no longer distract
dhāraṇā	choosing a focus and directing our attention there

dhyāna	focused and uninterrupted attention on a single place
samādhi	complete absorption of the heart-mind in the focus [ayaḥ subj pl m-i]
aṣṭau	eight [irregular subj pl n-p]
aṅga	limb, part [āni subj pl n-a]

1. The eight limbs are yama, niyama, āsana, prāṇāyāma, pratyāhāra, dhāraṇā, dhyāna, and samādhi.
2. The eight parts of yoga are social ethics, personal self-care, physical exercises, breath regulation, focusing attention away from external objects, choosing what to focus on, maintaining the focus, and assimilation of the object of focus.

अहिंसासत्यास्तेयब्रह्मचर्यापरिग्रहा यमाः ॥ २.३० ॥

2.30 ahiṃsāsatyāsteyabrahmacaryāparigrahā yamāḥ

ahiṃsā-satya-asteya-brahmacarya-aparigrahāḥ yamāḥ

ahiṃsā	nonviolence
satya	truthfulness
asteya	nonstealing
brahmacarya	conservation of vital energy; chaste studentship
aparigraha	nonpossessiveness [āḥ subj pl m-a]
yama	social ethics, interactions, "control, restraint" [āḥ subj pl m-a]

1. The yama-s are ahiṃsā, satya, asteya, brahmacarya, and aparigraha.
2. The social ethics are nonviolence, truthfulness, nonstealing, conservation of vital energy, and nonpossessiveness.

जातिदेशकालसमयानवच्छिन्नाः सर्वभौमा महाव्रतम् ॥ २.३१ ॥

2.31 jātideśakālasamayānavacchinnāḥ sarvabhaumā mahāvratam

jāti-deśa-kāla-samaya-anavacchinnāḥ sarvabhaumāḥ mahāvratam

jāti	birth class/condition/status; caste
deśa	place
kāla	time
samaya	circumstance
anavacchinna	not limited [āḥ subj pl m-a]
sarva-bhauma	all realms, all stages [āḥ subj pl m-a]
mahāvratam	great vow, promise to yourself—refers to each yama [am subj sg n-a]

1. A great vow that is universal and not limited by social class, place, time, or circumstance.

शौचसंतोषतपःस्वाध्यायेश्वरप्रणिधानानि नियमाः ॥ २.३२ ॥

2.32 śaucasantoṣatapaḥsvādhyāyeśvarapraṇidhānāni niyamāḥ

śauca-santoṣa-tapas-svādhyāya-īśvarapraṇidhānāni niyamāḥ

śauca	cleanliness, purity, personal hygiene
santoṣa	contentment
tapas	practice causing positive change
svādhyāya	self-study, self-observation, reciting one's mantra
īśvara-praṇidhāna	honoring the divine inner teacher [āni subj pl n-a]
niyama	personal practice or observance [āḥ subj pl m-a]

1. Niyama-s are śauca, santoṣa, tapas, svādhyāya, and īśvara-praṇidhāna.
2. Personal practices are cleanliness, contentment, practice causing positive change, self-study, and letting go.

वितर्कबाधने प्रतिपक्षभावनम् ॥ २.३३ ॥

2.33 vitarkabādhane pratipakṣabhāvanam

vitarka-bādhane pratipakṣa-bhāvanam

vitarka	antiyama, adverse to logic, negative thought or action
bādhana	troubling, disturbing, binding [e "in/upon" sg n-a]
pratipakṣa	"other wing," other side, opposite side
bhāvana	feeling, attitude, disposition; intention; cultivation [am subj sg n-a]

1. When disturbed by negative thoughts or events, cultivation of opposite thoughts or events.
2. When disturbed by an event opposed to the yama-s, we should cultivate an attitude that counteracts that (and act according to the yama-s).

वितर्का हिंसादयः कृतकारितानुमोदिता लोभक्रोधमोहपूर्वका मृदुमध्याधिमात्रा दुःखाज्ञानानन्तफला इति प्रतिपक्षभावनम् ॥ २.३४ ॥

2.34 vitarkā hiṃsādayaḥ kṛtakāritānumoditā lobhakrodhamohapūrvakā mṛdumadhyādhimātrā duḥkhājñānānantaphalā iti pratipakṣabhāvanam

vitarka	something that opposes the yama-s [āḥ subj pl m-a]
hiṃsā	violence
ādi	beginning with [ayaḥ subj pl m-i]
kṛta	done
kārita	caused to be done
anumodita	consented to [āḥ subj pl m-a]
lobha	greed
krodha	anger
moha	delusion

pūrvaka	preceded by [āḥ subj pl m-a]
mṛdu	mild
madhya	medium
adhimātra	excessive [āḥ subj pl m-a]
duḥkha	suffering, pain, discomfort
ajñāna	lack of knowledge
ananta	endless
phala	result [āḥ subj pl m-a]
iti	thus
pratipakṣa	"other wing," other side, opposite side
bhāvana	feeling, attitude, disposition; intention; cultivation [am subj sg n-a]

1. Vitarka-s, hiṃsā, etc., (meaning the opposite of all the yama-s) are done, caused, or consented to, whether mild, moderate, or excessive, are preceded by greed, anger, or delusion, and result in endless suffering and ignorance. Thus (incentive to practice) the opposite attitude.

अहिंसाप्रतिष्ठायां तत्संनिधौ वैरत्यागः ॥ २.३५ ॥

2.35 ahiṃsāpratiṣṭhāyāṃ tatsaṃnidhau vairatyāgaḥ

ahiṃsā-pratiṣṭhāyāṃ tad saṃnidhau vaira-tyāgaḥ

ahiṃsā	nonviolence, nonhurtfulness, kindness, compassion
pratiṣṭhā	being established in [āyām "in/upon" sg f-ā]
tad	(of) that, its [pronoun]
saṃnidhi	vicinity, presence [au "in/upon" sg m-i]
vaira	hostility
tyāga	relinquishing, abandoning [aḥ subj sg m-a]

1. When established in ahiṃsā, hostility is abandoned in its vicinity.
2. In the presence of one practicing nonviolence, hostility cannot exist.

सत्यप्रतिष्ठायां क्रियाफलाश्रयत्वम् ॥ २.३६ ॥

2.36 satyapratiṣṭhāyāṃ kriyāphalāśrayatvam

satya-pratiṣṭhāyāṃ kriyā-phala-āśrayatvam

satya	truthfulness
pratiṣṭhā	being established in [āyām "in/upon" sg f-ā]
kriyā	action
phala	results
āśrayatva	confidence, surity [am subj sg n-a]

1. When established in truthfulness, one can be sure of the results of action.
2. Truthfulness secures confidence in the results of an action.

अस्तेयप्रतिष्ठायां सर्वरत्नोपस्थानम् ॥ २.३७ ॥

2.37 asteyapratiṣṭhāyāṃ sarvaratnopasthānam

asteya-pratiṣṭhāyāṃ sarva-ratna-upasthānam

asteya	nonstealing, not taking
pratiṣṭhā	being established in [āyām "in/upon" sg f-ā]
sarva	all
ratna	jewels, wealth
upasthāna	close proximity [am subj sg n-a]

1. Established in nonstealing, all jewels come close.
2. Prosperity comes when we do not steal.

ब्रह्मचर्यप्रतिष्ठायां वीर्यलाभः ॥ २.३८ ॥

2.38 brahmacaryapratiṣṭhāyāṃ vīryalābhaḥ

brahmacarya-pratiṣṭhāyāṃ vīrya-lābhaḥ

brahmacarya	moving as Brahma, celibacy, conservation of sexual energy
pratiṣṭhā	being established in [āyām "in/upon" sg f-ā]
vīrya	vitality
lābha	obtainment [aḥ subj sg m-a]

1. When established in brahmacarya, vitality is obtained.
2. Vitality is gained when sexual energy is conserved and directed inward.

अपरिग्रहस्थैर्ये जन्मकथंतासंबोधः ॥ २.३९ ॥

2.39 aparigrahasthairye janmakathaṃtāsaṃbodhaḥ

aparigraha-sthairye janma-kathaṃtā-saṃbodhaḥ

aparigraha	nonpossessiveness, not being greedy
sthairya	being firm in [e "in/upon" sg m-a]
janma	birth
kathaṃtā	"how-ness," the reason for, what sort of manner
saṃbodha	complete knowledge [aḥ subj sg m-a]

1. When firm in aparigraha, complete knowledge of the reason one was born.
2. When no longer grasping for things, we discover why we were born.

शौचात्स्वाङ्गजुगुप्सा परैरसंसर्गः ॥ २.४० ॥

2.40 śaucātsvāṅgajugupsā parairasaṃsargaḥ

śaucāt svāṅga-jugupsā paraiḥ asaṃsargaḥ

śauca	cleanliness, purity of body, mind, and surroundings [āt "from/due to" sg m-a]
svāṅga	one's own limbs/body

jugupsā	disgust [ā subj sg f-ā]
para	another [aiḥ "by/with" sg m-p]
asaṃsarga	nonassociation, noncontact [aḥ subj sg m-a]

1. From cleanliness, aversion to our body (and) nonassociation with others.
2. From cleanliness, a disfavor with our body and of contact with other (bodies).

सत्त्वशुद्धिसौमनस्यैकाग्र्येन्द्रियजयात्मदर्शनयोग्यत्वानि च ॥ २.४१ ॥

2.41 sattvaśuddhisaumanasyaikāgryendriyajayātmadarśanayogyatvāni ca

sattva-śuddhi-saumanasya-ekāgrya-indriya-jaya-ātma-darśana-yogyatvāni ca

sattva	guṇa of light, intelligence, purity, goodness, etc.
śuddhi	purity
saumanasya	happy mind
ekāgrya	one-pointedness
indriya	sensory organ
jaya	victory, conquering, mastery
ātma	(inner) self
darśana	seeing, perceiving
yogyatva	fitness, readiness [āni subj pl n-a]
ca	and

1. And (from śauca) arises the purity of sattva, a happy mind, one-pointedness, mastery over the senses, and readiness for seeing the (inner) self.

सन्तोषादनुत्तमः सुखलाभः ॥ २.४२ ॥

2.42 santoṣādanuttamaḥ sukhalābhaḥ

santoṣāt anuttamaḥ sukha-lābhaḥ

santoṣa	contentment [āt "from/due to" sg m-a]
anuttama	unexcelled [aḥ subj sg m-a]
sukha	happiness
lābha	obtainment, attainment [aḥ subj sg m-a]

1. From santoṣa, (we) obtain unexcelled happiness.
2. When we are content with who we are, we become happy.

कायेन्द्रियसिद्धिरशुद्धिक्षयात्तपसः ॥ २.४३ ॥

2.43 kāyendriyasiddhiraśuddhikṣayāttapasaḥ

kāya-indriya-siddhiḥ aśuddhi-kṣayāt tapasaḥ

kāya	body
indriya	sensory organ
siddhi	perfection, power [iḥ subj sg f-i]

aśuddhi	impurity m-a
kṣaya	destruction [āt "from/due to" sg n-a]
tapas	practice causing positive change [aḥ "from/due to" sg n-cons]

1. Perfection of the body and sensory organs is from the destruction of impurities due to tapas.

स्वाध्यायादिष्टदेवतासंप्रयोगः ॥ २.४४ ॥

2.44 svādhyāyādiṣṭadevatāsaṃprayogaḥ

svādhyāyāt iṣṭa-devatā-saṃprayogaḥ

svādhyāya	self-study, self-observation [āt "from/due to" sg m-a]
iṣṭa-devatā	desired deity, something to look up to, strive for
saṃprayoga	communion [aḥ subj sg m-a]

1. From svādhyāya, communion with our desired deity.
2. By observing our self in action, we can connect with our higher truth.

समाधिसिद्धिरीश्वरप्रणिधानात् ॥ २.४५ ॥

2.45 samādhisiddhirīśvarapraṇidhānāt

samādhi-siddhiḥ īśvara-praṇidhānāt

samādhi	complete absorption of the heart-mind in the focus
siddhi	power [iḥ subj sg f-i]
īśvara-praṇidhāna	honoring the divine inner teacher [āt "from/due to" sg n-a]

1. The power of samādhi is due to īśvara-praṇidhāna.
2. Samādhi is experienced from surrendering the results of action to, and deeply respecting, the inner, universal light of knowledge.

स्थिरसुखमासनम् ॥ २.४६ ॥

2.46 sthirasukhamāsanam

sthira-sukham āsanam

sthira	stable, steady, firm, alert
sukha	comfortable, adaptable, relaxed [am subj sg n-a]
āsana	sitting, seat, posture [am subj sg n-a]

1. Āsana (sitting) is (should be) stable and comfortable.
2. Correct posture has a balance of firmness and pliability.

प्रयत्नशैथिल्यानन्तसमापत्तिभ्याम् ॥ २.४७ ॥

2.47 prayatnaśaithilyānantasamāpattibhyām

prayatna-śaithilya-ananta-samāpattibhyām

prayatna	proactive effort

śaithilya	relaxed
ananta	endless, infinite
samāpatti	saturation of the heart-mind with the focus (see samādhi) [ibhyām "from/due to" du f-i]

1. (Āsana becomes stable and comfortable) due to samāpatti on the infinite and relaxed effort.

ततो द्वन्द्वानभिघातः ॥ २.४८ ॥

2.48 tato dvandvānabhighātaḥ

tataḥ dvaṇdva-anabhighātaḥ

tataḥ	from that
dvandva	duality, pairs of opposites
anabhighāta	not distracted or disturbed; invulnerable [aḥ subj sg m-a]

1. From that (āsana), we are not distracted by the pairs of opposites (heat/cold, pleasure/pain, etc.).

तस्मिन्सति श्वासप्रश्वासयोर्गतिविच्छेदः प्राणायामः ॥ २.४९ ॥

2.49 tasminsati śvāsapraśvāsayorgativicchedaḥ prāṇāyāmaḥ

tasmin sati śvāsa-praśvāsayoḥ gati-vicchedaḥ prāṇāyāmaḥ

tasmin	upon that (āsana) [pronoun "on/upon/in" sg n-p]
sat	being present, existing [i "on/upon/in" sg n-c]
śvāsa	inhalation
praśvāsa	exhalation [ayoḥ "of" du m-a]
gati	movement, gait
viccheda	separation, cutting off [aḥ subj sg m-a]
prāṇāyāma	regulation of breath [aḥ subj sg m-a]

1. When that (āsana) is present, prāṇāyāma is breaking the (irregular) movements of inhalation and exhalation.
2. Once the sitting posture is (stable and comfortable), then the regulation of breath is cutting off the movements of inhalation and exhalation (so the breath is still).

बाह्याभ्यन्तरस्तम्भवृत्तिर्देशकालसंख्याभिः परिदृष्टो दीर्घसूक्ष्मः ॥ २.५० ॥

2.50 bāhyābhyantarastambhavṛttirdeśakālasaṃkhyābhiḥ paridṛṣṭo dīrghasūkṣmaḥ

bāhya-abhyantara-stambha-vṛttiḥ deśa-kāla-saṃkhyābhiḥ paridṛṣṭaḥ dīrgha-sūkṣmaḥ

bāhya	external
abhyantara	internal

stambha	suspended
vṛtti	fluctuation or activity in the heart-mind [iḥ subj sg m-i]
deśa	place, location
kāla	time, ratio
saṃkhyā	numbering [ābhiḥ "by/with" pl f-ā]
paridṛṣṭa	observed [aḥ subj sg m-a]
dīrgha	long, protracted
sūkṣma	subtle, smooth [aḥ subj sg m-a]

1. The external, internal, and suspended movements (of the breath), when observed as to location, duration, and number, (can become) long and subtle.

बाह्याभ्यन्तरविषयाक्षेपी चतुर्थः ॥ २.५१ ॥

2.51 bāhyābhyantaraviṣayākṣepī caturthaḥ

bāhya-abhyantara-viṣaya-ākṣepī caturthaḥ

bāhya	external
abhyantara	internal
viṣaya	sensory object
ākṣepin	transcending [ī subj sg m-in]
caturtha	fourth [aḥ subj sg m-a]

1. The fourth (kind of breathing) transcends external and internal objects.

ततः क्षीयते प्रकाशावरणम् ॥ २.५२ ॥

2.52 tataḥ kṣīyate prakāśāvaraṇam

tataḥ kṣīyate prakāśa-āvaraṇam

tataḥ	from that
kṣīyate	it disappears [passive verb 3rd person sg]
prakāśa	light, radiance, sattva
āvaraṇa	covering [am subj sg n-a]

1. From that (stillness of prāṇa), that which covers the light (avidyā) disappears.

धारणासु च योग्यता मनसः ॥ २.५३ ॥

2.53 dhāraṇāsu ca yogyatā manasaḥ

dhāraṇāsu ca yogyatā manasaḥ

dhāraṇā	choosing a focus and directing our attention there [āsu "in/upon" pl f-ā]
ca	and
yogyatā	fitness, readiness [ā subj sg f-ā]
manas	outer mind [aḥ "of" sg n-cons]

1. And readiness of the mind for dhāraṇā.

स्वविषयासंप्रयोगे चित्तस्य स्वरूपानुकार इवेन्द्रियाणां प्रत्याहारः ॥ २.५४ ॥

2.54 svaviṣayāsaṃprayoge cittasya svarūpānukāra ivendriyāṇāṃ pratyāhāraḥ

sva-viṣaya-asaṃprayoge cittasya svarūpa-anukāraḥ iva indriyāṇām pratyāhāraḥ

sva	own
viṣaya	sensory object
asaṃprayoga	not connecting [e "in/upon" sg m-a]
citta	heart-mind field of consciousness [asya "of" sg n-a]
svarūpa	true nature
anukāra	following, imitating [aḥ subj sg m-a]
iva	as if
indriya	sensory organ (see Sāṅkhya) [āṇām "of" pl n-a]
pratyāhāra	exclusion, turning off [aḥ subj sg m-a]

1. Pratyāhāra is when the sensory organs no longer connect with their own objects, as if following the true nature of citta.
2. Turning off sensory inputs is directing the attention inward following the true nature of the heart-mind, thus disconnecting with external objects.

ततः परमा वश्यतेन्द्रियाणाम् ॥ २.५५ ॥

2.55 tataḥ paramā vaśyatendriyāṇām

tataḥ paramā vaśyatā-indriyāṇām

tataḥ	from that
paramā	highest, perfect [ā subj sg f-ā]
vaśyatā	mastery [ā subj sg f-ā]
indriya	sensory organ [āṇām "of" pl n-a]

1. From that, perfect mastery of the sensory organs.

३. विभूतिपादः

VIBHŪTIPĀDAḤ

The Chapter on Extraordinary Abilities

देशबन्धश्चित्तस्य धारणा ॥ ३.१ ॥

3.1 deśabandhaścittasya dhāraṇā

deśa-bandhaḥ cittasya dhāraṇā

deśa	place, point, location
bandha	bound, fixed [aḥ subj sg m-a]
citta	heart-mind field of consciousness [asya "of" sg n-a]
dhāraṇā	establishing a locus [ā subj sg f-ā]

1. Dhāraṇā is the focus of citta at a locus.
2. Dhāraṇā is choosing a focus and directing the attention there.

तत्र प्रत्ययैकतानता ध्यानम् ॥ ३.२ ॥

3.2 tatra pratyayaikatānatā dhyānam

tatra pratyaya-eka-tānatā dhyānam

tatra	there
pratyaya	presented thought; current vṛtti directed toward an object
eka	one, single, uniform
tānatā	continuous flow, extension [ā subj sg f-ā]
dhyāna	focused and uninterrupted attention on a single place [am subj sg n-a]

1. There (in dhāraṇā), dhyāna is the continuous flow (of attention) on a single pratyaya.
2. Once dhāraṇā is in place, then when the heart-mind's focus on one object is uninterrupted, dhyāna occurs.

तदेवार्थमात्रनिर्भासं स्वरूपशून्यमिव समाधिः ॥ ३.३ ॥

3.3 tadevārthamātranirbhāsaṃ svarūpaśūnyamiva samādhiḥ

tat eva artha-mātra-nirbhāsaṃ svarūpa-śūnyam iva samādhiḥ

tat	that [pronoun subj sg n-p]
eva	indeed
artha	purpose

mātra	alone
nirbhāsa	shining forth, apparent [am subj sg n-a]
svarūpa	own form
śūnya	void, empty [am subj sg n-a]
iva	like, as
samādhi	complete absorption of the heart-mind in the focus [iḥ subj sg m-i]

1. That (dhyāna) is samādhi (when) the object alone shines forth (in the citta) as if devoid of its own form.
2. Meditation becomes complete absorption when the object alone is reflected in the heart-mind and subject and object seem the same.

त्रयमेकत्र संयमः ॥ ३.४ ॥

3.4 trayamekatra saṃyamaḥ

trayam ekatra saṃyamaḥ

traya	triad [am subj sg n-a]
ekatra	a single place
saṃyama	turning the attention inward toward a focus [aḥ subj sg m-a]

1. Saṃyama is the (previous) three (focused in) one place.
2. Complete control (of attention) is dhāraṇā, dhyāna, and samādhi directed toward the same place or object.

तज्जयात्प्रज्ञालोकः ॥ ३.५ ॥

3.5 tajjayātprajñālokaḥ

tad-jayāt prajñā-lokaḥ

tad	(of) that [pronoun stem]
jaya	victory, conquest, mastery [āt "from" sg m-a]
prajñā	deep insight
āloka	radiance, splendor [aḥ subj sg m-a]

1. Due to mastery of that (saṃyama), the splendor of deep insight.

तस्य भूमिषु विनियोगः ॥ ३.६ ॥

3.6 tasya bhūmiṣu viniyogaḥ

tasya bhūmiṣu viniyogaḥ

tasya	of that [pronoun "of" sg m-p]
bhūmi	stage, plane, phase [iṣu "on/upon/in" pl f-i]
viniyoga	application [aḥ subj sg m-a]

1. The application of that (saṃyama) occurs in (sequential) stages.

त्रयमन्तरङ्गं पूर्वेभ्यः ॥ ३.७ ॥

3.7 trayamantaraṅgaṃ pūrvebhyaḥ

trayam antar-aṅgaṃ pūrvebhyaḥ

traya	threefold, triad [am subj sg n-a]
antar	inner
aṅga	limb, part [am subj sg n-a]
pūrva	previous [ebhyaḥ "from/than" pl m-p]

1. (This) triad (saṃyama) is an inner limb (relative) to the previous (five limbs).

तदपि बहिरङ्गं निर्बीजस्य ॥ ३.८ ॥

3.8 tadapi bahiraṅgaṃ nirbījasya

tad api bahir-aṅgaṃ nirbījasya

tad	that [pronoun subj sg n-p]
api	also, even
bahir	outer, external
aṅga	limb, part [am subj sg n-a]
nirbīja	without seed (see samādhi) [asya "of" sg m-a]

1. Even that (saṃyama) is an outer limb relative to the seedless (nirbīja-samādhi). (This shows that saṃyama is associated with sabīja-samādhi.)

व्युत्थाननिरोधसंस्कारयोरभिभवप्रादुर्भावौ निरोधक्षणचित्तान्वयो निरोधपरिणामः ॥ ३.९ ॥

3.9 vyutthānanirodhasaṃskārayorabhibhavaprādurbhāvau nirodhakṣaṇacittānvayo nirodhapariṇāmaḥ

vyutthāna-nirodha-saṃskārayoḥ abhibhava-prādur-bhāvau nirodha-kṣaṇa-citta-anvayaḥ nirodha-pariṇāmaḥ

vyutthāna	activity
nirodha	stillness
saṃskāra	strong impression in memory causing a habitual tendency [ayoḥ "of/on/upon" du m-a]
abhibhava	subduing
prādur-bhāva	arising, emergence [au subj du m-a]
nirodha	stillness
kṣaṇa	moment
citta	heart-mind field of consciousness
anvaya	association, connection [aḥ subj sg m-a]
nirodha	stillness
pariṇāma	transformation, change, mutation [aḥ subj sg m-a]

1. When the saṃskāra-s fueling an active heart-mind are subdued, and the saṃskāra-s helping a still mind arise, the association of the heart-mind with the moment of stillness is nirodha-pariṇāma.

तस्य प्रशान्तवाहिता संस्कारात् ॥ ३.१० ॥

3.10 tasya praśāntavāhitā saṃskārāt

tasya praśānta-vāhitā saṃskārāt

tasya	of that [pronoun "of" sg m-p]
praśānta	tranquil, calm
vāhitā	flow [ā subj sg f-ā]
saṃskāra	strong impression in memory causing a habitual tendency [āt "from" sg m-a]

1. The tranquil flow of that (heart-mind in stillness) is from the saṃskāra (of nirodha).

सर्वार्थतैकाग्रतयोः क्षयोदयौ चित्तस्य समाधिपरिणामः ॥ ३.११ ॥

3.11 sarvārthataikāgratayoḥ kṣayodayau cittasya samādhipariṇāmaḥ

sarva-arthatā-ekāgratayoḥ kṣaya-udayau cittasya samādhi-pariṇāmaḥ

sarva	all
arthatā	objectness
ekāgratā	one-pointedness [ayoḥ "of/in" du f-ā]
kṣaya	destruction, disappearance
udaya	arising, emergence [au subj du m-a]
citta	heart-mind field of consciousness [asya "of" sg n-a]
samādhi	complete absorption of the heart-mind in the focus
pariṇāma	transformation, change, mutation [aḥ subj sg m-a]

1. The elimination of (attention toward) all objects (and) the emergence of one-pointedness are the transformation into samādhi of the heart-mind.
2. As attention toward all objects decreases and a one-pointed state of mind arises, the transformation into samādhi takes place.

ततः पुनः शान्तोदितौ तुल्यप्रत्ययौ चित्तस्यैकाग्रतापरिणामः ॥ ३.१२ ॥

3.12 tataḥ punaḥ śāntoditau tulyapratyayau cittasyaikāgratāpariṇāmaḥ

tataḥ punar śānta-uditau tulya-pratyayau cittasya ekāgratā-pariṇāmaḥ

tataḥ	from that
punar	again
śānta	quieted, calmed, receded
udita	arisen [au subj du m-a]
tulya	same

pratyaya presented thought; current vṛtti directed toward an object [au subj du m-a]
citta heart-mind field of consciousness [asya "of" sg m-a]
ekāgratā one-pointedness
pariṇāma transformation, change, mutation [aḥ subj sg m-a]

1. From that again, when the quieted and the arising pratyaya-s are the same, the transformation into a one-pointed heart-mind occurs.
2. When the past pratyaya-s are the same as the present pratyaya-s, the transformation into a one-pointed heart-mind occurs.

एतेन भूतेन्द्रियेषु धर्मलक्षणावस्थापरिणामा व्याख्याताः ॥ ३.१३ ॥

3.13 etena bhūtendriyeṣu dharmalakṣaṇāvasthāpariṇāmā vyākhyātāḥ

etena bhūta-indriyeṣu dharma-lakṣaṇa-avasthā-pariṇāmāḥ vyākhyātāḥ

etena by this [pronoun "by/with" sg n-p]
bhūta fundamental element (earth, water, fire, air, and space)
indriya sensory organ [eṣu "on/upon/in" pl n-a]
dharma characteristic form
lakṣaṇa temporal characteristic, feature, marker; changes over time
avasthā state at any moment; current situation or condition
pariṇāma transformation, change, mutation [āḥ subj pl m-a]
vyākhyāta explained [āḥ subj pl m-a]

1. By this are explained the transformations of dharma, lakṣaṇa, and avasthā in the sensory organs and gross elements.
2. This explains the changes taking place in gross matter (sensory organs and elements) in terms of characteristic form, time, and outward condition of the form.

शान्तोदिताव्यपदेश्यधर्मानुपाती धर्मी ॥ ३.१४ ॥

3.14 śāntoditāvyapadeśyadharmānupātī dharmī

śānta-udita-avyapadeśya-dharma-anupātī dharmī

śānta quieted, calmed; *past*
udita arisen; *present*
avyapadeśya dormant, not manifested yet; potential, *future*
dharma characteristic form
anupātin follows [ī subj sg m-in]
dharmin substratum [ī subj sg m-in]

1. That which follows (continues unchanged) through past, present, and future characteristic forms is the substratum.

2. The substratum remains the same no matter what different forms it takes over time.

क्रमान्यत्वं परिणामान्यत्वे हेतुः ॥ ३.१५ ॥

3.15 kramānyatvaṃ pariṇāmānyatve hetuḥ

krama-anyatvaṃ pariṇāma-anyatve hetuḥ

krama	sequence
anyatva	separateness, otherness [am subj sg n-a]
pariṇāma	transformation, change, mutation
anyatva	separateness, otherness [e "on/upon/in" sg n-a]
hetu	cause [uḥ subj sg m-u]

1. The difference in sequence is the reason for the difference in transformations.
2. Changes occur parallel to the sequential progression over time.

परिणामत्रयसंयमादतीतानागतज्ञानम् ॥ ३.१६ ॥

3.16 pariṇāmatrayasaṃyamādatītānāgatajñānam

pariṇāma-traya-saṃyamāt atītānāgata-jñānam

pariṇāma	transformation, change, mutation
traya	threefold, triad
saṃyama	turning the attention inward toward a focus [āt "from" sg m-a]
atīta	past, "gone"
anāgata	future, "not come"
jñāna	knowledge [am subj sg n-a]

1. From saṃyama on the three transformations (see 3.13), knowledge of past and future.

शब्दार्थप्रत्ययानामितरेतराध्यासात्सङ्करस्तत्प्रविभागसंयमात्सर्वभूतरुतज्ञानम् ॥ ३.१७ ॥

3.17 śabdārthapratyayānāmitaretarādhyāsātsaṅkarastatpravibhāga-saṃyamātsarvabhūtarutajñānam

śabda-artha-pratyayānām itara-itara-adhyāsāt saṅkaraḥ tat-pravibhāga-saṃyamāt sarva-bhūta-ruta-jñānam

śabda	word, sound
artha	meaning, purpose, object
pratyaya	idea; presented thought; current vṛtti directed toward an object [ānām "of" pl m-a]
itara-itara	one upon the other, overlapping
adhyāsa	false attribution, wrong assumption [āt "from" sg m-a]

saṇkara	mixing up, confusing [aḥ subj sg m-a]
tat	(of) those [pronoun stem]
pravibhāga	difference, distinction
saṃyama	turning the attention inward toward a focus [āt "from" sg m-a]
sarva	all
bhūta	being
ruta	sound, language
jñāna	knowledge [am subj sg n-a]

1. The confusion of words, objects, and ideas is from wrongly overlapping one upon the other. From saṃyama on the distinction among those, knowledge of the language of all beings.
2. Our perception of an object is based on a word or label, what we think it means, and our ideas about it.

संस्कारसाक्षात्करणात्पूर्वजातिज्ञानम् ॥ ३.१८ ॥

3.18 saṃskārasākṣātkaraṇātpūrvajātijñānam

saṃskāra-sākṣāt karaṇāt pūrva-jāti-jñānam

saṃskāra	strong impression in memory causing a habitual tendency
sākṣāt	direct [āt "from" sg m-a]
karaṇa	doing, perception [āt "from" sg n-a]
pūrva	previous
jāti	birth class/condition/status; caste
jñāna	knowledge [am subj sg n-a]

1. From direct perception of past impressions (saṃskāra-s), knowledge of previous births.

प्रत्ययस्य परचित्तज्ञानम् ॥ ३.१९ ॥

3.19 pratyayasya paracittajñānam

pratyayasya para-citta-jñānam

pratyaya	presented thought; current vṛtti directed toward an object [asya "of" sg m-a]
para	another
citta	heart-mind field of consciousness
jñāna	knowledge [am subj sg n-a]

1. From direct perception of a current thought (pratyaya), knowledge of another's heart-mind.

न च तत्सालम्बनं तस्याविषयीभूतत्वात् ॥ ३.२० ॥

3.20 na ca tatsālambanaṃ tasyāviṣayībhūtatvāt*

na ca tat sālambanaṃ tasya aviṣayī-bhūtatvāt

na	not
ca	and
tat	that [pronoun stem]
sālambana	with support [am subj sg n-a]
tasya	of that [pronoun "of" sg n-p]
aviṣayī	has no object, without an object
bhūtatva	existence, nature of being [āt "from" sg n-a]

1. And the supporting object of that (thought of another) is not (known because of) its (citta's) nature of being without an object.
2. The supporting object of that thought (of another) is not known because it was not the object of concentration. The knowledge of another's heart-mind does not extend to the object (of another's heart-mind) itself.

*3.20 is absent in some versions

कायरूपसंयमात्तद्ग्राह्यशक्तिस्तम्भे चक्षुःप्रकाशासंप्रयोगे ऽन्तर्धानम् ॥ ३.२१ ॥

3.21 kāyarūpasaṃyamāttadgrāhyaśaktistambhe cakṣuḥprakāśāsaṃprayoge 'ntardhānam*

kāya-rūpa-saṃyamāt tad-grāhya-śakti-stambhe cakṣus-prakāśā-asaṃprayoge antar-dhānam

kāya	body
rūpa	form
saṃyama	turning the attention inward toward a focus [āt "from" sg m-a]
tad	(of) that, its [pronoun stem]
grāhya	graspable, seeable
śakti	power
stambha	suspension, stopping [e "on/upon/in" sg m-a]
cakṣus	eye
prakāśa	light
asaṃprayoga	disconnecting, disengaging, break [e "on/upon/in" sg m-a]
antar	inner
dhāna	placing [am subj sg n-a]
antar-dhanam	"invisibility"

1. From saṃyama on the form of the body, when its ability to be seen is suspended (and) light is cut off from the eyes, invisibility.
2. From saṃyama on the form of the body, invisibility.

* 3.21.5—etena sabdādyantardhānamuktam—is added in some versions after 3.21.

सोपक्रमं निरुपक्रमं च कर्म तत्संयमादपरान्तज्ञानमरिष्टेभ्यो वा ॥ ३.२२ ॥

3.22 sopakramaṃ nirupakramaṃ ca karma tatsaṃyamādaparāntajñānamariṣṭebhyo vā

sopakramaṃ nirupakramaṃ ca karma tat-saṃyamāt aparānta-jñānam ariṣṭebhyaḥ vā

sopakrama	with momentum, already started, fast [am subj sg n-a]
nirupakrama	without momentum, not started yet, slow [am subj sg n-a]
ca	and
karma	action [a subj sg n-an]
tad	(upon) that [pronoun stem]
saṃyama	turning the attention inward toward a focus [āt "from" sg m-a]
aparānta	death, "other end"
jñāna	knowledge [am subj sg n-a]
ariṣṭa	sign, omen, clue [ebhyaḥ "from" pl m-a]
vā	or

1. Karma either has momentum or does not. From saṃyama on that, or by omens, knowledge of time of death.
2. From saṃyama on how fast karma bears fruit, or by omens, knowledge of time of death.

मैत्र्यादिषु बलानि ॥ ३.२३ ॥

3.23 maitryādiṣu balāni

maitrī-ādiṣu balāni

maitrī	friendship
ādi	beginning with [iṣu "on/upon/in" pl m-i]
bala	strength [āni subj pl n-a]

1. (From saṃyama) on friendship, etc., (see 1.33), strengths.

बलेषु हस्तिबलादीनि ॥ ३.२४ ॥

3.24 baleṣu hastibalādīni

baleṣu hasti-bala-ādīni

bala	strength [eṣu "on/upon/in" pl n-a]
hasti	elephant
bala	strength
ādi	beginning with [īni subj pl n-i]

1. (From saṃyama) on strengths (3.23), the strengths, etc., of an elephant. Because it says "strengths, etc." we can assume other characteristics like endurance and power.

प्रवृत्त्यालोकन्यासात्सूक्ष्मव्यवहितविप्रकृष्टज्ञानम् ॥ ३.२५ ॥

3.25 pravṛttyālokanyāsātsūkṣmavyavahitaviprakṛṣṭajñānam

pravṛtti-āloka-nyāsāt sūkṣma-vyavahita-viprakṛṣṭa-jñānam

pravṛtti	activity of refined sensory perception
āloka	radiance, light
nyāsa	projection [āt "from" sg m-a]
sūkṣma	subtle
vyavahita	hidden, concealed, obscure
viprakṛṣṭa	distant, remote
jñāna	knowledge [am subj sg n-a]

1. By projecting the light of pravṛtti (1.36), knowledge of objects subtle, hidden, or distant.

भुवनज्ञानं सूर्ये संयमात् ॥ ३.२६ ॥

3.26 bhuvanajñānaṃ sūrye saṃyamāt

bhuvana-jñānaṃ sūrye saṃyamāt

bhuvana	realms, planes, worlds
jñāna	knowledge [am subj sg n-a]
sūrya	sun [e "on/upon/in" sg m-a]
saṃyama	turning the attention inward toward a focus [āt "from" sg m-a]

1. From saṃyama on the sun, knowledge of all realms.

चन्द्रे ताराव्यूहज्ञानम् ॥ ३.२७ ॥

3.27 candre tārāvyūhajñānam

candre tārā-vyūha-jñānam

candra	moon [e "on/upon/in" sg m-a]
tārā	star
vyūha	organization
jñāna	knowledge [am subj sg n-a]

1. (From saṃyama) on the moon, knowledge of organization of the stars.

ध्रुवे तद्गतिज्ञानम् ॥ ३.२८ ॥

3.28 dhruve tadgatijñānam

dhruve tad-gati-jñānam

dhruva	pole star [e "on/upon/in" sg m-a]
tad	(of) them, their [pronoun stem]
gati	motion, gait
jñāna	knowledge [am subj sg n-a]

1. (From saṃyama) on the pole star, knowledge of the motion (of other stars).

नाभिचक्रे कायव्यूहज्ञानम् ॥ ३.२९ ॥

3.29 nābhicakre kāyavyūhajñānam

nābhi-cakre kāya-vyūha-jñānam

nābhi	navel area
cakra	energy center [e "on/upon/in" sg n-a]
kāya	body
vyūha	organization
jñāna	knowledge [am subj sg n-a]

1. (From saṃyama) on the navel cakra, knowledge of organization of the body.

कण्ठकूपे क्षुत्पिपासानिवृत्तिः ॥ ३.३० ॥

3.30 kaṇṭhakūpe kṣutpipāsānivṛttiḥ

kaṇṭha-kūpe kṣut-pipāsā-nivṛttiḥ

kaṇṭha	throat
kūpa	a hollow, pit, well [e "on/upon/in" sg m-a]
kṣut	hunger
pipāsā	thirst
nivṛtti	ending, alleviating [iḥ subj sg f-i]

1. (From saṃyama) on the hollow in the throat, ending of hunger and thirst.

कूर्मनाड्यां स्थैर्यम् ॥ ३.३१ ॥

3.31 kūrmanāḍyāṃ sthairyam

kūrma-nāḍyāṃ sthairyam

kūrma	tortoise
nāḍī	energy channel [yām "on/upon/in" sg f-ī]
sthairya	steadiness [am subj sg n-a]

1. (From saṃyama) on the tortoise energy channel, steadiness.

मूर्धज्योतिषि सिद्धदर्शनम् ॥ ३.३२ ॥

3.32 mūrdhajyotiṣi siddhadarśanam

mūrdha-jyotiṣi siddha-darśanam

mūrdha	crown of the head
jyotis	light [i "on/upon/in" sg n-is]
siddha	power, accomplishment, perfected
darśana	seeing [am subj sg n-a]

1. (From saṃyama) on the light at top of head, vision of a perfected being.

प्रातिभाद्वा सर्वम् ॥ ३.३३ ॥

3.33 prātibhādvā sarvam

prātibhāt vā sarvam

prātibha	intuitive flash of brilliance [āt "from" sg m-a]
vā	or
sarva	all [am subj sg n-p]

1. Or from an intuitive flash, all (knowledge).

हृदये चित्तसंवित् ॥ ३.३४ ॥

3.34 hṛdaye cittasaṃvit

hṛdaye citta-saṃvit

hṛdaya	heart [e "on/upon/in" sg n-a]
citta	heart-mind field of consciousness
saṃvit	complete knowledge [subj sg f-cons]

1. (From saṃyama) on the heart, complete knowledge of the heart-mind.

सत्त्वपुरुषयोरत्यन्तासंकीर्णयोः
प्रत्ययाविशेषो भोगः परार्थत्वात्स्वार्थसंयमात्पुरुषज्ञानम् ॥ ३.३५ ॥

3.35 sattvapuruṣayoratyantāsaṃkīrṇayoḥ pratyayāviśeṣo bhogaḥ parārthatvātsvārthasaṃyamātpuruṣajñānam

sattva-puruṣayoḥ atyantā-saṃkīrṇayoḥ pratyaya-aviśeṣaḥ bhogaḥ para-arthatvāt sva-artha-saṃyamāt puruṣa-jñānam

sattva	guṇa of light, intelligence, purity, goodness, etc.
puruṣa	the inner light of awareness, the observer [ayoḥ "of" du m-a]
atyanta	absolutely
asaṃkīrṇa	distinct, "not mixed together" [ayoḥ "of" du m-a]
pratyaya	presented thought; current vṛtti directed toward an object
aviśeṣa	not distinguishing [aḥ subj sg m-a]
bhoga	experience (of pleasure or pain) [aḥ subj sg m-a]
para	other
arthatva	purposefulness, meaningfulness [āt "from" sg m-a]
svārtha	"own-purpose"
saṃyama	turning the attention inward toward a focus [āt "from" sg m-a]
puruṣa	the inner light of awareness, the observer
jñāna	knowledge [am subj sg n-a]

1. Experience is a pratyaya that does not distinguish between sattva (a sattvic buddhi) and Puruṣa, (which are) absolutely distinct. From saṃyama on that which has its own purpose (Puruṣa), as opposed to that whose purpose is for another (sattva), knowlege of Puruṣa.

2. Understanding Puruṣa, the inner Self, requires understanding the difference between a heart-mind that is sattvic (yet still changeable) and the Puruṣa, which never changes. The Puruṣa needs nothing, but Prakṛti cannot exist without Puruṣa. Remember that Prakṛti's purpose is to provide something for Puruṣa to witness.

ततः प्रातिभश्रावणवेदनादर्शास्वादवार्त्ता जायन्ते ॥ ३.३६ ॥

3.36 tataḥ prātibhaśrāvaṇavedanādarśāsvādavārttā jāyante

tataḥ prātibha-śrāvaṇa-vedana-ādarśa-āsvāda-vārttāḥ jāyante

tataḥ	from that
prātibha	intuitive flash of brilliance
śrāvaṇa	suprasensory hearing
vedana	suprasensory touch
ādarśa	suprasensory sight
āsvāda	suprasensory taste
vārtta	suprasensory smell [āḥ subj pl f-ā]
jāyante	are born [verb 3rd person pl verb-atm]

1. From that (knowledge of Puruṣa—3.35), flash of illumination and suprasensory hearing, touch, sight, taste, and smell.

ते समाधावुपसर्गा व्युत्थाने सिद्धयः ॥ ३.३७ ॥

3.37 te samādhāvupasargā vyutthāne siddhayaḥ

te samādhau upasargāḥ vyutthāne siddhayaḥ

te	those [pronoun subj pl m-p]
samādhi	complete absorption of the heart-mind in the focus [au "in reference to" sg m-i]
upasarga	obstacle [āḥ subj pl m-a]
vyutthāna	outward, active, externalized (lower) state of mind [e "on/upon/in" sg n-a]
siddhi	power, accomplishment [ayaḥ subj pl f-i]

1. These are obstacles to samādhi (though) accomplishments to a very active state of mind.

बन्धकारणशैथिल्यात्प्रचारसंवेदनाच्च चित्तस्य परशरीरावेशः ॥ ३.३८ ॥

3.38 bandhakāraṇaśaithilyātpracārasaṃvedanācca cittasya paraśarīrāveśaḥ

bandha-kāraṇa-śaithilyāt pracāra-saṃvedanāt ca cittasya para-śarīra-āveśaḥ

bandha	bondage
kāraṇa	cause

śaithilya	relaxation [āt "from/due to" sg m-a]
pracāra	circulation, flow
saṃvedana	complete experience/feeling/knowledge [āt "from/due to" sg n-a]
ca	and
citta	heart-mind field of consciousness [asya "of" sg m-a]
para	another
śarīra	body
āveśa	entry into, possession [aḥ subj sg m-a]

1. From loosening the cause of bondage (to the body) and experiencing (how the energy) of the heart-mind circulates, entry into (possession of) another body.

उदानजयाज्जलपङ्ककण्टकादिष्वसङ्ग उत्क्रान्तिश्च ॥ ३.३९ ॥

3.39 udānajayājjalapaṅkakaṇṭakādiṣvasaṅga utkrāntiśca

udāna-jayāt jala-paṅka-kaṇṭaka-ādiṣu asaṅgaḥ utkrāntiḥ ca

udāna	upward moving energy
jaya	victory, conquest [āt "from/due to" sg m-a]
jala	water
paṅka	mud
kaṇṭaka	thorn(s)
ādi	etc. [iṣu "on/upon/in" pl n-i]
asaṅga	noncontact, not getting attached to/stuck in
utkrānti	ascent, rising above, levitation, ability to die at will [iḥ subj sg f-i]
ca	and

1. From mastery of udāna (upward-moving energy in the body), not getting stuck in water, mud, thorns, etc., and the ability to die at will.

समानजयाज्ज्वलनम् ॥ ३.४० ॥

3.40 samānajayājjvalanam

samāna-jayāt jvalanam

samāna	energy of homeostasis in the body, "equalizing air"
jaya	victory, conquest [āt "from/due to" sg m-a]
jvalana	radiance [am subj sg n-a]

1. From mastery of samāna (energy that maintains equilibrium in the body), radiance.

श्रोत्राकाशयोः संबन्धसंयमाद्दिव्यं श्रोत्रम् ॥ ३.४१ ॥

3.41 śrotrākāśayoḥ saṃbandhasaṃyamāddivyaṃ śrotram

śrotra-ākāśayoḥ saṃbandha-saṃyamāt divyaṃ śrotram

śrotra	hearing
ākāśa	space [ayoḥ "on/upon/in" du m-a]
saṃbandha	relationship
saṃyama	turning the attention inward toward a focus [āt "from/due to" sg m-a]
divya	divine [am subj sg n-a]
śrotram	hearing [am subj sg n-a]

1. From saṃyama on the relationship between hearing and space, divine hearing.

कायाकाशयोः संबन्धसंयमाल्लघुतूलसमापत्तेश्चाकाशगमनम् ॥ ३.४२ ॥

3.42 kāyākāsayoḥ saṃbandhasaṃyamāllaghutūlasamāpatteś cākāśagamanam

kāya-ākāsayoḥ saṃbandha-saṃyamāt laghu-tūla-samāpatteḥ ca ākāśa-gamanam

kāya	body
ākāśa	space [ayoḥ "on/upon/in" du m-a]
saṃbandha	relationship
saṃyama	turning the attention inward toward a focus [āt "from/due to" sg m-a]
laghu	lightweight
tūla	cotton
samāpatti	saturation of the heart-mind with the focus (see samādhi) [eḥ "from/due to" sg f-i]
ca	and
ākāśa	space
gamana	going, moving [am subj sg n-a]

1. From saṃyama on the relationship between body and space, and samāpatti with lightweight cotton, travel through space.
2. By completely focusing on the relationship between the physical body and space, and visualizing ourself as light as cotton, we defy gravity and are able to travel through space.

बहिरकल्पिता वृत्तिर्महाविदेहा ततः प्रकाशावरणक्षयः ॥ ३.४३ ॥

3.43 bahirakalpitā vṛttirmahāvidehā tataḥ prakāśāvaraṇakṣayaḥ

bahir akalpitā vṛttiḥ mahā-videhā tataḥ prakāsa-́āvaraṇa-kṣayaḥ

bahis	external, outer
akalpitā	real, unimagined [ā subj sg f-ā]
vṛtti	fluctuation or activity in the heart-mind [iḥ subj sg f-i]
mahā	great, large
videhā	out-of-body state [ā subj sg f-ā]
tataḥ	from that [aḥ "from" sg m-cons]
prakāśa	light (of knowledge/Puruṣa)
āvaraṇa	covering
kṣaya	destruction, removal [aḥ subj sg m-a]

1. Mahā-videha is a vṛtti. From saṃyama on mahāvideha, removing the covering of light (avidyā).
2. From saṃyama on the great out-of-body state, which is a real, external vṛtti, avidyā (the covering over light) is removed.

स्थूलस्वरूपसूक्ष्मान्वयार्थवत्त्वसंयमाद्भूतजयः ॥ ३.४४ ॥

3.44 sthūlasvarūpasūkṣmānvayārthavattvasaṃyamādbhūtajayaḥ

sthūla-svarūpa-sūkṣma-anvaya-arthavattva-saṃyamāt bhūta-jayaḥ

sthūla	gross, coarse, dense
svarūpa	"own form," essential nature
sūkṣma	subtle
anvaya	relationship, guṇa composition
arthavattva	sense of purpose
saṃyama	turning the attention inward toward a focus [āt "from" sg m-a]
bhūta	fundamental element (earth, water, fire, air, and space)
jaya	victory, conquest [aḥ subj sg m-a]

1. From saṃyama on (all five elements') gross form, essential nature, subtle form (tanmātra), guṇa composition, and purposefulness, mastery of the (five) elements.

ततो ऽणिमादिप्रादुर्भावः कायसंपत्तद्धर्मानभिघातश्च ॥ ३.४५ ॥

3.45 tato 'ṇimādiprādurbhāvaḥ kāyasaṃpattaddharmānabhighātaśca

tataḥ aṇima-ādi-prādur-bhāvaḥ kāya-saṃpat tad-dharma-anabhighātaḥ ca

tataḥ	from that [aḥ "from" sg m-cons]
aṇima	power to become tiny
ādi	etc.
prādurbhāva	arising, emergence; attainment [aḥ subj sg m-a]
kāya	body
saṃpat	perfection [subj sg f-c]
tad	(of) that, its [pronoun stem]

dharma	constituents, functions
anabhighāta	not distracted or disturbed; unaffected; invulnerable [aḥ subj sg m-a]
ca	and

1. From that (mastery of the five elements—3.44), attainment of the power to become small, etc., perfection of the body (so that) its functions are unaffected (by anything).
2. Mastery over the five elements develops many extraordinary powers including the ability to become small, and also perfects the body so it becomes resistant to external forces.

रूपलावण्यबलवज्रसंहननत्वानि कायसंपत् ॥ ३.४६ ॥

3.46 rūpalāvaṇyabalavajrasaṃhananatvāni kāyasaṃpat

rūpa-lāvaṇya-bala-vajra-saṃhananatvāni kāya-saṃpat

rūpa	form
lāvaṇya	gracefulness
bala	strength
vajra	diamond, thunderbolt
saṃhananatva	firmness [āni subj pl n-a]
kāya	body
saṃpat	perfection [subj sg f-cons]

1. Perfection of the body consists of beauty, gracefulness, strength, and diamondlike firmness.

ग्रहणस्वरूपास्मितान्वयार्थवत्त्वसंयमादिन्द्रियजयः ॥ ३.४७ ॥

3.47 grahaṇasvarūpāsmitānvayārthavattvasaṃyamādindriyajayaḥ

grahaṇa-svarūpa-asmitā-anvaya-arthavattva-saṃyamāt indriya-jayaḥ

grahaṇa	grasping, perceiving
svarūpa	"own form," true nature
asmitā	ego
anvaya	relationship, guṇa composition
arthavattva	sense of purpose
saṃyama	turning the attention inward toward a focus [āt "from" sg m-a]
indriya	sensory organ
jaya	victory, conquest, mastery [aḥ subj sg m-a]

1. From saṃyama on (all five sensory organs') process of perception, essential nature, individuality, guṇa composition, and purposefulness, mastery of the sensory organs.

ततो मनोजवित्वं विकरणभावः प्रधानजयश्च ॥ ३.४८ ॥

3.48 tato manojavitvaṃ vikaraṇabhāvaḥ pradhānajayaśca

tataḥ manas-javitvaṃ vikaraṇa-bhāvaḥ pradhāna-jayaḥ ca

tataḥ	from that
manas	outer mind
javitva	swiftness, speed [am subj sg n-a]
vikaraṇa	independent of instruments (sensory organs)
bhāva	state, feeling [aḥ subj sg m-a]
pradhāna	Prakṛti, the phenomenal world
jaya	victory, conquest, mastery [aḥ subj sg m-a]
ca	and

1. From that, quickness of the mind, a state independent of sensory organs, and mastery over Prakṛti.
2. Free from the burden of the sensory organs, the senses move as quickly as thought in the mind, thereby gaining mastery over the phenomenal world.

सत्त्वपुरुषान्यताख्यातिमात्रस्य सर्वभावाधिष्ठातृत्वं सर्वज्ञातृत्वं च ॥ ३.४९ ॥

3.49 sattvapuruṣānyatākhyātimātrasya sarvabhāvādhiṣṭhātṛtvaṃ sarvajñātṛtvaṃ ca

sattva-puruṣa-anyatā-khyāti-mātrasya sarva-bhāva-adhiṣṭhātṛtvaṃ sarva-jñātṛtvaṃ ca

sattva	guṇa of light, intelligence, purity, goodness, etc.
puruṣa	the inner light of awareness, the observer
anyatā	distinction, separateness
khyāti	awareness, realization, understanding, identification
mātra	only, just [asya "of" sg n-a]
sarva	all
bhāva	state
adhiṣṭhātṛtva	supremacy [am subj sg n-a]
sarva	all
jñātṛtva	understandability [am subj sg n-a]
sarva-jñātṛtva	having complete knowledge of the heart-mind
ca	and

1. One who just identifies the distinction between Puruṣa and sattva, (attains) supremacy over all states and full knowledge of the heart-mind.
2. When we can understand the difference between the pure, inner awareness and a sattvic heart-mind, then all states of existence are understood and surmounted.

तद्वैराग्यादपि दोषबीजक्षये कैवल्यम् ॥ ३.५० ॥

3.50 tadvairāgyādapi doṣabījakṣaye kaivalyam

tad-vairāgyāt api doṣa-bīja-kṣaye kaivalyam

tad	(of) that [pronoun stem]
vairāgya	unattached awareness, noninvolvement, noninterference [āt "from/due to" sg n-a]
api	also, even
doṣa	defective, detrimental
bīja	seed
kṣaya	destruction, removal [e "on/upon/in" sg m-a]
kaivalya	final emancipation [am subj sg n-a]

1. Due to vairāgya of even that (3.49), upon the destruction of the detrimental seeds (kleśa-s), kaivalya.
2. When we are not attached even to understanding the phenomenal world completely, then the kleśa-seeds die out, leaving us to experience the oneness of kaivalya, liberation.

स्थान्युपनिमन्त्रणे सङ्गस्मयाकरणं पुनरनिष्टप्रसङ्गात् ॥ ३.५१ ॥

3.51 sthānyupanimantraṇe saṅgasmayākaraṇaṃ punaraniṣṭaprasaṅgāt

sthāni-upanimantraṇe saṅga-smaya-akaraṇaṃ punar-aniṣṭa-prasaṅgāt

sthānin	elevated being, astral energy
upanimantraṇa	invitation, admiration, beckoning, temptation [e "on/upon/in" sg n-a]
saṅga	attachment, contact, allured
smaya	pride, flattery, smiling proudly
akaraṇa	no cause [am subj sg n-a]
punar	again, renewal
aniṣṭa	not desired
prasaṅga	possibility of attachment, opportunity [āt "from/due to" sg m-a]

1. Upon admiration by higher beings there (should be) no reason for pride or allurement due to the possibility of reattachment again to the undesirable.
2. When a heart-mind has reached this high state of consciousness, astral energies may approach and attempt to sway the heart-mind away from its focus. This is the time to maintain focus and ignore those distractions.

क्षणतत्क्रमयोः संयमाद्विवेकजं ज्ञानम् ॥ ३.५२ ॥

3.52 kṣaṇatatkramayoḥ saṃyamādvivekajaṃ jñānam

kṣaṇa-tad-kramayoḥ saṃyamāt vivekajaṃ jñānam

kṣaṇa	moment
tad	(of) that, its [pronoun stem]
krama	sequence [ayoḥ "of/on/upon/in" du m-a]
saṃyama	turning the attention inward toward a focus [āt "from" sg m-a]
vivekaja	born of discernment [am subj sg n-a]
jñāna	knowledge [am subj sg n-a]

1. Due to saṃyama on a moment and its sequence, knowledge born of discernment.
2. When the heart-mind is focused completely on the present moment and where it stands in the ongoing succession of moments called time, then knowledge from discernment arises.

जातिलक्षणदेशैरन्यतानवच्छेदात्तुल्ययोस्ततः प्रतिपत्तिः ॥ ३.५३ ॥

3.53 jātilakṣaṇadeśairanyatānavacchedāttulyayostataḥ pratipattiḥ

jāti-lakṣaṇa-deśaiḥ anyatā-anavacchedāt tulyayoḥ tataḥ pratipattiḥ

jāti	birth class/condition/status; caste; species, category of object
lakṣaṇa	temporal characteristic, feature, marker
deśa	place, location, position in space [aiḥ "by/with" pl m-a]
anyatā	distinction, separateness, otherwise
anavaccheda	not limited, indistinguishable [āt "from/due to" sg m-a]
tulya	identical, similar, like [ayoḥ "of" du m-a]
tataḥ	from that
pratipatti	ascertainment, ability to perceive [iḥ subj sg f-i]

1. From that (3.52), the ability to perceive (a difference) between two seemingly identical (objects) that are otherwise indistinguishable by position in space, time, and species.
2. From perceiving the minutest moments of time (3.52), subtle differences can be perceived in space-time between two objects that appear the same.

तारकं सर्वविषयं सर्वथाविषयमक्रमं चेति विवेकजं ज्ञानम् ॥ ३.५४ ॥

3.54 tārakaṃ sarvaviṣayaṃ sarvathāviṣayamakramaṃ ceti vivekajaṃ jñānam

tārakaṃ sarva-viṣayaṃ sarvathā-viṣayam akramaṃ ca iti vivekajaṃ jñānam

tāraka	transcendant, crossing over [am subj sg n-a]
sarva	all
viṣaya	sensory object [am subj sg n-a]
sarvathā	all ways, all conditions
viṣaya	sensory object [am subj sg n-a]
akrama	without sequence [am subj sg n-a]

ca and
iti thus
vivekaja born of discernment [am subj sg n-a]
jñāna knowledge [am subj sg n-a]

1. Transcending all objects in all conditions, and without regard to their sequential appearance, thus the knowledge born of viveka.
2. When objects are understood on the subtlest level, true discernment is attained.

सत्त्वपुरुषयोः शुद्धिसाम्ये कैवल्यम् ॥ ३.५५ ॥

3.55 sattvapuruṣayoḥ śuddhisāmye kaivalyam

sattva-puruṣayoḥ śuddhi-sāmye kaivalyam

sattva guṇa of light, intelligence, purity, goodness, etc.
puruṣa the inner light of awareness, the observer [ayoḥ "of" du m-a]
śuddhi purity
sāmya equal, same [e "on/upon/in" sg m-a]
kaivalya final emancipation [am subj sg n-a]

1. Upon the equal purity of Puruṣa and sattva (buddhi), kaivalya.
2. When the heart-mind is transparent, still and pure as the inner Self, then kaivalya is experienced.

४. कैवल्यपादः

KAIVALYAPĀDAḤ

The Chapter on Permanent Oneness

जन्मौषधिमन्त्रतपःसमाधिजाः सिद्धयः ॥ ४.१ ॥

4.1 janmauṣadhimantratapaḥsamādhijāḥ siddhayaḥ

janma-auṣadhi-mantra-tapaḥ-samādhijāḥ siddhayaḥ

janma birth
auṣadhi herb, medicine
mantra sound causing a specific effect
tapas practice causing positive change
samādhija produced from samādhi [āḥ subj pl f-ā]

siddhi a power, accomplishment [ayaḥ subj pl f-i]

1. The siddhi-s are produced from innate abilities, herbal medicine, mantra, tapas, and samādhi.
2. The special abilities (partially listed in chapter 3) can be attained from genetic inheritance, herbal medicine, chanting sounds with specific effects, practicing with effort, and by samādhi (same as saṃyama here). This sūtra mentions other ways of achieving the powers described in chapter 3.

जात्यन्तरपरिणामः प्रकृत्यापूरात् ॥ ४.२ ॥

4.2 jātyantarapariṇāmaḥ prakṛtyāpūrāt

jāti-antara-pariṇāmaḥ prakṛti-āpūrāt

jāti birth class/condition/status; caste; category of existence
antara other
pariṇāma transformation, change, mutation [aḥ subj sg m-a]
prakṛti phenomenal/manifest world
āpūra overflow, adjustment [āt "from/due to" sg m-a]

1. The change into another category of existence is due to the overflow of natural forces.
2. Matter changes from one state into another state from the abundant flow of nature's forces.

निमित्तमप्रयोजकं प्रकृतीनां वरणभेदस्तु ततः क्षेत्रिकवत् ॥ ४.३ ॥

4.3 nimittamaprayojakaṃ prakṛtīnāṃ varaṇabhedastu tataḥ kṣetrikavat

nimittam aprayojakaṃ prakṛtīnāṃ varaṇa-bhedaḥ tu tataḥ kṣetrikavat

nimitta proximate cause, catalyst [am subj sg n-a]
aprayojaka noninitiator, nondriver, nonmotivator [am subj sg n-a]
prakṛti natural processes [īnām "of" pl f-i]
varaṇa covering, obstacle
bheda separate, divide, part (in order to clear a path) [aḥ subj sg m-a]
tu but
tataḥ from that
kṣetrikavat like a farmer

1. The cause is not the initiator of natural processes, but rather separates the obstacles, like a farmer (who divides the earth so the water can flow to irrigate his field).
2. The causes of natural processes do not of themselves drive change, but cause obstacles to part so everything will flow without resistance.

निर्माणचित्तान्यस्मितामात्रात् ॥ ४.४ ॥

4.4 nirmāṇacittānyasmitāmātrāt

nirmāṇa-cittāni asmitā-mātrāt

nirmāṇa	fabricating, constructing, shaping, forming
citta	heart-mind field of consciousness [āni subj pl n-a]
asmitā	ego
mātra	alone, only [āt "from/due to" sg m-a]

1. Individually fabricated heart-minds (come) only from asmitā.
2. Individual heart-minds are molded by our own sense of identity and by other personalities we come into contact with.

प्रवृत्तिभेदे प्रयोजकं चित्तमेकमनेकेषाम् ॥ ४.५ ॥

4.5 pravṛttibhede prayojakaṃ cittamekamanekeṣām

pravṛtti-bhede prayojakaṃ cittam ekam anekeṣām

pravṛtti	activity of refined sensory organs
bheda	division, separation [e "on/upon/in" sg m-a]
prayojaka	initiator, motivator, director [am subj sg n-a]
citta	heart-mind field of consciousness [am subj sg n-a]
eka	one, single [am subj sg n-p]
aneka	many [eṣām "of" pl n-p]

1. While separate activities (occur in different heart-minds), one heart-mind is the director of many (individual heart-minds).
2. One person can influence many other people, and the same thought, word, or deed may affect people in different ways.

तत्र ध्यानजमनाशयम् ॥ ४.६ ॥

4.6 tatra dhyānajamanāśayam

tatra dhyānajam anāśayam

tatra	there
dhyānaja	born of dhyāna (continuous meditation) [am subj sg n-a]
anāśaya	no accumulation, nothing deposited in the karmāśaya [am subj sg n-a]

1. There (the heart-mind) produced in dhyāna (leaves) no residual impressions (saṃskāra-s or vāsanā-s).
2. A heart-mind focused in meditation does not produce any subconscious impressions.

कर्माशुक्लाकृष्णं योगिनस्त्रिविधमितरेषाम् ॥ ४.७ ॥

4.7 karmāśuklākṛṣṇaṃ yoginastrividhamitareṣām

karma-aśukla-akṛṣṇaṃ yoginaḥ trividham itareṣām

karma	action
aśukla	not white
akṛṣṇa	not black [am subj sg n-a]
yogin	one who practices yoga as defined in 1.2 [aḥ "of" sg m-in]
trividha	threefold [am subj sg n-a]
itara	other [eṣām "of" pl m-p]

1. The actions of a yogin are neither white nor black. (The actions) of others are threefold.
2. Actions of nonyogins are threefold: white (positive/good/right), black (negative/bad/wrong), or gray (neutral). The actions of a yogin transcend good or bad, right or wrong.

ततस्तद्विपाकानुगुणानामेवाभिव्यक्तिर्वासनानाम् ॥ ४.८ ॥

4.8 tatastadvipākānuguṇānāmevābhivyaktirvāsanānām

tataḥ tad-vipāka-anuguṇānām eva abhivyaktiḥ vāsanānām

tataḥ	from that, therefore
tad	(of) those [pronoun stem]
vipāka	ripening, fruition
anuguṇa	corresponding, following in qualities [ānām "of" pl f-ā]
eva	specifically
abhivyakti	manifestation [iḥ subj sg f-i]
vāsanā	subtle saṃskāra, propensity, or trait [ānām "of" pl f-ā]

1. Therefore the manifestation of vāsanā-s corresponds specifically to the fruition of those (threefold actions).
2. The three kinds of actions (karma-s) performed by a nonyogin leave a subtle residue that influences how future actions will play out according to the qualities of the actions (proportion of sattva, rajas, and tamas).

जातिदेशकालव्यवहितानामप्यानन्तर्यं स्मृतिसंस्कारयोरेकरूपत्वात् ॥ ४.९ ॥

4.9 jātideśakālavyavahitānāmapyānantaryaṃ smṛtisaṃskārayorekarūpatvāt

jāti-deśa-kāla-vyavahitānām api ānantaryaṃ smṛti-saṃskārayoḥ eka-rūpatvāt

jāti	birth class/condition/status; caste
deśa	place, location
kāla	time
vyavahita	separated by anything intervening, "placed apart" [ānām "of" pl f-ā]

api	also, even
ānantarya	uninterrupted, continuous [am subj sg n-a]
smṛti	memory
saṃskāra	strong impression in memory causing a habitual tendency [ayoḥ "of" du m-a]
eka-rūpatva	affinity, uniformity [āt "from/due to" sg n-a]

1. The affinity between saṃskāra and memory is continuous, even of those (vāsanā-s) separated by birth-class, place, or time.
2. Saṃskāra-s are stored in memory (in the karmāśaya—see appendix F, figure 3) and can affect what is remembered from an experience.

तासामनादित्वं चाशिषो नित्यत्वात् ॥ ४.१० ॥

4.10 tāsāmanāditvaṃ cāśiṣo nityatvāt

tāsām anāditvaṃ ca āśiṣaḥ nityatvāt

tāsām	of those [pronoun "of" sg f-ā]
anāditva	without beginning, "beginninglessness" [am subj sg n-a]
ca	and
āśis	desire to live, will to survive (see abhiniveṣa-kleśa) [aḥ "of" sg m-cons]
nityatva	eternalness, perpetuity [āt "from/due to" sg n-a]

1. And the beginninglessness of those (vāsanā-s) is due to the eternality of the desire to live.
2. Those vāsanā-s have always existed, due to the never-ending will to live.

हेतुफलाश्रयालम्बनैः संगृहीतत्वादेषामभावे तदभावः ॥ ४.११ ॥

4.11 hetuphalāśrayālambanaiḥ saṃgṛhītatvādeṣāmabhāve tadabhāvaḥ

hetu-phala-āśraya-ālambanaiḥ saṃgṛhītatvāt eṣām abhāve tad-abhāvaḥ

hetu	cause
phala	result, effect
āśraya	substratum
ālambana	supporting [aiḥ "by/with" pl n-a]
saṃgṛhītatva	"held-together-ness" [āt "from/due to" sg n-a]
eṣām	of these [pronoun "of" pl n-p]
abhāva	absence, disappearance [e "on/upon/in" sg m-a]
tad	(of) those [pronoun stem]
abhāva	absence, disappearance [aḥ subj sg m-a]

1. Because of being held together by cause, effect, and supporting substratum (citta), upon the disappearance of these (three components), the disappearance of those (vāsanā-s).

2. Cause (here, avidyā), resulting effect (memory formed), container (citta), and supporting objects all contribute to the continuation of vāsanā-s. When these go away, so do the vāsanā-s.

अतीतानागतं स्वरूपतो ऽस्त्यध्वभेदाद्धर्माणाम् ॥ ४.१२ ॥

4.12 atītānāgataṃ svarūpato 'styadhvabhedāddharmāṇām

atīta-anāgātaṃ svarūpataḥ asti adhva-bhedāt dharmāṇām

atīta	past, "gone"
anāgata	future, "not come" [am subj sg n-a]
svarūpata	fundamental form [aḥ "from/due to/of" sg]
asti	is [verb 3rd sg root as]
adhva	path, journey, course, way
bheda	separate, different [āt "from/due to" sg m-a]
dharma	characteristic form (see pariṇāma-s) [ānām "of" pl m-a]

1. Past and future are present (in their) fundamental forms due to the different paths of dharma-s.
2. With regard to changes in form, the past exists as memories and the future exists as potential.

ते व्यक्तसूक्ष्मा गुणात्मानः ॥ ४.१३ ॥

4.13 te vyaktasūkṣmā guṇātmānaḥ

te vyakta-sūkṣmāḥ guṇa-ātmānaḥ

te	those [pronoun subj pl m-p]
vyakta	manifested
sūkṣma	subtle [āḥ subj pl m-a]
guṇa	quality of nature
ātman	composed of, having the nature of (as a suffix) [ānaḥ subj pl m-an]

1. Those (dharma-s—4.12) are subtle or manifest (and) are composed of the guṇa-s (sattva, rajas, and tamas).

परिणामैकत्वाद्वस्तुतत्त्वम् ॥ ४.१४ ॥

4.14 pariṇāmaikatvādvastutattvam

pariṇāma-ekatvāt vastu-tattvam

pariṇāma	transformation, change, mutation
ekatva	oneness, uniqueness [āt "from/due to" sg n-a]
vastu	object
tattva	essence, "that-ness" [am subj sg n-a]

1. The essence of an object is due to the uniqueness of (its) transformations.

2. Every object is a unique combination of guṇa-s at a particular moment in space-time due to the continuous changes occuring in matter.

वस्तुसाम्ये चित्तभेदात्तयोर्विभक्तः पन्थाः ॥ ४.१५ ॥

4.15 vastusāmye cittabhedāttayorvibhaktaḥ panthāḥ

vastu-sāmye citta-bhedāt tayoḥ vibhaktaḥ panthāḥ

vastu	object
sāmya	sameness [e "on/upon/in" pl m-p]
citta	heart-mind field of consciousness
bheda	difference, division [āt "from/due to" sg m-a]
tayoḥ	of those, of both [pronoun "of" du m-p]
vibhakta	distinct, different [aḥ subj sg m-a]
panthin	path, way [āḥ subj sg m-cons-in-irreg]

1. Even though objects are actually the same, because of separate heart-minds, the way an object *is* may be different from what the heart-mind thinks it is.
2. Objects are perceived differently by different people because of the conditioning present in their heart-minds.

न चैकचित्ततन्त्रं चेद्वस्तु तदप्रमाणकं तदा किं स्यात् ॥ ४.१६ ॥

4.16 na caikacittatantraṃ cedvastu tadapramāṇakaṃ tadā kiṃ syāt

na ca eka-citta-tantraṃ ced vastu tad-apramāṇakaṃ tadā kiṃ syāt

na	not
ca	and
eka	one, single
citta	heart-mind field of consciousness
tantra	dependent [am subj sg n-a]
ced	if
vastu	object [u subj sg n-p]
tat	that [pronoun subj sg n-p]
apramāṇaka	not depending on [am subj sg n-a]
tadā	then
kiṃ	what? [interrogative pronoun subj sg n-p]
syāt	might be [verb 3rd sg root as]

1. And if an object is not dependent on (its perception by) a single heart-mind, (for if this were so) and that (heart-mind) is not perceiving (the object) correctly, then what would (the object) be?
2. If an object was dependent on one individual heart-mind, and that heart-mind was not correctly evaluating the object, then what would the object become?

तदुपरागापेक्षित्वाच्चित्तस्य वस्तु ज्ञाताज्ञातम् ॥ ४.१७ ॥

4.17 taduparāgāpekṣitvāccittasya vastu jñātājñātam

tad-uparāga-apekṣitvāt cittasya vastu jñāta-ajñātam

tad	(of) that, its [pronoun stem]
uparāga	reflected color
apekṣitva	necessity [āt "from/due to" sg n-a]
citta	heart-mind field of consciousness [asya "of" sg n-a]
vastu	object [u subj sg n-u]
jñāta	known
ajñāta	unknown [am subj sg n-a]

1. Because of the heart-mind being dependent on its reflected color, an object is either known or unknown.
2. We visually know an object based on the color of light reflected off it. If no reflection is there, we do not see it and therefore it is unknown to us.

सदा ज्ञाताश्चित्तवृत्तयस्तत्प्रभोः पुरुषस्यापरिणामित्वात् ॥ ४.१८ ॥

4.18 sadā jñātāścittavṛttayastatprabhoḥ puruṣasyāpariṇāmitvāt

sadā jñātāḥ citta-vṛttayaḥ tad-prabhoḥ puruṣasya-apariṇāmitvāt

sadā	always
jñāta	known [āḥ subj pl f-a]
citta	heart-mind field of consciousness
vṛtti	fluctuation or activity in the heart-mind [ayaḥ subj pl f-i]
tad	(of) those, their [pronoun stem]
prabhu	master, lord, "exists in front of" [oḥ "of" sg m-u]
puruṣa	the inner light of awareness, the observer [asya "of" sg m-a]
apariṇāmitva	changelessness [āt "from/due to" sg n-a]

1. The citta-vṛtti-s are always known due to the changelessness of their master, Puruṣa.
2. From the point of stillness the Puruṣa can see the fluctuations happening in the heart-mind.

न तत्स्वाभासं दृश्यत्वात् ॥ ४.१९ ॥

4.19 na tatsvābhāsaṃ dṛśyatvāt

na tat svābhāsaṃ dṛśyatvāt

na	not
tat	that [pronoun subj sg n-p]
svābhāsa	self-luminous, "own radiance" [am subj sg n-a]
dṛśyatva	seeableness, nature of being part of Prakṛti (dṛśya) [āt "from/due to" sg n-a]

1. That (citta) is not self-luminous due to (its being) a seeable object.
2. The light of Puruṣa (draṣṭṛ=seer) illuminates all objects in Prakṛti (dṛśya=seeable) including the heart-mind (citta). Only the seer is self-luminous.

एकसमये चोभयानवधारणम् ॥ ४.२० ॥

4.20 ekasamaye cobhayānavadhāraṇam

eka-samaye ca ubhaya-anavadhāraṇam

eka	one, single
samaya	time [e "on/upon/in" sg m-a]
ca	and
ubhaya	both
anavadhāraṇa	not cognized [am subj sg n-a]

1. And both are not cognized at the same time.
2. The citta and its object cannot be cognized (by the citta) simultaneously.

चित्तान्तरदृश्ये बुद्धिबुद्धेरतिप्रसङ्गः स्मृतिसंकरश्च ॥ ४.२१ ॥

4.21 cittāntaradṛśye buddhibuddheratiprasaṅgaḥ smṛtisaṃkaraśca

citta-antara-dṛśye buddhi-buddheḥ atiprasaṅgaḥ smṛti-saṃkaraḥ ca

citta	heart-mind field of consciousness
antara	another
dṛśya	seeable [e "on/upon/in" sg n-a]
buddhi	intellect; decision-making part of the heart-mind
buddhi	same as above [eḥ "from/due to" sg f-i]
atiprasaṅga	infinite regression [aḥ subj sg m-a]
smṛti	memory
saṃkara	mixing up, confusing [aḥ subj sg m-a]
ca	and

1. (If one) citta was perceivable (illuminated) by another citta, (it would result in) an infinite regression of buddhi upon buddhi, and confusion of memories.
2. If one heart-mind could illuminate another heart-mind, this would go on ad infinitum, from one intellect to another, causing intermixture of memory and thus no way to clearly apprehend any single memory. This provides evidence that only Puruṣa illuminates the heart-mind.

चितेरप्रतिसंक्रमायास्तदाकारापत्तौ स्वबुद्धिसंवेदनम् ॥ ४.२२ ॥

4.22 citerapratisaṃkramāyāstadākārāpattau svabuddhisaṃvedanam

citeḥ apratisaṃkramāyāḥ tad-ākāra-āpattau sva-buddhi-saṃvedanam

citi	unconditioned heart-mind, pure awareness [eḥ "from/due to" sg f-i]
apratisaṃkramā	unchanging, lacking sequential changes [āyāḥ "from/due to" sg f-ā]
tad	(in) that [pronoun stem]
ākāra	shape, form
āpatti	appearance [au "on/upon/in" sg f-i]
sva-buddhi	"own buddhi"
saṃvedana	complete experience/feeling/knowledge [am subj sg n-a]

1. Because pure awareness is changeless, it has an experience of the buddhi when a form appears in it.
2. When the buddhi part of citta reflects the form of an object, the seer (Puruṣa) is aware of the change because of its changeless nature.

द्रष्टृदृश्योपरक्तं चित्तं सर्वार्थम् ॥ ४.२३ ॥

4.23 draṣṭṛdṛśyoparaktaṃ cittaṃ sarvārtham

draṣṭṛ-dṛśya-uparaktaṃ cittaṃ sarva-artham

draṣṭṛ	pure awareness, "seer" = Puruṣa
dṛśya	the manifest world, "seeable" = Prakṛti
uparakta	colored through reflection [am subj sg n-a]
citta	heart-mind field of consciousness [am subj sg n-a]
sarva	all
artha	object [am subj sg n-a]

1. The citta, colored by the seeable and the seer, (serves) the purpose of all.
2. The heart-mind is affected by sensory objects (when it acts as the subject and receives sensory input). From the other direction the heart-mind's buddhi reflects the light of pure awareness (the seer) as its object. Therefore the heart-mind is both subject and object, and serves the purpose of all aspects of one's psyche.

तदसंख्येयवासनाभिश्चित्रमपि परार्थं संहत्यकारित्वात् ॥ ४.२४ ॥

4.24 tadasaṃkhyeyavāsanābhiścitramapi parārthaṃ saṃhatyakāritvāt

tat asaṃkhyeya-vāsanābhiḥ citram api parārthaṃ saṃhatya-kāritvāt

tat	that [pronoun subj sg n-p]
asaṃkhyeya	uncountable, countless, innumerable
vāsanā	subtle saṃskāra, propensity or trait [ābhiḥ "by/with" pl f-ā]
citra	manifold, variegated, varicolored [am subj sg n-a]
api	also, even, even though
parārtha	purpose of another [am subj sg n-a]

saṃhatya collaboration, association
kāritva activity [āt "from/due to" sg n-a]

1. That (citta), even though varicolored by countless vāsanā-s, (exists for) the purpose of another because of its activity of collaboration.
2. The heart-mind coordinates the functions of the various components of our psyche, while also being influenced by the subtle impressions that develop and manifest through action. All this is done for the sake of another, the pure awareness.

विशेषदर्शिन आत्मभावभावनानिवृत्तिः ॥ ४.२५ ॥

4.25 viśeṣadarśina ātmabhāvabhāvanānivṛttiḥ

viśeṣa-darśinaḥ ātma-bhāva-bhāvanā-nivṛttiḥ

viśeṣa distinct
darśin one who can see/perceive [aḥ "of" sg m-in]
ātma self
bhāva sense, nature, appearance
bhāvanā existing, feeling,
nivṛtti ceasing, ending of activity [iḥ subj sg f-i]

1. For one who can perceive the distinction (between a sattvic buddhi and Puruṣa), the feeling of the sense of self ceases.

तदा विवेकनिम्नं कैवल्यप्राग्भारं चित्तम् ॥ ४.२६ ॥

4.26 tadā vivekanimnaṃ kaivalyaprāgbhāraṃ cittam

tadā viveka-nimnaṃ kaivalya-prāgbhāraṃ cittam

tadā then
viveka discernment
nimna deep, slope, incline, oriented toward [am subj sg n-a]
kaivalya final emancipation
prāgbhāra gravitation, "weighted in the front" [am subj sg n-a]
citta heart-mind field of consciousness [am subj sg n-a]

1. Then the citta, oriented toward discernment, gravitates toward kaivalya.
2. Then the heart-mind, (while in the) depths of clear discernment, goes deeper toward kaivalya.

तच्छिद्रेषु प्रत्ययान्तराणि संस्कारेभ्यः ॥ ४.२७ ॥

4.27 tacchidreṣu pratyayāntarāṇi saṃskārebhyaḥ

tat chidreṣu pratyaya-antarāṇi saṃskārebhyaḥ

tat (of) that [pronoun stem]
chidra interval, gap [eṣu "on/upon/in" pl m-a]

pratyaya	presented thought; current vṛtti directed toward an object
antara	another [āṇi subj pl n-a]
saṃskāra	habitual tendency memory caused by a strong impression [ebhyaḥ "from/due to" pl m-a]

1. In the intervals of that (citta), other pratyaya come from saṃskāra-s.
2. In between the times of clear discernment, other heart-mind activities (intervening thoughts) are only due to (previously developed) habitual tendencies.

हानमेषां क्लेशवदुक्तम् ॥ ४.२८ ॥

4.28 hānameṣāṃ kleśavaduktam

hānam eṣāṃ kleśavat uktam

hāna	ending, removing, destroying [am subj sg n-a]
eṣāṃ	of those [pronoun "of" pl m-p]
kleśavat	like the kleśa-s
ukta	said, described [am subj sg n-a]

1. Ending these (saṃskāra-s) is said to be like (the process of ending) the kleśa-s (i.e., by pratiprasava—2.10–11).
2. The saṃskāra-s that cause intervening thoughts to appear can be ended by pratiprasava.

प्रसंख्याने ऽप्यकुसीदस्य सर्वथा विवेकख्यातेर्धर्ममेघः समाधिः ॥ ४.२९ ॥

4.29 prasaṃkhyāne 'pyakusīdasya sarvathā vivekakhyāterdharmameghaḥ samādhiḥ

prasaṃkhyāne api akusīdasya sarvathā viveka-khyāteḥ dharma-meghaḥ samādhiḥ

prasaṃkhyāna	higher state [e "on/upon/in" sg m-a]
api	also, even
akusīda	disinterested [asya "of" sg m-a]
sarvathā	in all ways, in every way, totally, continuously
viveka	wise discernment
khyāti	awareness, realization, understanding, identification [eḥ "of" sg f-i]
dharma	virtue
megha	cloud [aḥ subj sg m-a]
samādhi	complete absorption of the heart-mind in the focus [iḥ subj sg m-i]

1. Of one who is disinterested even in a higher state due to continuous and total viveka-khyāti, dharma-megha samādhi (arises).

2. Perpetual discernment (without any intervening thoughts because the saṃskāra-s that cause them are gone) causes us not to seek enlightenment anymore, since we are indifferent even to that. This kind of samādhi, when our heart-mind is completely absorbed in viveka-khyāti, results in virtue (dharma) raining down on us as if from a virtue-laden cloud.

ततः क्लेशकर्मनिवृत्तिः ॥ ४.३० ॥

4.30 tataḥ kleśakarmanivṛttiḥ

tataḥ kleśa-karma-nivṛttiḥ

tataḥ	from that [pronoun]
kleśa	deep emotional affliction
karma	action
nivṛtti	turning back, ceasing [iḥ subj sg f-i]

1. From that, the termination of karma-s and kleśa-s.

तदा सर्वावरणमलापेतस्य ज्ञानस्यानन्त्याज्ज्ञेयमल्पम् ॥ ४.३१ ॥

4.31 tadā sarvāvaraṇamalāpetasya jñānasyānantyājjñeyamalpam

tadā sarva-āvaraṇa-mala-apetasya jñānasya ānantyāt jñeyam alpam

tadā	then
sarva	all
āvaraṇa	covering
mala	impurity
apeta	removal [asya "of" sg n-a]
jñāna	knowledge [asya "of" sg n-a]
ānantya	eternality [āt "from" sg n-a]
jñeya	knowable [am subj sg n-a]
alpa	little, small [am subj sg n-a]

1. Then due to the eternality of knowledge because of the removal of impurities covering everything, little (more) is to be known.
2. Knowledge that is free of the coatings of karma-s, kleśa-s, and saṃskāra-s is thus unfiltered, clear, and almost unlimited.

ततः कृतार्थानां परिणामक्रमसमाप्तिर्गुणानाम् ॥ ४.३२ ॥

4.32 tataḥ kṛtārthānāṃ pariṇāmakramasamāptirguṇānām

tataḥ kṛta-arthānāṃ pariṇāma-krama-samāptiḥ guṇānām

tataḥ	from that
kṛta	done, achieved
artha	purpose, object [ānām "of" pl m-a]
pariṇāma	transformation, change, mutation

krama sequence
samāpti finish, conclusion, end [iḥ subj sg f-i]
guṇa quality of nature [ānām "of" pl m-a]

1. From that, the conclusion of the sequential changes of the guṇa-s whose purpose is done.
2. From dharma-megha-samādhi, the guṇa-s, having served their purpose (of experience), end their movement, causing the transformations to end as well.

क्षणप्रतियोगी परिणामापरान्तनिर्ग्राह्यः क्रमः ॥ ४.३३ ॥

4.33 kṣaṇapratiyogī pariṇāmāparāntanirgrāhyaḥ kramaḥ

kṣaṇa-pratiyogī pariṇāma-aparānta-nirgrāhyaḥ kramaḥ

kṣaṇa moment
pratiyogin corresponding [ī subj sg m-in]
pariṇāma transformation, change, mutation
apara nothing higher; other
anta end
aparānta culmination, "other end"
nirgrāhya apprehensible, understandable [aḥ subj sg m-a]
krama sequence [aḥ subj sg m-a]

1. The sequence, corresponding to each moment in time, is grasped at the very end of the transformations.
2. The sequential progression of changes over time is finally understood now that the changes have ended.

पुरुषार्थशून्यानां गुणानां प्रतिप्रसवः कैवल्यं स्वरूपप्रतिष्ठा वा चितिशक्तिरिति ॥ ४.३४ ॥

4.34 puruṣārthaśūnyānāṃ guṇānāṃ pratiprasavaḥ kaivalyaṃ svarūpapratiṣṭhā vā citiśaktiriti

puruṣa-artha-śūnyānāṃ guṇānāṃ pratiprasavaḥ kaivalyaṃ
svarūpa-pratiṣṭhā vā citi-śaktiḥ iti

puruṣa the inner light of awareness, the observer
artha object, purpose
śūnya empty, devoid of [ānām "of" pl m-a]
guṇa quality of nature [ānām "of" pl m-a]
pratiprasava returning back to the origin [aḥ subj sg m-a]
kaivalya final emancipation [am subj sg n-a]
svarūpa true nature, "own form"
pratiṣṭhā established [ā subj sg f-ā]
vā and

citi	unconditioned consciousness
śakti	power, ability [iḥ subj sg f-i]
iti	thus

1. The pratiprasava of the guṇa-s, empty of their purpose for Puruṣa, is kaivalya. In other words, the power of unconditioned consciousness is established in its own true nature.
2. Once the basic qualities of nature have been fully understood, the true operations behind Prakṛti are revealed, leaving Puruṣa standing alone in its own brilliance.

part 4

The Yoga Sutras for Chanting

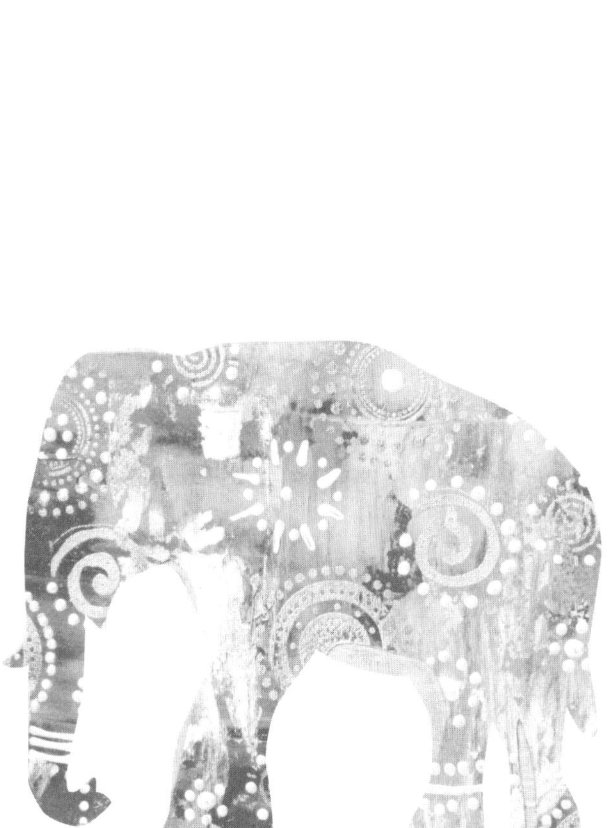

This format of the *Yoga Sūtra-s* is for learning how to chant through the sūtra-s one after the other. You may choose to deepen your oral practice with the addition of *The Yoga Sutras* original audio program. The font is larger and there are marks to indicate whether the syllable is a lower, middle, or upper tone. The notations of the *Yoga Sūtra-s* as presented here are based on a system designed and taught by the late T. K. V. Desikachar. A vertical line above a syllable indicates a high tone, a horizontal line beneath a syllable represents a low tone, and no marking represents a middle tone. These marks are the same as the ones seen in Vedic texts, and are used here to make it easier to follow along.

PĀTAÑJALAYOGADARŚANAM

SAMĀDHIPĀDAḤ

atha yogānuśāsanam | 1.1 |

yogaścittavṛttinirodhaḥ | 1.2 |

tadā draṣṭuḥ svarūpe 'vasthānam | 1.3 |

vṛttisārūpyamitaratra | 1.4 |

vṛttayaḥ pañcatayyaḥ kliṣṭākliṣṭāḥ | 1.5 |

pramāṇaviparyayavikalpanidrāsmṛtayaḥ | 1.6 |

pratyakṣānumānāgamāḥ pramāṇāni | 1.7 |

viparyayo mithyājñānamatadrūpapratiṣṭham | 1.8 |

śabdajñānānupātī vastuśūnyo vikalpaḥ | 1.9 |

abhāvapratyayālambanā tamovṛttirnidrā | 1.10 |

anubhūtaviṣayāsaṃpramoṣaḥ smṛtiḥ | 1.11 |

abhyāsavairāgyābhyāṃ tannirodhaḥ | 1.12 |

tatra sthitau yatno 'bhyāsaḥ | 1.13 |

sa tu dīrghakālanairantaryasatkārādarāsevito dṛḍhabhūmiḥ | 1.14 |

dṛṣṭānuśravikaviṣayavitṛṣṇasya vaśīkārasaṃjñā vairāgyam | 1.15 |

tatparaṃ puruṣakhyāterguṇavaitṛṣṇyam | 1.16 |

vitarkavicārānandāsmitārūpānugamātsaṃprajñātaḥ | 1.17 |

virāmapratyayābhyāsapūrvaḥ saṃskāraśeṣo 'nyaḥ | 1.18 |

bhavapratyayo videhaprakṛtilayānām | 1.19 |

śraddhāvīryasmṛtisamādhiprajñāpūrvaka itareṣām | 1.20 |

tīvrasaṃvegānāmāsannaḥ | 1.21 |

mṛdumadhyādhimātratvāttato 'pi viśeṣaḥ | 1.22 |

īśvarapraṇidhānādvā | 1.23 |

kleśakarmavipākāśayairaparāmṛṣṭaḥ puruṣaviśeṣa īśvaraḥ | 1.24 |

tatra niratiśayaṃ sarvajñabījam | 1.25 |

sa eṣa pūrveṣāmapi guruḥ kālenānavacchedāt | 1.26 |

tasya vācakaḥ praṇavaḥ | 1.27 |

tajjapastadarthabhāvanam | 1.28 |

tataḥ pratyakcetanādhigamo 'pyantarāyābhāvaśca | 1.29 |

vyādhistyānasaṃśayapramādālasyāviratibhrāntidarśanālabdha-bhūmikatvānavasthitatvāni cittavikṣepāste antarāyāḥ | 1.30 |

duḥkhadaurmanasyāṅgamejayatvaśvāsapraśvāsā vikṣepasahabhuvaḥ | 1.31 |

tatpratiṣedhārthamekatattvābhyāsaḥ | 1.32 |

maitrīkaruṇāmuditopekṣāṇāṃ sukhaduḥkhapuṇyāpuṇyaviṣayāṇāṃ bhāvanātaścittaprasādanam | 1.33 |

pracchardhanavidhāraṇābhyāṃ vā prāṇasya | 1.34 |

viṣayavatī vā pravṛttirutpannā manasaḥ sthitinibandhinī | 1.35 |

viśokā vā jyotiṣmatī | 1.36 |

vītarāgaviṣayaṃ vā cittam | 1.37 |

svapnanidrājñānālambanaṃ vā | 1.38 |

yathābhimatadhyānādvā | 1.39 |

paramāṇuparamamahattvānto 'sya vaśīkāraḥ | 1.40 |

kṣīṇavṛtterabhijātasyeva manergrahītṛgrahaṇagrāhyeṣu tatsthatadañjanatā samāpattiḥ | 1.41 |

tatra śabdārthajñānavikalpaiḥ saṃkīrṇā savitarkā samāpattiḥ | 1.42 |

smṛtipariśuddhau svarūpaśūnyevārthamātranirbhāsā nirvitarkā | 1.43 |

etayaiva savicārā nirvicārā ca sūkṣmaviṣayā vyākhyātā | 1.44 |

sūkṣmaviṣayatvaṃ cāliṅgaparyavasānam | 1.45 |

tā eva sabījaḥ samādhiḥ | 1.46 |

nirvicāravaiśāradye 'dhyātmaprasādaḥ | 1.47 |

ṛtambharā tatra prajñā | 1.48 |

śrutānumānaprajñābhyāmanyaviṣayā viśeṣārthatvāt | 1.49 |

tajjaḥ saṃskāro 'nyasaṃskārapratibandhī | 1.50 |

tasyāpi nirodhe sarvanirodhānnirbījaḥ samādhiḥ | 1.51 |

SĀDHANAPĀDAḤ

tapaḥsvādhyāyeśvarapraṇidhānāni kriyāyogaḥ | 2.1 |

samādhibhāvanārthaḥ kleśatanūkaraṇārthaśca | 2.2 |

avidyāsmitārāgadveṣābhiniveśāḥ kleśāḥ | 2.3 |

avidyā kṣetramuttareṣāṃ prasuptatanuvicchinnodārāṇām | 2.4 |

anityāśuciduḥkhānātmasu nityaśucisukhātmakhyātiravidyā | 2.5 |

dṛgdarśanaśaktyorekātmatevāsmitā | 2.6 |

sukhānuśayī rāgaḥ | 2.7 |

duḥkhānuśayī dveṣaḥ | 2.8 |

svarasavāhī viduṣo 'pi samārūḍho 'bhiniveśaḥ | 2.9 |

te pratiprasavaheyāḥ sūkṣmāḥ | 2.10 |

dhyānaheyāstadvṛttayaḥ | 2.11 |

kleśamūlaḥ karmāśayo dṛṣṭādṛṣṭajanmavedanīyaḥ | 2.12 |

sati mūle tadvipāko jātyāyurbhogāḥ | 2.13 |

te hlādaparitāpaphalāḥ puṇyāpuṇyahetutvāt | 2.14 |

pariṇāmatāpasaṃskāraduḥkhairguṇavṛttivirodhācca duḥkhameva sarvaṃ vivekinaḥ | 2.15 |

heyaṃ duḥkhamanāgatam | 2.16 |

draṣṭṛdṛśyayoḥ saṃyogo heyahetuḥ | 2.17 |

prakāśakriyāsthitiśīlaṃ bhūtendriyātmakaṃ bhogāpavargārthaṃ dṛśyam | 2.18 |

viśeṣāviśeṣaliṅgamātrāliṅgāni guṇaparvāṇi | 2.19 |

draṣṭā dṛśimātraḥ śuddho 'pi pratyayānupaśyaḥ | 2.20 |

tadartha eva dṛṣyasyātmā | 2.21 |

kṛtārthaṃ pratinaṣṭamapyanaṣṭaṃ tadanyasādhāraṇatvāt | 2.22 |

svasvāmiśaktyoḥ svarūpopalabdhihetuḥ saṃyogaḥ | 2.23 |

tasya heturavidyā | 2.24 |

tadabhāvātsaṃyogābhāvo hānaṃ taddṛśeḥ kaivalyam | 2.25 |

vivekakhyātiraviplavā hānopāyaḥ | 2.26 |

tasya saptadhā prāntabhūmiḥ prajñā | 2.27 |

yogāṅgānuṣṭhānādaśuddhikṣaye jñānadīptirāvivekakhyāteḥ | 2.28 |

yamaniyamāsanaprāṇāyāmapratyāhāradhāraṇādhyānasamādhayo 'ṣṭāvaṅgāni | 2.29 |

ahiṃsāsatyāsteyabrahmacaryāparigrahā yamāḥ | 2.30 |

jātideśakālasamayānavacchinnāḥ sarvabhaumā mahāvratam | 2.31 |

śaucasaṃtoṣatapaḥsvādhyāyeśvarapraṇidhānāni niyamāḥ | 2.32 |

vitarkabādhane pratipakṣabhāvanam | 2.33 |

vitarkā hiṃsādayaḥ kṛtakāritānumoditā lobhakrodhamohapūrvakā mṛdumadhyādhimātrā duḥkhājñānānantaphalā iti pratipakṣabhāvanam | 2.34 |

ahiṃsāpratiṣṭhāyāṃ tatsaṃnidhau vairatyāgaḥ | 2.35 |

satyapratiṣṭhāyāṃ kriyāphalāśrayatvam | 2.36 |

asteyapratiṣṭhāyāṃ sarvaratnopasthānam | 2.37 |

brahmacaryapratiṣṭhāyāṃ vīryalābhaḥ | 2.38 |

aparigrahasthairye janmakathaṃtāsaṃbodhaḥ | 2.39 |

śaucātsvāṅgajugupsā parairasaṃsargaḥ | 2.40 |

sattvaśuddhisaumanasyaikāgryendriyajayātmadarśanayogyatvāni ca | 2.41 |

saṃtoṣādanuttamaḥ sukhalābhaḥ | 2.42 |

kāyendriyasiddhiraśuddhikṣayāttapasaḥ | 2.43 |

svādhyāyādiṣṭadevatāsaṃprayogaḥ | 2.44 |

samādhisiddhirīśvarapraṇidhānāt | 2.45 |

sthirasukhamāsanam | 2.46 |

prayatnaśaithilyānantasamāpattibhyām | 2.47 |

tato dvandvānabhighātaḥ | 2.48 |

tasminsati śvāsapraśvāsayorgativicchedaḥ prāṇāyāmaḥ | 2.49 |

bāhyābhyantarastambhavṛttirdeśakālasaṃkhyābhiḥ paridṛṣṭo dīrghasūkṣmaḥ | 2.50 |

bāhyābhyantaraviṣayākṣepī caturthaḥ | 2.51 |

tataḥ kṣīyate prakāśāvaraṇam | 2.52 |

dhāraṇāsu ca yogyatā manasaḥ | 2.53 |

svaviṣayāsaṃprayoge cittasya svarūpānukāra ivendriyāṇāṃ pratyāhāraḥ | 2.54 |

tataḥ paramā vaśyatendriyāṇām | 2.55 |

VIBHŪTIPĀDAḤ

deśabandhaścittasya dhāraṇā | 3.1 |

tatra pratyayaikatānatā dhyānam | 3.2 |

tadevārthamātranirbhāsaṃ svarūpaśūnyamiva samādhiḥ | 3.3 |

trayamekatra saṃyamaḥ | 3.4 |

tajjayātprajñālokaḥ | 3.5 |

tasya bhūmiṣu viniyogaḥ | 3.6 |

trayamantaraṅgaṃ pūrvebhyaḥ | 3.7 |

tadapi bahiraṅgaṃ nirbījasya | 3.8 |

vyutthānanirodhasaṃskārayorabhibhavaprādurbhāvau nirodhakṣaṇacittānvayo nirodhapariṇāmaḥ | 3.9 |

tasya praśāntavāhitā saṃskārāt | 3.10 |

sarvārthataikāgratayoḥ kṣayodayau cittasya samādhipariṇāmaḥ | 3.11 |

tataḥ punaḥ śāntoditau tulyapratyayau cittasyaikāgratāpariṇāmaḥ | 3.12 |

etena bhūtendriyeṣu dharmalakṣaṇāvasthāpariṇāmā vyākhyātāḥ | 3.13 |

śāntoditāvyapadeśyadharmānupātī dharmī | 3.14 |

kramānyatvaṃ pariṇāmānyatve hetuḥ | 3.15 |

pariṇāmatrayasaṃyamādatītānāgatajñānam | 3.16 |

śabdārthapratyayānāmitaretarādhyāsātsaṅkarastatpravibhāga-saṃyamātsarvabhūtarutajñānam | 3.17 |

saṃskārasākṣātkaraṇātpūrvajātijñānam | 3.18 |

pratyayasya paracittajñānam | 3.19 |

na ca tatsālambanaṃ tasyāviṣayībhūtatvāt | 3.20 |

kāyarūpasaṃyamāttadgrāhyaśaktistambhe cakṣuḥprakāśāsaṃprayoge antardhānam | 3.21 |

sopakramaṃ nirupakramaṃ ca karma tatsaṃyamādaparāntajñānamariṣṭebhyo vā | 3.22 |

maitryādiṣu balāni | 3.23 |

baleṣu hastibalādīni | 3.24 |

pravṛttyālokanyāsātsūkṣmavyavahitaviprakṛṣṭajñānam | 3.25 |

bhuvanajñānaṃ sūrye saṃyamāt | 3.26 |

candre tārāvyūhajñānam | 3.27 |

dhruve tadgatijñānam | 3.28 |

nābhicakre kāyavyūhajñānam | 3.29 |

kaṇṭhakūpe kṣutpipāsānivṛttiḥ | 3.30 |

kūrmanāḍyāṃ sthairyam | 3.31 |

mūrdhajyotiṣi siddhadarśanam | 3.32 |

prātibhādvā sarvam | 3.33 |

hṛdaye cittasaṃvit | 3.34 |

sattvapuruṣayoratyantāsaṃkīrṇayoḥ pratyayāviśeṣo bhogaḥ parārthatvātsvārthasaṃyamātpuruṣajñānam | 3.35 |

tataḥ prātibhaśrāvaṇavedanādarśāsvādavārttā jāyante | 3.36 |

te samādhāvupasargā vyutthāne siddhayaḥ | 3.37 |

bandhakāraṇaśaithilyātpracārasaṃvedanācca cittasya paraśarīrāveśaḥ | 3.38 |

udānajayājjalapaṅkakaṇṭakādiṣvasaṅga utkrāntiśca | 3.39 |

samānajayājjvalanam | 3.40 |

śrotrākāśayoḥ saṃbandhasaṃyamāddivyaṃ śrotram | 3.41 |

kāyākāśayoḥ saṃbandhasaṃyamāllaghutūlasamāpatteś cākāśagamanam | 3.42 |

bahirakalpitā vṛttirmahāvidehā tataḥ prakāśāvaraṇakṣayaḥ | 3.43 |

sthūlasvarūpasūkṣmānvayārthavattvasaṃyamādbhūtajayaḥ | 3.44 |

tato 'ṇimādiprādurbhāvaḥ kāyasaṃpattaddharmānabhighātaśca | 3.45 |

rūpalāvaṇyabalavajrasaṃhananatvāni kāyasaṃpat | 3.46 |

grahaṇasvarūpāsmitānvayārthavattvasaṃyamādindriyajayaḥ | 3.47 |

tato manojavitvaṃ vikaraṇabhāvaḥ pradhānajayaśca | 3.48 |

sattvapuruṣānyatākhyātimātrasya sarvabhāvādhiṣṭhātṛtvaṃ sarvajñātṛtvaṃ ca | 3.49 |

tadvairāgyādapi doṣabījakṣaye kaivalyam | 3.50 |

sthānyupanimantraṇe saṅgasmayākaraṇaṃ punaraniṣṭaprasaṅgāt | 3.51 |

kṣaṇatatkramayoḥ saṃyamādvivekajaṃ jñānam | 3.52 |

jātilakṣaṇadeśairanyatānavacchedāttulyayostataḥ pratipattiḥ | 3.53 |

tārakaṃ sarvaviṣayaṃ sarvathāviṣayamakramaṃ ceti vivekajaṃ jñānam | 3.54 |

sattvapuruṣayoḥ śuddhisāmye kaivalyam | 3.55 |

KAIVALYAPĀDAḤ

janmauṣadhimantratapaḥsamādhijāḥ siddhayaḥ | 4.1 |

jātyantarapariṇāmaḥ prakṛtyāpūrāt | 4.2 |

nimittamaprayojakaṃ prakṛtīnāṃ varaṇabhedastu tataḥ kṣetrikavat | 4.3 |

nirmāṇacittānyasmitāmātrāt | 4.4 |

pravṛttibhede prayojakaṃ cittamekamanekeṣām | 4.5 |

tatra dhyānajamanāśayam | 4.6 |

karmāśuklākṛṣṇaṃ yoginastrividhamitareṣām | 4.7 |

tatastadvipākānuguṇānāmevābhivyaktirvāsanānām | 4.8 |

jātideśakālavyavahitānāmapyānantaryaṃ smṛtisaṃskārayorekarūpatvāt | 4.9 |

tāsāmanāditvaṃ cāśiṣo nityatvāt | 4.10 |

hetuphalāśrayālambanaiḥ saṃgṛhītatvādeṣāmabhāve tadabhāvaḥ | 4.11 |

atītānāgataṃ svarūpato ‘styadhvabhedāddharmāṇām | 4.12 |

te vyaktasūkṣmā guṇātmānaḥ | 4.13 |

pariṇāmaikatvādvastutattvam | 4.14 |

vastusāmye cittabhedāttayorvibhaktaḥ panthāḥ | 4.15 |

na caikacittatantraṃ cedvastu tadapramāṇakaṃ tadā kiṃ syāt | 4.16 |

taduparāgāpekṣitvāccittasya vastu jñātājñātam | 4.17 |

sadā jñātāścittavṛttayastatprabhoḥ puruṣasyāpariṇāmitvāt | 4.18 |

na tatsvābhāsaṃ dṛśyatvāt | 4.19 |

ekasamaye cobhayānavadhāraṇam | 4.20 |

cittāntaradṛśye buddhibuddheratiprasaṅgaḥ smṛtisaṃkaraśca | 4.21 |

citerapratisaṃkramāyāstadākārāpattau svabuddhisaṃvedanam | 4.22 |

draṣṭṛdṛśyoparaktaṃ cittaṃ sarvārtham | 4.23 |

tadasaṃkhyeyavāsanābhiścitramapi parārthaṃ saṃhatyakāritvāt | 4.24 |

viśeṣadarśina ātmabhāvabhāvanānivṛttiḥ | 4.25 |

tadā vivekanimnaṃ kaivalyaprāgbhāraṃ cittam | 4.26 |

tacchidreṣu pratyayāntarāṇi saṃskārebhyaḥ | 4.27 |

hānameṣāṃ kleśavaduktam | 4.28 |

prasaṃkhyāne 'pyakusīdasya sarvathā vivekakhyāterdharmameghaḥ samādhiḥ | 4.29 |

tataḥ kleśakarmanivṛttiḥ | 4.30 |

tadā sarvāvaraṇamalāpetasya jñānasyānantyājjñeyamalpam | 4.31 |

tataḥ kṛtārthānāṃ pariṇāmakramasamāptirguṇānām | 4.32 |

kṣaṇapratiyogī pariṇāmāparāntanirgrāhyaḥ kramaḥ | 4.33 |

puruṣārthaśūnyānāṃ guṇānāṃ pratiprasavaḥ kaivalyaṃ svarūpapratiṣṭhā vā citiśaktiriti | 4.34 |

Acknowledgments

First, I would like to thank Sonia Nelson, David Frawley (Vāmadeva Śāstri), and Vyaas Houston, who selflessly shared their knowledge and experience with me for many years. I am very grateful to you all.

Thanks are also due to those who took the time to proofread the text: Tias Little, Linda Spackman, and Sean Tebor.

And a special thank you to my wife, Margo, who not only proofread the text, but did anything and everything to support me through to completion.

Appendix A

THE *YOGA SŪTRA-S*
Translation Outline

This format allows us to see a bird's eye view of the text. Sūtra-s are grouped and indented so we can quickly ascertain what each section of the text is about.

Chapter 1
COMPLETE ATTENTION

Yoga

1 Here begins the instruction of yoga.
2 Yoga is the stilling (nirodha) of fluctuations (vṛtti-s) in the heart-mind (citta).
3 Then (in the state of yoga) the radiant seer (is seen clearly) resting in its own form.
4 Otherwise (not in yoga) we are identified with the fluctuations (vṛtti-s).

Vṛtti-s

5 Fluctuations (vṛtti-s) are fivefold (and can be) afflicting or nonafflicting.
6 They are correct evaluation, misperception, imagination, sleep, and the act of memory.
7 Pramāṇa: The correct ways to evaluate what we perceive are direct experience, inference, and reliable testimony.
8 Viparyaya: Misperception is perceiving an object incorrectly, thinking it is something else.
9 Vikalpa: Imagination is without an object, relying on knowledge from words or language.
10 Nidrā: Sleep is a tamasic mental activity supported by the absence of presented thoughts.
11 Smṛti: The act of memory is the retention of an experienced object.

Abhyāsa and Vairāgya

12 The stilling (nirodha) of those (vṛtti-s) is due to diligent practice (abhyāsa) and unattached awareness (vairāgya).
13 Abhyāsa is the effort put forth to maintain a point of focus.
14 Abhyāsa becomes firmly established when pursued with eagerness, sincerity, and continuity for a long time.
15 Vairāgya is a state in which the heart-mind no longer thirsts for objects perceivable by the senses, heard about, or read.
16 The higher (and more subtle vairāgya) is the nonclinging to the guṇa-s due to the realization of one's individual Self.

Samādhi

17 Saṃprajñāta-samādhi (complete mastery of an object) occurs from comprehending it on four levels:
Vitarka: Logical reasoning
Vicāra: Subtle reflection
Ānanda: The joy of deeper understanding
Asmitā: Completely identifying with it (knowing it "in your bones").
18 Asaṃprajñāta-samādhi (beyond saṃprajñāta) is preceded by diligent practice (abhyāsa) on the cessation of presented thoughts (pratyaya), and still contains residual saṃskāra-s.

19 For those who innately know yoga, it is also preceded by one's inclination toward existing.
20 For most people, it is also preceded by faith, vitality, (strong and sustained) memory, samādhi, then deep insight.
21 Intense momentum of practice and faith accelerate them toward samādhi.
22 Their level of practice or faith (mild, medium or extraordinary) also makes a difference.
23 Or because of īśvara-praṇidhāna (seeing the same light of knowledge in all beings).

Īśvara

24 Īśvara is a distinct (and separate) Puruṣa, in no way connected to the storehouse of ripened karma-s and kleśa-s.
25 There, the seed of all-knowing is beyond compare.
26 Īśvara represents the eternal teachings, available to those in the past, present, and future.
27 The spoken expression of Īśvara is praṇava.
28 Repeating that (praṇava) leads us to understand the meaning of Īśvara.
29 From that our consciousness goes inward and the distractions to practice (antarāya-s) disappear.

Antarāya-s

30 The obstacles to practice are
Disease
Apathy
Doubt
Carelessness
Lethargy
Temptation
Erroneous Views
Ungroundedness
Regression
31 The accompanying disruptions are
Suffering
Negative thinking
Trembling of the body
(Disturbed) inhalation and exhalation
32 The obstacles and their effects can be prevented by diligent practice (abhyāsa) focused on one thing (tattva).

Citta-Prasādana

33 The purification of our heart-mind field of consciousness (citta) occurs from an attitude of
Friendship when encountering happiness
Compassion when encountering suffering
Gladness when encountering virtue
Neutrality when encountering vice
34 Or from exhalation and retention of the prāṇa (through prāṇāyāma).
35 Or from the development of finer sensory perceptions (results in) maintaining steadiness of mind.
36 Or from perception that is free from sorrow and filled with light (sattvic).
37 Or when the heart-mind (is focused on) an object without rāga (the kleśa).
38 Or when focused on an object supported by the knowledge from dreams or deep sleep.
39 Or due to dhyāna (meditation) on whatever we like (and has the sattva quality).
40 Once the heart-mind is clarified, its realm of perception spans the smallest objects to the largest.

Samāpatti—Stages of Sabīja-Samādhi

41 When the (heart-mind's) vṛtti-s have been reduced, (it acts) like a flawless gemstone in terms of the perceiver, act of perceiving, and the object of perception. Samāpatti is the (gradual) saturation of that (heart-mind) due to focusing on that (object).
42 Savitarka "with thought"
Mixed with words, meaning, and conceptual knowledge
43 Nirvitarka "beyond thought"
When the memory has been completely purified, the object alone appears (as a reflection in the heart-mind, which is) as if empty of its own form
44 Savicāra "with inward reflection"
Same as savitarka, but for subtle objects
Nirvicāra "beyond inward reflection"
Same as nirvitarka, but for subtle objects
45 The subtlety of objects traces back to unmanifest matter (aliṅga).
46 Only those (aforementioned kinds of samāpatti constitute) sabīja-samādhi (samādhi involving an object).

Nirvicāra-Samāpatti

47 Purity of the inner instruments of perception. (Sattva predominates over rajas and tamas in the buddhi.)
48 Prajñā (deep insight) bears the actual truth. We see all aspects of the object clearly and accurately.
49 The scope of this prajñā is much broader and involves direct perception (pratyakṣa) rather than inference or testimony.

50 The saṃskāra born from that (prajñā) inhibits other saṃskāra-s.

Nirbīja-Samādhi

51 Seedless samādhi occurs when nirodha of even that (saṃskāra of prajñā) happens due to the nirodha of all (saṃskāra-s).

Chapter 2
PRACTICE

Kriyā-Yoga

1 Kriyā-yoga consists of tapas, svādhyāya, and īśvara-praṇidhāna.
2 Purpose is to weaken the mental/emotional afflictions (kleśa-s) and experience samādhi.

Kleśa-s

3 The kleśa-s are
Avidyā (unawareness)
Asmitā (egotism)
Rāga (clinging to past pleasure)
Dveṣa (clinging to past pain)
Abhiniveśa (fear of death)
4 Avidyā is a field for the others, which can be dormant, weakly active, intermittent, or strongly active.
5 (Avidyā is falsely) identifying the impermanent, impure, suffering nonself (which constitutes Prakṛti) as the permanent, pure, happy Self (which describes Puruṣa).
6 Asmitā, "I am-ness," makes us think that our decision-making power is the same as the unchanging witness consciousness.
7 Rāga is holding on to past pleasure.
8 Dveṣa is holding on to past pain.
9 Abhiniveśa (fear of death) is strong in everyone, as our essence of experience is carried along from lifetime to lifetime.

Overcoming the Kleśa-s

10 Those (kleśa-s), when subtle, are to be removed by pratiprasava (the reverse of how they were produced).
11 The vṛtti-s of those kleśa-s (kliṣṭa-vṛtti-s) are to be overcome by dhyāna (meditation).

Cause and Effects of the Kleśa-s

12 The source of the kleśa-s is the karmāśaya (collection of past impressions resulting from past actions), experienced in seen and unseen births.
13 When the karmāśaya is present, it ripens as our birth class, life span, and life experience.
14 Those (birth class, life span, and life experience) result in joy or sorrow, depending on whether they result in actions that are virtuous (positive/helpful) or nonvirtuous (negative/harmful).

Duḥkha (Suffering)

15 To a person with discrimination, everything in the manifest world is painful (duḥkha) [compared to the unchanging inner light of awareness] due to the naturally conflicting activities of the guṇa-s and through the suffering caused by (unintended) change, craving, or habitual patterns.
16 Future suffering is avoidable.

Draṣṭṛ and Dṛśya (Seer and Seeable)

17 The false identification of the seer as the seeable causes suffering.
18 The seeable has the (dual) purpose of experience and emancipation, consists of the elements and sensory organs, and has the qualities of light (sattva-guṇa), activity (rajas-guṇa), and inertia (tamas-guṇa).
19 The stages of the guṇa-s are specific (five elements, five sense organs, five action organs, and the mind), non-specific (five sense objects, ego, and buddhi), primary matter (mahat), and unmanifest (Prakṛti).
20 The seer only sees, and remains pure even when watching thoughts in the buddhi.
21 The seeable exists only for the purpose of that (seer).
22 For one whose purpose is done (awareness of their inner Puruṣa is present), (the seeable seems to) disappear, even though it does not actually disappear since it is common to others.
23 Saṃyoga (thinking that what changes is the same as what does not change) causes suffering that leads us to inquire as to the true nature of each.
24 Lack of awareness (avidyā) is the cause of saṃyoga.
25 When avidyā goes away, saṃyoga disappears, and kaivalya (aloneness) happens.

Viveka-Khyāti
(Discriminating Perception)

26 Mindful and continuous discriminating perception (viveka-khyāti) is the way to the goal (kaivalya).

27 Prajñā (insight) of that (viveka-khyāti) is the final, sevenfold stage.

28 From practicing the (eight) limbs of yoga, when impurities are eliminated, (we experience) the light of knowledge leading to viveka-khyāti.

Eight Limbs of Yoga

29 The eight limbs are
Yama (social ethics)
Niyama (personal self-care)
Āsana (physical exercises)
Prāṇāyāma (breath regulation)
Pratyāhāra (focusing attention away from external objects)
Dhāraṇā (choosing what to focus on)
Dhyāna (maintaining the focus)
Samādhi (assimilation of the object of focus)

30 Yama-s:
Ahiṃsā (nonviolence)
Satya (truthfulness)
Asteya (not taking from others)
Brahmacarya (conservation of vital energy)
Aparigraha (nonhoarding)

31 They are a great vow that is universal and not limited by social class, place, time, or circumstance.

32 Niyama-s:
Śauca (cleanliness)
Santoṣa (contentment)
Tapas (practice causing positive change)
Svādhyāya (study by and of oneself)
Īśvara-praṇidhāna (humility and faith)

33 Pratipakṣa-Bhāvana
When disturbed by thoughts or events opposed to the yama-s, we should act according to the yama-s.

34 Vitarka-s, violence, etc. (the opposites of all the yama-s) whether done, caused, or consented to, whether mild, moderate, or excessive, are preceded by greed, anger, or delusion, and result in endless suffering and ignorance. Thus (incentive to practice) the opposite attitude.

Results of Yama-s

35 Ahiṃsā: In the presence of one practicing nonviolence, hostility cannot exist.

36 Satya: Truthfulness secures confidence in the results of an action.

37 Asteya: Prosperity comes when we do not steal.

38 Brahmacarya: Vitality is gained when sexual energy is conserved and directed inward.

39 Aparigraha: When no longer grasping for things, we discover why we were born.

Results of Niyama-s

40 Śauca: From cleanliness, a disfavor of our body and of contact with other (bodies) and

41 The purity of sattva, a happy mind, one-pointedness, mastery over the senses, and readiness for seeing the (inner) self.

42 Santoṣa: From contentment, unexcelled happiness.

43 Tapas: Perfection of the body and sensory organs is from the destruction of impurities due to tapas.

44 Svādhyāya: By observing ourself in action, we can connect with their higher truth (iṣṭa-devatā).

45 Īśvara-praṇidhāna: samādhi is experienced from surrendering the results of action to, and deeply respecting, the inner, universal light of knowledge.

Āsana

46 Āsana (sitting) is (should be) stable and comfortable.

47 Becomes stable and comfortable due to samāpatti on the infinite and relaxed effort.

48 Then we are not distracted by the pairs of opposites (heat/cold, pleasure/pain, etc.).

Prāṇayāma

49 Once the sitting posture is stable and comfortable, then the regulation of breath is cutting off the movements of inhalation and exhalation (so the breath is still).

50 The external, internal, and suspended movements (of the breath), when observed as to location, duration, and number, (can become) long and subtle.

51 The fourth (kind of breathing) transcends external and internal objects.

52 From the stillness of prāṇa, that which covers the light (avidyā) disappears.

53 And readiness of the mind for dhāraṇā.

Pratyāhāra

54 Turning off sensory inputs is disconnecting with external objects by directing the attention inward, following the true nature of the heart-mind.

55 From that, perfect mastery of the sensory organs.

Chapter 3
EXTRAORDINARY POWERS

Dhāraṇā (choosing a place of focus)

1 Dhāraṇā is choosing a focus and directing the attention there.

Dhyāna (continuously focusing)

2 There (in dhāraṇā), dhyāna is the continuous flow (of attention) on a single thought (pratyaya).

Samādhi (complete attention)

3 That (dhyāna) becomes samādhi when the object alone is reflected in the heart-mind and subject and object seem the same.

Saṃyama (turning inward)

4 Saṃyama is the (previous) three (focused in) one place.
5 Mastery leads to the splendor of deep insight.
6 Its application occurs in (sequential) stages.
7 Is an inner limb (relative) to the previous (five limbs).
8 Is an outer limb relative to the seedless (nirbīja-samādhi).

Pariṇāma-s (transformations)

9 When the saṃskāra-s fueling an active heart-mind are subdued, and the saṃskāra-s helping a still mind arise, the association of the heart-mind with the moment of stillness is nirodha-pariṇāma.
10 The tranquil flow of that (heart-mind in stillness) is from the saṃskāra (of nirodha).
11 As attention toward all objects decreases and a one-pointed state of mind arises, the transformation into samādhi takes place.
12 When the past thoughts (pratyaya-s) are the same as the present thoughts, the transformation into a one-pointed heart-mind occurs.
13 This explains the changes taking place in gross matter (sensory organs and elements) in terms of characteristic form, time, and outward condition of the form.
14 That which continues unchanged through past, present, and future characteristic forms is the substratum.
15 The difference in sequence is the reason for the difference in transformations.

Powers from Saṃyama

16 From saṃyama on the three transformations (3.13)
Knowledge of past and future.
17 The confusion of words, objects, and ideas is from wrongly overlapping one upon the other. From saṃyama on the distinction among those
Knowledge of the language of all beings.
18 From direct perception of past impressions
Knowledge of previous births.
19 From direct perception of a current thought (pratyaya)
Knowledge of another's heart-mind.
20 The supporting object of that thought (of another) is not known because it was not the object of concentration.
21 From saṃyama on the form of the body, when its ability to be seen is suspended (and) light is cut off from the eyes
Invisibility.
22 From saṃyama on how fast karma bears fruit, or by omens
Knowledge of time of death.
23 (From saṃyama) on friendship, etc. (1.33)
Strengths
24 (From saṃyama) on strengths (3.23)
The strengths, etc. of an elephant.
25 By projecting the light of pravṛtti (1.36)
Knowledge of objects subtle, hidden, or distant.
26 From saṃyama on the sun
Knowledge of all realms.
27 (From saṃyama) on the moon
Knowledge of organization of the stars.
28 (From saṃyama) on the pole star
Knowledge of the motion (of other stars).
29 (From saṃyama) on the navel cakra
Knowledge of organization of the body.
30 (From saṃyama) on the hollow in the throat.
Ending of hunger and thirst.
31 (From saṃyama) on the tortoise energy channel
Steadiness.
32 (From saṃyama) on the light at top of head
Vision of a perfected being.
33 *Or* from an intuitive flash
All (knowledge).
34 (From saṃyama) on the heart
Complete knowledge of the heart-mind.

35 Experience is a pratyaya that does not distinguish between sattva (a sattvic buddhi) and Puruṣa, (which are) absolutely distinct. From saṃyama on that which has its own purpose (Puruṣa), as opposed to that whose purpose is for another (sattva)
Knowledge of Puruṣa.

36 From that (knowledge of Puruṣa—3.35)
Flash of illumination and suprasensory hearing, touch, sight, taste, and smell.

37 These are obstacles to samādhi (though) accomplishments to a very active state of mind.

38 From loosening the cause of bondage (to the body) and experiencing (how the energy) of the heart-mind circulates
Entry into (possession of) another body.

39 From mastery of udāna (upward-moving energy in the body)
Not getting stuck in water, mud, thorns, etc., and the ability to die at will.

40 From mastery of samāna (energy that maintains equilibrium in the body)
Radiance.

41 From saṃyama on the relationship between hearing and space
Divine hearing.

42 From saṃyama on the relationship between body and space, and samāpatti with lightweight cotton
Travel through space.

43 From saṃyama on the great out-of-body state, which is a real, external vṛtti
Avidyā (the covering of light) is removed.

44 From saṃyama on (all five elements)
Gross form
Essential nature
Subtle form (tanmātra)
Guṇa composition
Purposefulness
Mastery of the five elements.

45 *Attainment of the power to become small, etc. Perfection of the body (so that) its functions are unaffected (by anything).*

46 Perfection of the body consists of beauty, gracefulness, strength, and diamond-like firmness.

47 From saṃyama on (all five sensory organs)
Process of perception
Essential nature
Individuality
Guṇa composition
Purposefulness
Mastery of the sensory organs.

48 *Quickness of the mind*
A state independent of sensory organs
Mastery over Prakṛti.

Viveka with Saṃyama

49 When we identify the distinction between Puruṣa and sattva
Supremacy over all states
Full knowledge of the heart-mind.

50 Due to vairāgya of even that distinction (3.49), upon the destruction of the detrimental seeds (kleśa-s)
Kaivalya.

51 When a heart-mind has reached this high state of consciousness, astral energies may approach and attempt to sway the heart-mind away from its focus. This is the time to maintain focus and ignore those distractions.

52 From saṃyama on a moment and its sequence

53 *Knowledge born of discernment.*
And the ability to perceive (a difference) between two seemingly identical (objects) that are otherwise indistinguishable by position in space, time, and species.

54 Transcending all objects in all conditions, without regard to their sequential appearance, true discernment is attained.

55 Upon the equal purity of Puruṣa and sattva (buddhi), kaivalya.

Chapter 4
PERMANENT ONENESS

Other Ways to Attain Powers

1 The siddhi-s (special abilities from chapter 3) can be attained from
Genetic inheritance
Herbal medicine
Mantra (chanting sounds with specific effects)
Tapas (practicing with effort)
Samādhi (same as saṃyama here).

Change (Pariṇāma)

2 Matter changes from one state into another state from the abundant flow of nature's forces.

3 The causes of natural processes do not of themselves drive change, but cause obstacles to part so everything will flow without resistance.

Citta (Heart-mind Field)

4 Individual heart-minds are molded by our sense of identity (asmitā) and by other personalities we contact.

5 While separate activities (occur in different heart-minds), one heart-mind is the director of many (individual ones).

6 A heart-mind focused in meditation (dhyāna) does not produce any habitual impressions (saṃskāra-s).

Karma, Saṃskāra, Vāsanā

7 The actions of a yogin are neither white nor black (i.e., transcend good or bad, right or wrong). (The actions) of others are threefold:
White (positive/good/right)
Black (negative/bad/wrong)
Gray (neutral).

8 From the fruition of those threefold actions
subtle residue (vāsanā-s)

9 Saṃskāra and memory are forever linked, even as vāsanā-s through birth class, place, or time.

10 Those vāsanā-s have always existed, due to the never-ending will to live.

11 Vāsanā-s continue due to
Cause (avidyā)
Resulting effect (memory formed)
Container (citta)
Supporting objects

12 Past (as memories) and future (as potential) exist in their fundamental forms due to the different paths of dharma-s.

13 Those forms (dharma-s) are subtle or manifest (and) are composed of the guṇa-s (sattva, rajas, and tamas).

14 The essence of an object is due to the uniqueness of (its) transformations.

Mechanics of the Citta

15 Even though objects are actually the same, because of separate heart-minds, the way an object *is* may be different from what the heart-mind thinks it is.

16 If an object was dependent on one individual heart-mind, and that heart-mind was not correctly evaluating the object, then what would the object become?

17 Because the heart-mind's perception of an object is dependent on the object's reflected color, an object is either known or unknown.

18 The citta-vṛtti-s are always known due to the changelessness of their master, Puruṣa, who is quietly witnessing.

19 That (citta) is not self-luminous due to (its being) a seeable object. Only the seer is self-luminous.

20 The citta and its object cannot be cognized (by the citta) simultaneously.

21 (If one) citta was perceivable (illuminated) by another citta, (it would result in) an infinite regression of buddhi upon buddhi, and confusion of memories.

22 When the buddhi part of citta reflects the form of an object, the seer (Puruṣa) is aware of the change because of its changeless nature.

23 The citta acts as a middleman, colored by the seeable and the seer, thus serving the purpose of all.

24 That (citta), even though varicolored by countless vāsanā-s, (exists for) the purpose of another because of its activity of collaboration.

Steps Leading to Kaivalya

25 For one who can perceive the distinction (between a sattvic buddhi and Puruṣa)
The feeling of the sense of self ceases.

26 Then the citta, oriented toward discernment, gravitates toward kaivalya.

27 In between the times of clear discernment, other heart-mind activities (intervening thoughts) are only due to (previously developed) habitual tendencies.

28 The saṃskāra-s that cause intervening thoughts to appear can be ended by pratiprasava.

29 When we are disinterested even in a higher state due to continuous and total viveka-khyāti
Dharma-megha samādhi (arises)

30 *The termination of karma-s and kleśa-s*

31 Knowledge that is free of the coatings of karma-s, kleśa-s, and saṃskāra-s, is thus unfiltered, clear, and almost unlimited.

32 The guṇa-s, having served their purpose (of experience), end their movement, causing the transformations to end as well.

33 The sequential progression of changes over time is finally understood now that the changes have ended.

34 The pratiprasava of the guṇa-s, empty of their purpose for Puruṣa, is kaivalya. In other words, the power of unconditioned consciousness is established in its own true nature.

Appendix B

THE *YOGA SŪTRA-S*
English Alphabetical Order

This format is for finding a sūtra quickly by knowing its first few syllables. When we learn the sound of each sūtra (see part 4), we can find each one easily here.

abhāvapratyayālambanā tamovṛttirnidrā | | 1.10 | |
abhyāsavairāgyābhyāṃ tannirodhaḥ | | 1.12 | |
ahiṃsāpratiṣṭhāyāṃ tatsaṃnidhau vairatyāgaḥ | | 2.35 | |
ahiṃsāsatyāsteyabrahmacaryāparigrahā yamāḥ | | 2.30 | |
anityāśuciduḥkhānātmasu nityaśucisukhātmakhyātiravidyā | | 2.5 | |
anubhūtaviṣayāsaṃpramoṣaḥ smṛtiḥ | | 1.11 | |
aparigrahasthairye janmakathaṃtāsaṃbodhaḥ | | 2.39 | |
asteyapratiṣṭhāyāṃ sarvaratnopasthānam | | 2.37 | |
atha yogānuśāsanam | | 1.1 | |
atītānāgātaṃ svarūpato 'styadhvabhedāddharmāṇām | | 4.12 | |
avidyā kṣetramuttareṣāṃ prasuptatanuvicchinnodārāṇām | | 2.4 | |
avidyāsmitārāgadveṣābhiniveśāḥ kleśāḥ | | 2.3 | |
bahirakalpitā vṛttirmahāvidehā tataḥ prakāśāvaraṇakṣayaḥ | | 3.43 | |
bāhyābhyantarastambhavṛttirdeśakālasaṃkhyābhiḥ paridṛṣṭo dīrghasūkṣmaḥ | | 2.50 | |
bāhyābhyantaraviṣayākṣepī caturthaḥ | | 2.51 | |
baleṣu hastibalādīni | | 3.24 | |
bandhakāraṇaśaithilyātpracārasaṃvedanācca cittasya paraśarīrāveśaḥ | | 3.38 | |
bhavapratyayo videhaprakṛtilayānām | | 1.19 | |
bhuvanajñānaṃ sūrye saṃyamāt | | 3.26 | |
brahmacaryapratiṣṭhāyāṃ vīryalābhaḥ | | 2.38 | |
candre tārāvyūhajñānam | | 3.27 | |
citerapratisaṃkramāyāstadākārāpattau svabuddhisaṃvedanam | | 4.22 | |
cittāntaradṛśye buddhibuddheratiprasaṅgaḥ smṛtisaṃkaraśca | | 4.21 | |
deśabandhaścittasya dhāraṇā | | 3.1 | |
dhāraṇāsu ca yogyatā manasaḥ | | 2.53 | |
dhruve tadgatijñānam | | 3.28 | |
dhyānaheyāstadvṛttayaḥ | | 2.11 | |
draṣṭā dṛśimātraḥ śuddho 'pi pratyayānupaśyaḥ | | 2.20 | |
draṣṭṛdṛśyayoḥ saṃyogo heyahetuḥ | | 2.17 | |
draṣṭṛdṛśyoparaktaṃ cittaṃ sarvārtham | | 4.23 | |
dṛgdarśanaśaktyorekātmatevāsmitā | | 2.6 | |
dṛṣṭānuśravikaviṣayavitṛṣṇasya vaśīkārasaṃjñā vairāgyam | | 1.15 | |
duḥkhānuśayī dveṣaḥ | | 2.8 | |
duḥkhadaurmanasyāṅgamejayatvaśvāsapraśvāsā vikṣepasahabhuvaḥ | | 1.31 | |

ekasamaye cobhayānavadhāraṇam | | 4.20 | |
etayaiva savicārā nirvicārā ca sūkṣmaviṣayā vyākhyātā | | 1.44 | |
etena bhūtendriyeṣu dharmalakṣaṇāvasthāpariṇāmā vyākhyātāḥ | | 3.13 | |
grahaṇasvarūpāsmitānvayārthavattvasaṃyamādindriyajayaḥ | | 3.47 | |
hānameṣāṃ kleśavaduktam | | 4.28 | |
hetuphalāśrayālambanaiḥ saṃgṛhītatvādeṣāmabhāve tadabhāvaḥ | | 4.11 | |
heyaṃ duḥkhamanāgatam | | 2.16 | |
hṛdaye cittasaṃvit | | 3.34 | |
īśvarapraṇidhānādvā | | 1.23 | |
janmauṣadhimantratapaḥsamādhijāḥ siddhayaḥ | | 4.1 | |
jātideśakālasamayānavacchinnāḥ sarvabhaumā mahāvratam | | 2.31 | |
jātideśakālavyavahitānāmapyānantaryaṃ smṛtisaṃskārayorekarūpatvāt | | 4.9 | |
jātilakṣaṇadeśairanyatānavacchedāttulyayostataḥ pratipattiḥ | | 3.53 | |
jātyantarapariṇāmaḥ prakṛtyāpūrāt | | 4.2 | |
kaṇṭhakūpe kṣutpipāsānivṛttiḥ | | 3.30 | |
karmāśuklākṛṣṇaṃ yoginastrividhamitareṣām | | 4.7 | |
kāyākāsayoḥ saṃbandhasaṃyamāllaghutūlasamāpatteścākāśagamanam | | 3.42 | |
kāyarūpasaṃyamāttadgrāhyaśaktistambhe cakṣuḥprakāśāsaṃprayoge 'ntardhānam | | 3.21 | |
kāyendriyasiddhiraśuddhikṣayāttapasaḥ | | 2.43 | |
kleśakarmavipākāśayairaparāmṛṣṭaḥ puruṣaviśeṣa īśvaraḥ | | 1.24 | |
kleśamūlaḥ karmāśayo dṛṣṭādṛṣṭajanmavedanīyaḥ | | 2.12 | |
kramānyatvaṃ pariṇāmānyatve hetuḥ | | 3.15 | |
kṛtārthaṃ prati naṣṭamapyanaṣṭaṃ tadanyasādhāraṇatvāt | | 2.22 | |
kṣaṇapratiyogī pariṇāmāparāntanirgrāhyaḥ kramaḥ | | 4.33 | |
kṣaṇatatkramayoḥ saṃyamādvivekajaṃ jñānam | | 3.52 | |
kṣīṇavṛtterabhijātasyeva maṇergrahītṛgrahaṇagrāhyeṣu tatsthatadañjanatā samāpattiḥ | | 1.41 | |
kūrmanāḍyāṃ sthairyam | | 3.31 | |
maitrīkaruṇāmuditopekṣāṇāṃ sukhaduḥkhapuṇyāpuṇyaviṣayāṇāṃ bhāvanātaścittaprasādanam | | 1.33 | |
maitryādiṣu balāni | | 3.23 | |
mṛdumadhyādhimātratvāttato 'pi viśeṣaḥ | | 1.22 | |
mūrdhajyotiṣi siddhadarśanam | | 3.32 | |
na ca tatsālambanaṃ tasyāviṣayībhūtatvāt | | 3.20 | |
na caikacittatantraṃ cedvastu tadapramāṇakaṃ tadā kiṃ syāt | | 4.16 | |
na tatsvābhāsaṃ dṛśyatvāt | | 4.19 | |
nābhicakre kāyavyūhajñānam | | 3.29 | |
nimittamaprayojakaṃ prakṛtīnāṃ varaṇabhedastu tataḥ kṣetrikavat | | 4.3 | |
nirmāṇacittānyasmitāmātrāt | | 4.4 | |
nirvicāravaiśāradye 'dhyātmaprasādaḥ | | 1.47 | |
paramāṇuparamamahattvānto 'sya vaśīkāraḥ | | 1.40 | |
pariṇāmaikatvādvastutattvam | | 4.14 | |
pariṇāmatāpasaṃskāraduḥkhairguṇavṛttivirodhācca duḥkhameva sarvaṃ vivekinaḥ | | 2.15 | |
pariṇāmatrayasaṃyamādatītānāgatajñānam | | 3.16 | |
pracchardhanavidhāraṇābhyāṃ vā prāṇasya | | 1.34 | |
prakāśakriyāsthitiśīlaṃ bhūtendriyātmakaṃ bhogāpavargārthaṃ dṛśyam | | 2.18 | |
pramāṇaviparyayavikalpanidrāsmṛtayaḥ | | 1.6 | |
prasaṃkhyāne 'pyakusīdasya sarvathā vivekakhyāterdharmameghaḥ samādhiḥ | | 4.29 | |
prātibhādvā sarvam | | 3.33 | |
pratyakṣānumānāgamāḥ pramāṇāni | | 1.7 | |
pratyayasya paracittajñānam | | 3.19 | |
pravṛttibhede prayojakaṃ cittamekamanekeṣām | | 4.5 | |
pravṛttyālokanyāsātsūkṣmavyavahitaviprakṛṣṭajñānam | | 3.25 | |
prayatnaśaithilyānantasamāpattibhyām | | 2.47 | |
puruṣārthaśūnyānāṃ guṇānāṃ pratiprasavaḥ kaivalyaṃ svarūpapratiṣṭhā vā citiśaktiriti | | 4.34 | |
ṛtambharā tatra prajñā | | 1.48 | |
rūpalāvaṇyabalavajrasaṃhananatvāni kāyasaṃpat | | 3.46 | |
sa eṣa pūrveṣāmapi guruḥ kālenānavacchedāt | | 1.26 | |

sa tu dīrghakālanairantaryasatkārādarāsevito dṛḍhabhūmiḥ || 1.14 ||
śabdajñānānupātī vastuśūnyo vikalpaḥ || 1.9 ||
śabdārthapratyayānāmitaretarādhyāsātsaṅkarastatpravibhāgasaṃyamātsarvabhūtarutajñānam || 3.17 ||
sadā jñātāścittavṛttayastatprabhoḥ puruṣasyāpariṇāmitvāt || 4.18 ||
samādhibhāvanārthaḥ kleśatanūkaraṇārthaśca || 2.2 ||
samādhisiddhirīśvarapraṇidhānāt || 2.45 ||
samānajayājjvalanam || 3.40 ||
saṃskārasākṣātkaraṇātpūrvajātijñānam || 3.18 ||
śāntoditāvyapadeśyadharmānupātī dharmī || 3.14 ||
santoṣādanuttamaḥ sukhalābhaḥ || 2.42 ||
sarvārthataikāgratayoḥ kṣayodayau cittasya samādhipariṇāmaḥ || 3.11 ||
sati mūle tadvipāko jātyāyurbhogāḥ || 2.13 ||
sattvapuruṣānyatākhyātimātrasya sarvabhāvādhiṣṭhātṛtvaṃ sarvajñātṛtvaṃ ca || 3.49 ||
sattvapuruṣayoḥ śuddhisāmye kaivalyam || 3.55 ||
sattvapuruṣayoratyantāsaṃkīrṇayoḥ pratyayāviśeṣo bhogaḥ parārthatvātsvārthasaṃyamātpuruṣajñānam || 3.35 ||
sattvaśuddhisaumanasyaikāgryendriyajayātmadarśanayogyatvāni ca || 2.41 ||
satyapratiṣṭhāyāṃ kriyāphalāśrayatvam || 2.36 ||
śaucasantoṣatapaḥsvādhyāyeśvarapraṇidhānāni niyamāḥ || 2.32 ||
śaucātsvāṅgajugupsā parairasaṃsargaḥ || 2.40 ||
smṛtipariśuddhau svarūpaśūnyevārthamātranirbhāsā nirvitarkā || 1.43 ||
sopakramaṃ nirupakramaṃ ca karma tatsaṃyamādaparāntajñānamariṣṭebhyo vā || 3.22 ||
śraddhāvīryasmṛtisamādhiprajñāpūrvaka itareṣām || 1.20 ||
śrotrākāśayoḥ saṃbandhasaṃyamāddivyaṃ śrotram || 3.41 ||
śrutānumānaprajñābhyāmanyaviṣayā viśeṣārthatvāt || 1.49 ||
sthānyupanimantraṇe saṅgasmayākaraṇaṃ punaraniṣṭaprasaṅgāt || 3.51 ||
sthirasukhamāsanam || 2.46 ||
sthūlasvarūpasūkṣmānvayārthavattvasaṃyamādbhūtajayaḥ || 3.44 ||
sukhānuśayī rāgaḥ || 2.7 ||
sūkṣmaviṣayatvaṃ cāliṅgaparyavasānam || 1.45 ||
svādhyāyādiṣṭadevatāsaṃprayogaḥ || 2.44 ||
svapnanidrājñānālambanaṃ vā || 1.38 ||
svarasavāhī viduṣo 'pi samārūḍho 'bhiniveśaḥ || 2.9 ||
svasvāmiśaktyoḥ svarūpopalabdhihetuḥ saṃyogaḥ || 2.23 ||
svaviṣayāsaṃprayoge cittasya svarūpānukāra ivendriyāṇāṃ pratyāhāraḥ || 2.54 ||
tā eva sabījaḥ samādhiḥ || 1.46 ||
tacchidreṣu pratyayāntarāṇi saṃskārebhyaḥ || 4.27 ||
tadā draṣṭuḥ svarūpe 'vasthānam || 1.3 ||
tadā sarvāvaraṇamalāpetasya jñānasyānantyājjñeyamalpam || 4.31 ||
tadā vivekanimnaṃ kaivalyaprāgbhāraṃ cittam || 4.26 ||
tadabhāvātsaṃyogābhāvo hānaṃ taddṛśeḥ kaivalyam || 2.25 ||
tadapi bahiraṅgaṃ nirbījasya || 3.8 ||
tadartha eva dṛṣyasyātmā || 2.21 ||
tadasaṃkhyeyavāsanābhiścitramapi parārthaṃ saṃhatyakāritvāt || 4.24 ||
tadevārthamātranirbhāsaṃ svarūpaśūnyamiva samādhiḥ || 3.3 ||
taduparāgāpekṣitvāccittasya vastu jñātājñātam || 4.17 ||
tadvairāgyādapi doṣabījakṣaye kaivalyam || 3.50 ||
tajjaḥ saṃskāro 'nyasaṃskārapratibandhī || 1.50 ||
tajjapastadarthabhāvanam || 1.28 ||
tajjayātprajñālokaḥ || 3.5 ||
tapaḥsvādhyāyeśvarapraṇidhānāni kriyāyogaḥ || 2.1 ||
tārakaṃ sarvaviṣayaṃ sarvathāviṣayamakramaṃ ceti vivekajaṃ jñānam || 3.54 ||
tāsāmanāditvaṃ cāśiṣo nityatvāt || 4.10 ||
tasminsati śvāsapraśvāsayorgativicchedaḥ prāṇāyāmaḥ || 2.49 ||
tasya bhūmiṣu viniyogaḥ || 3.6 ||
tasya heturavidyā || 2.24 ||

tasya praśāntavāhitā saṃskārāt || 3.10 ||
tasya saptadhā prāntabhūmiḥ prajñā || 2.27 ||
tasya vācakaḥ praṇavaḥ || 1.27 ||
tasyāpi nirodhe sarvanirodhānnirbījaḥ samādhiḥ || 1.51 ||
tataḥ kleśakarmanivṛttiḥ || 4.30 ||
tataḥ kṛtārthānāṃ pariṇāmakramasamāptirguṇānām || 4.32 ||
tataḥ kṣīyate prakāśāvaraṇam || 2.52 ||
tataḥ paramā vaśyatendriyāṇām || 2.55 ||
tataḥ prātibhaśrāvaṇavedanādarśāsvādavārttā jāyante || 3.36 ||
tataḥ pratyakcetanādhigamo 'pyantarāyābhāvaśca || 1.29 ||
tataḥ punaḥ śāntoditau tulyapratyayau cittasyaikāgratāpariṇāmaḥ || 3.12 ||
tatastadvipākānuguṇānāmevābhivyaktirvāsanānām || 4.8 ||
tato dvandvānabhighātaḥ || 2.48 ||
tato 'ṇimādiprādurbhāvaḥ kāyasaṃpattaddharmānabhighātaśca || 3.45 ||
tato manojavitvaṃ vikaraṇabhāvaḥ pradhānajayaśca || 3.48 ||
tatparaṃ puruṣakhyāterguṇavaitṛṣṇyam || 1.16 ||
tatpratiṣedhārthamekatattvābhyāsaḥ || 1.32 ||
tatra dhyānajamanāśayam || 4.6 ||
tatra niratiśayaṃ sarvajñabījam || 1.25 ||
tatra pratyayaikatānatā dhyānam || 3.2 ||
tatra śabdārthajñānavikalpaiḥ saṃkīrṇā savitarkā samāpattiḥ || 1.42 ||
tatra sthitau yatno 'bhyāsaḥ || 1.13 ||
te hlādaparitāpaphalāḥ puṇyāpuṇyahetutvāt || 2.14 ||
te pratiprasavaheyāḥ sūkṣmāḥ || 2.10 ||
te samādhāvupasargā vyutthāne siddhayaḥ || 3.37 ||
te vyaktasūkṣmā guṇātmānaḥ || 4.13 ||
tīvrasaṃvegānāmāsannaḥ || 1.21 ||
trayamantaraṅgaṃ pūrvebhyaḥ || 3.7 ||
trayamekatra saṃyamaḥ || 3.4 ||
udānajayājjalapaṅkakaṇṭakādiṣvasaṅga utkrāntiśca || 3.39 ||
vastusāmye cittabhedāttayorvibhaktaḥ panthāḥ || 4.15 ||
viparyayo mithyājñānamatadrūpapratiṣṭham || 1.8 ||
virāmapratyayābhyāsapūrvaḥ saṃskāraśeṣo 'nyaḥ || 1.18 ||
viṣayavatī vā pravṛttirutpannā manasaḥ sthitinibandhinī || 1.35 ||
viśeṣadarśina ātmabhāvabhāvanānivṛttiḥ || 4.25 ||
viśeṣāviśeṣaliṅgamātrāliṅgāni guṇaparvāṇi || 2.19 ||
viśokā vā jyotiṣmatī || 1.36 ||
vītarāgaviṣayaṃ vā cittam || 1.37 ||
vitarkā hiṃsādayaḥ kṛtakāritānumoditā lobhakrodhamohapūrvakā mṛdumadhyādhimātrā duḥkhājñānānantaphalā iti pratipakṣabhāvanam || 2.34 ||
vitarkabādhane pratipakṣabhāvanam || 2.33 ||
vitarkavicārānandāsmitārūpānugamātsaṃprajñātaḥ || 1.17 ||
vivekakhyātiraviplavā hānopāyaḥ || 2.26 ||
vṛttayaḥ pañcatayyaḥ kliṣṭākliṣṭāḥ || 1.5 ||
vṛttisārūpyamitaratra || 1.4 ||
vyādhistyānasaṃśayapramādālasyāviratibhrāntidarśanālabdhabhūmikatvānavasthitatvāni cittavikṣepāste 'ntarāyāḥ || 1.30 ||
vyutthānanirodhasaṃskārayorabhibhavaprādurbhāvau nirodhakṣaṇacittānvayo nirodhapariṇāmaḥ || 3.9 ||
yamaniyamāsanaprāṇāyāmapratyāhāradhāraṇādhyānasamādhayo 'ṣṭāvaṅgāni || 2.29 ||
yathābhimatadhyānādvā || 1.39 ||
yogāṅgānuṣṭhānādaśuddhikṣaye jñānadīptirāvivekakhyāteḥ || 2.28 ||
yogaścittavṛttinirodhaḥ || 1.2 ||

Appendix C

THE *YOGA SŪTRA-S*
Original Sanskrit Script

This shows the *Yoga Sūtra-s* in their original state, written in the Sanskrit script called Devanāgarī.

पातञ्जलयोगदर्शनम्

१. समाधिपादः

अथ योगानुशासनम् ॥ १.१ ॥

योगश्चित्तवृत्तिनिरोधः ॥ १.२ ॥

तदा द्रष्टुः स्वरूपे ऽवस्थानम् ॥ १.३ ॥

वृत्तिसारूप्यमितरत्र ॥ १.४ ॥

वृत्तयः पञ्चतय्यः क्लिष्टाक्लिष्टाः ॥ १.५ ॥

प्रमाणविपर्ययविकल्पनिद्रास्मृतयः ॥ १.६ ॥

प्रत्यक्षानुमानागमाः प्रमाणानि ॥ १.७ ॥

विपर्ययो मिथ्याज्ञानमतद्रूपप्रतिष्ठम् ॥ १.८ ॥

शब्दज्ञानानुपाती वस्तुशून्यो विकल्पः ॥ १.९ ॥

अभावप्रत्ययालम्बना तमोवृत्तिर्निद्रा ॥ १.१० ॥

अनुभूतविषयासंप्रमोषः स्मृतिः ॥ १.११ ॥

अभ्यासवैराग्याभ्यां तन्निरोधः ॥ १.१२ ॥

तत्र स्थितौ यत्नो ऽभ्यासः ॥ १.१३ ॥

स तु दीर्घकालनैरन्तर्यसत्कारादरासेवितो दृढभूमिः ॥ १.१४ ॥

दृष्टानुश्रविकविषयवितृष्णस्य वशीकारसंज्ञा वैराग्यम् ॥ १.१५ ॥

तत्परं पुरुषख्यातेर्गुणवैतृष्ण्यम् ॥ १.१६ ॥

वितर्कविचारानन्दास्मितारूपानुगमात्संप्रज्ञातः ॥ १.१७ ॥

विरामप्रत्ययाभ्यासपूर्वः संस्कारशेषो ऽन्यः ॥ १.१८ ॥

भवप्रत्ययो विदेहप्रकृतिलयानाम् ॥ १.१९ ॥

श्रद्धावीर्यस्मृतिसमाधिप्रज्ञापूर्वक इतरेषाम् ॥ १.२० ॥

तीव्रसंवेगानामासन्नः ॥ १.२१ ॥

मृदुमध्याधिमात्रत्वात्ततो ऽपि विशेषः ॥ १.२२ ॥

ईश्वरप्रणिधानाद्वा ॥ १.२३ ॥

क्लेशकर्मविपाकाशयैरपरामृष्टः पुरुषविशेष ईश्वरः ॥ १.२४ ॥

तत्र निरतिशयं सर्वज्ञबीजम् ॥ १.२५ ॥

स एष पूर्वेषामपि गुरुः कालेनानवच्छेदात् ॥ १.२६ ॥

तस्य वाचकः प्रणवः ॥ १.२७ ॥

तज्जपस्तदर्थभावनम् ॥ १.२८ ॥

ततः प्रत्यक्चेतनाधिगमो ऽप्यन्तरायाभावश्च ॥ १.२९ ॥

व्याधिस्त्यानसंशयप्रमादालस्याविरति-
भ्रान्तिदर्शनालब्धभूमिकत्वानवस्थितत्वानि चित्तविक्षेपास्ते
ऽन्तरायाः ॥ १.३० ॥

दुःखदौर्मनस्याङ्गमेजयत्वश्वासप्रश्वासा विक्षेपसहभुवः ॥ १.३१ ॥

तत्प्रतिषेधार्थमेकतत्त्वाभ्यासः ॥ १.३२ ॥

मैत्रीकरुणामुदितोपेक्षाणां सुखदुःखपुण्यापुण्यविषयाणां
भावनातश्चित्तप्रसादनम् ॥ १.३३ ॥

प्रच्छर्धनविधारणाभ्यां वा प्राणस्य ॥ १.३४ ॥

विषयवती वा प्रवृत्तिरुत्पन्ना मनसः स्थितिनिबन्धिनी ॥ १.३५ ॥

विशोका वा ज्योतिष्मती ॥ १.३६ ॥

वीतरागविषयं वा चित्तम् ॥ १.३७ ॥

स्वप्ननिद्राज्ञानालम्बनं वा ॥ १.३८ ॥

यथाभिमतध्यानाद्वा ॥ १.३९ ॥

परमाणुपरममहत्त्वान्तो ऽस्य वशीकारः ॥ १.४० ॥

क्षीणवृत्तेरभिजातस्येव मणेर्ग्रहीतृग्रहणग्राह्येषु तत्स्थतदञ्जनता समापत्तिः ॥ १.४१ ॥

तत्र शब्दार्थज्ञानविकल्पैः संकीर्णा सवितर्का समापत्तिः ॥ १.४२ ॥

स्मृतिपरिशुद्धौ स्वरूपशून्येवार्थमात्रनिर्भासा निर्वितर्का ॥ १.४३ ॥

एतयैव सविचारा निर्विचारा च सूक्ष्मविषया व्याख्याता ॥ १.४४ ॥

सूक्ष्मविषयत्वं चालिङ्गपर्यवसानम् ॥ १.४५ ॥

ता एव सबीजः समाधिः ॥ १.४६ ॥

निर्विचारवैशारद्ये ऽध्यात्मप्रसादः ॥ १.४७ ॥

ऋतम्भरा तत्र प्रज्ञा ॥ १.४८ ॥

श्रुतानुमानप्रज्ञाभ्यामन्यविषया विशेषार्थत्वात् ॥ १.४९ ॥

तज्जः संस्कारो ऽन्यसंस्कारप्रतिबन्धी ॥ १.५० ॥

तस्यापि निरोधे सर्वनिरोधान्निर्बीजः समाधिः ॥ १.५१ ॥

२. साधनपादः

तपःस्वाध्यायेश्वरप्रणिधानानि क्रियायोगः ॥ २.१ ॥

समाधिभावनार्थः क्लेशतनूकरणार्थश्च ॥ २.२ ॥

अविद्यास्मितारागद्वेषाभिनिवेशाः क्लेशाः ॥ २.३ ॥

अविद्या क्षेत्रमुत्तरेषां प्रसुप्ततनुविच्छिन्नोदाराणाम् ॥ २.४ ॥

अनित्याशुचिदुःखानात्मसु नित्यशुचिसुखात्मख्यातिरविद्या ॥ २.५ ॥

दृग्दर्शनशक्त्योरेकात्मतेवास्मिता ॥ २.६ ॥

सुखानुशयी रागः ॥ २.७ ॥

दुःखानुशयी द्वेषः ॥ २.८ ॥

स्वरसवाही विदुषो ऽपि समारूढो ऽभिनिवेशः ॥ २.९ ॥

ते प्रतिप्रसवहेयाः सूक्ष्माः ॥ २.१० ॥

ध्यानहेयास्तद्वृत्तयः ॥ २.११ ॥

क्लेशमूलः कर्माशयो दृष्टादृष्टजन्मवेदनीयः ॥ २.१२ ॥

सति मूले तद्विपाको जात्यायुर्भोगाः ॥ २.१३ ॥

ते ह्लादपरितापफलाः पुण्यापुण्यहेतुत्वात् ॥ २.१४ ॥

परिणामतापसंस्कारदुःखैर्गुणवृत्तिविरोधाच्च दुःखमेव सर्वं विवेकिनः ॥ २.१५ ॥

हेयं दुःखमनागतम् ॥ २.१६ ॥

द्रष्टृदृश्ययोः संयोगो हेयहेतुः ॥ २.१७ ॥

प्रकाशक्रियास्थितिशीलं भूतेन्द्रियात्मकं भोगापवर्गार्थं दृश्यम् ॥ २.१८ ॥

विशेषाविशेषलिङ्गमात्रालिङ्गानि गुणपर्वाणि ॥ २.१९ ॥

द्रष्टा दृशिमात्रः शुद्धो ऽपि प्रत्ययानुपश्यः ॥ २.२० ॥

तदर्थ एव दृष्यस्यात्मा ॥ २.२१ ॥

कृतार्थं प्रति नष्टमप्यनष्टं तदन्यसाधारणत्वात् ॥ २.२२ ॥

स्वस्वामिशक्त्योः स्वरूपोपलब्धिहेतुः संयोगः ॥ २.२३ ॥

तस्य हेतुरविद्या ॥ २.२४ ॥

तदभावात्संयोगाभावो हानं तद्दृशेः कैवल्यम् ॥ २.२५ ॥

विवेकख्यातिरविप्लवा हानोपायः ॥ २.२६ ॥

तस्य सप्तधा प्रान्तभूमिः प्रज्ञा ॥ २.२७ ॥

योगाङ्गानुष्ठानादशुद्धिक्षये ज्ञानदीप्तिराविवेकख्यातेः ॥ २.२८ ॥

यमनियमासनप्राणायामप्रत्याहारधारणाध्यानसमाधयो ऽष्टावङ्गानि ॥ २.२९ ॥

अहिंसासत्यास्तेयब्रह्मचर्यापरिग्रहा यमाः ॥ २.३० ॥

जातिदेशकालसमयानवच्छिन्नाः सर्वभौमा महाव्रतम् ॥ २.३१ ॥

शौचसंतोषतपःस्वाध्यायेश्वरप्रणिधानानि नियमाः ॥ २.३२ ॥

वितर्कबाधने प्रतिपक्षभावनम् ॥ २.३३ ॥

वितर्का हिंसादयः कृतकारितानुमोदिता लोभक्रोधमोहपूर्वका मृदुमध्याधिमात्रा दुःखाज्ञानानन्तफला इति प्रतिपक्षभावनम् ॥ २.३४ ॥

अहिंसाप्रतिष्ठायां तत्संनिधौ वैरत्यागः ॥ २.३५ ॥

सत्यप्रतिष्ठायां क्रियाफलाश्रयत्वम् ॥ २.३६ ॥

अस्तेयप्रतिष्ठायां सर्वरत्नोपस्थानम् ॥ २.३७ ॥

ब्रह्मचर्यप्रतिष्ठायां वीर्यलाभः ॥ २.३८ ॥

अपरिग्रहस्थैर्ये जन्मकथंतासंबोधः ॥ २.३९ ॥

शौचात्स्वाङ्गजुगुप्सा परैरसंसर्गः ॥ २.४० ॥

सत्त्वशुद्धिसौमनस्यैकाग्र्येन्द्रियजयात्मदर्शनयोग्यत्वानि च ॥ २.४१ ॥

सन्तोषादनुत्तमः सुखलाभः ॥ २.४२ ॥

कायेन्द्रियसिद्धिरशुद्धिक्षयात्तपसः ॥ २.४३ ॥

स्वाध्यायादिष्टदेवतासंप्रयोगः ॥ २.४४ ॥

समाधिसिद्धिरीश्वरप्रणिधानात् ॥ २.४५ ॥

स्थिरसुखमासनम् ॥ २.४६ ॥

प्रयत्नशैथिल्यानन्तसमापत्तिभ्याम् ॥ २.४७ ॥

ततो द्वन्द्वानभिघातः ॥ २.४८ ॥

तस्मिन्सति श्वासप्रश्वासयोर्गतिविच्छेदः प्राणायामः ॥ २.४९ ॥

बाह्याभ्यन्तरस्तम्भवृत्तिर्देशकालसंख्याभिः परिदृष्टो दीर्घसूक्ष्मः ॥ २.५० ॥

बाह्याभ्यन्तरविषयाक्षेपी चतुर्थः ॥ २.५१ ॥

ततः क्षीयते प्रकाशावरणम् ॥ २.५२ ॥

धारणासु च योग्यता मनसः ॥ २.५३ ॥

स्वविषयासंप्रयोगे चित्तस्य स्वरूपानुकार इवेन्द्रियाणां प्रत्याहारः ॥ २.५४ ॥

ततः परमा वश्यतेन्द्रियाणाम् ॥ २.५५ ॥

३. विभूतिपादः

देशबन्धश्चित्तस्य धारणा ॥ ३.१ ॥

तत्र प्रत्ययैकतानता ध्यानम् ॥ ३.२ ॥

तदेवार्थमात्रनिर्भासं स्वरूपशून्यमिव समाधिः ॥ ३.३ ॥

त्रयमेकत्र संयमः ॥ ३.४ ॥

तज्जयात्प्रज्ञालोकः ॥ ३.५ ॥

तस्य भूमिषु विनियोगः ॥ ३.६ ॥

त्रयमन्तरङ्गं पूर्वेभ्यः ॥ ३.७ ॥

तदपि बहिरङ्गं निर्बीजस्य ॥ ३.८ ॥

व्युत्थाननिरोधसंस्कारयोरभिभवप्रादुर्भावौ निरोधक्षणचित्तान्वयो निरोधपरिणामः ॥ ३.९ ॥

तस्य प्रशान्तवाहिता संस्कारात् ॥ ३.१० ॥

सर्वार्थतैकाग्रतयोः क्षयोदयौ चित्तस्य समाधिपरिणामः ॥ ३.११ ॥

ततः पुनः शान्तोदितौ तुल्यप्रत्ययौ चित्तस्यैकाग्रतापरिणामः ॥ ३.१२ ॥

एतेन भूतेन्द्रियेषु धर्मलक्षणावस्थापरिणामा व्याख्याताः ॥ ३.१३ ॥

शान्तोदिताव्यपदेश्यधर्मानुपाती धर्मी ॥ ३.१४ ॥

क्रमान्यत्वं परिणामान्यत्वे हेतुः ॥ ३.१५ ॥

परिणामत्रयसंयमादतीतानागतज्ञानम् ॥ ३.१६ ॥

शब्दार्थप्रत्ययानामितरेतराध्यासात्सङ्करस्तत्प्रविभाग संयमात्सर्वभूतरुतज्ञानम् ॥ ३.१७ ॥

संस्कारसाक्षात्करणात्पूर्वजातिज्ञानम् ॥ ३.१८ ॥

प्रत्ययस्य परचित्तज्ञानम् ॥ ३.१९ ॥

न च तत्सालम्बनं तस्याविषयीभूतत्वात् ॥ ३.२० ॥

कायरूपसंयमात्तद्ग्राह्यशक्तिस्तम्भे चक्षुःप्रकाशासंप्रयोगे ऽन्तर्धानम् ॥ ३.२१ ॥

सोपक्रमं निरुपक्रमं च कर्म तत्संयमादपरान्तज्ञानमरिष्टेभ्यो वा ॥ ३.२२ ॥

मैत्र्यादिषु बलानि ॥ ३.२३ ॥

बलेषु हस्तिबलादीनि ॥ ३.२४ ॥

प्रवृत्त्यालोकन्यासात्सूक्ष्मव्यवहितविप्रकृष्टज्ञानम् ॥ ३.२५ ॥

भुवनज्ञानं सूर्ये संयमात् ॥ ३.२६ ॥

चन्द्रे ताराव्यूहज्ञानम् ॥ ३.२७ ॥

ध्रुवे तद्गतिज्ञानम् ॥ ३.२८ ॥

नाभिचक्रे कायव्यूहज्ञानम् ॥ ३.२९ ॥

कण्ठकूपे क्षुत्पिपासानिवृत्तिः ॥ ३.३० ॥

कूर्मनाड्यां स्थैर्यम् ॥ ३.३१ ॥

मूर्धज्योतिषि सिद्धदर्शनम् ॥ ३.३२ ॥

प्रातिभाद्वा सर्वम् ॥ ३.३३ ॥

हृदये चित्तसंवित् ॥ ३.३४ ॥

सत्त्वपुरुषयोरत्यन्तासंकीर्णयोः प्रत्ययाविशेषो भोगः परार्थत्वात्स्वार्थसंयमात्पुरुषज्ञानम् ॥ ३.३५ ॥

ततः प्रातिभश्रावणवेदनादर्शास्वादवार्त्ता जायन्ते ॥ ३.३६ ॥

ते समाधावुपसर्गा व्युत्थाने सिद्धयः ॥ ३.३७ ॥

बन्धकारणशैथिल्यात्प्रचारसंवेदनाच्च चित्तस्य परशरीरावेशः ॥ ३.३८ ॥

उदानजयाज्जलपङ्ककण्टकादिष्वसङ्ग उत्क्रान्तिश्च ॥ ३.३९ ॥

समानजयाज्ज्वलनम् ॥ ३.४० ॥

श्रोत्राकाशयोः संबन्धसंयमाद्दिव्यं श्रोत्रम् ॥ ३.४१ ॥

कायाकाशयोः संबन्धसंयमल्लघुतूलसमापत्तेश्चाकाशगमनम् ॥ ३.४२ ॥

बहिरकल्पिता वृत्तिर्महाविदेहा ततः प्रकाशावरणक्षयः ॥ ३.४३ ॥

स्थूलस्वरूपसूक्ष्मान्वयार्थवत्त्वसंयमाद्भूतजयः ॥ ३.४४ ॥

ततो ऽणिमादिप्रादुर्भावः कायसंपत्तद्धर्मानभिघातश्च ॥ ३.४५ ॥

रूपलावण्यबलवज्रसंहननत्वानि कायसंपत् ॥ ३.४६ ॥

ग्रहणस्वरूपास्मितान्वयार्थवत्त्वसंयमादिन्द्रियजयः ॥ ३.४७ ॥

ततो मनोजवित्वं विकरणभावः प्रधानजयश्च ॥ ३.४८ ॥

सत्त्वपुरुषान्यताख्यातिमात्रस्य सर्वभावाधिष्ठातृत्वं सर्वज्ञातृत्वं च ॥ ३.४९ ॥

तद्वैराग्यादपि दोषबीजक्षये कैवल्यम् ॥ ३.५० ॥

स्थान्युपनिमन्त्रणे सङ्गस्मयाकरणं पुनरनिष्टप्रसङ्गात् ॥ ३.५१ ॥

क्षणतत्क्रमयोः संयमाद्विवेकजं ज्ञानम् ॥ ३.५२ ॥

जातिलक्षणदेशैरन्यतानवच्छेदात्तुल्ययोस्ततः प्रतिपत्तिः ॥ ३.५३ ॥

तारकं सर्वविषयं सर्वथाविषयमक्रमं चेति विवेकजं ज्ञानम् ॥ ३.५४ ॥

सत्त्वपुरुषयोः शुद्धिसाम्ये कैवल्यम् ॥ ३.५५ ॥

४. कैवल्यपादः

जन्मौषधिमन्त्रतपःसमाधिजाः सिद्धयः ॥ ४.१ ॥

जात्यन्तरपरिणामः प्रकृत्यापूरात् ॥ ४.२ ॥

निमित्तमप्रयोजकं प्रकृतीनां वरणभेदस्तु ततः क्षेत्रिकवत् ॥ ४.३ ॥

निर्माणचित्तान्यस्मितामात्रात् ॥ ४.४ ॥

प्रवृत्तिभेदे प्रयोजकं चित्तमेकमनेकेषाम् ॥ ४.५ ॥

तत्र ध्यानजमनाशयम् ॥ ४.६ ॥

कर्माशुक्लाकृष्णं योगिनस्त्रिविधमितरेषाम् ॥ ४.७ ॥

ततस्तद्विपाकानुगुणानामेवाभिव्यक्तिर्वासनानाम् ॥ ४.८ ॥

जातिदेशकालव्यवहितानामप्यानन्तर्यं स्मृतिसंस्कारयोरेकरूपत्वात् ॥ ४.९ ॥

तासामनादित्वं चाशिषो नित्यत्वात् ॥ ४.१० ॥

हेतुफलाश्रयालम्बनैः संगृहीतत्वादेषामभावे तदभावः ॥ ४.११ ॥

अतीतानागतं स्वरूपतो ऽस्त्यध्वभेदाद्धर्माणाम् ॥ ४.१२ ॥

ते व्यक्तसूक्ष्मा गुणात्मानः ॥ ४.१३ ॥

परिणामैकत्वाद्वस्तुतत्त्वम् ॥ ४.१४ ॥

वस्तुसाम्ये चित्तभेदात्तयोर्विभक्तः पन्थाः ॥ ४.१५ ॥

न चैकचित्ततन्त्रं चेद्वस्तु तदप्रमाणकं तदा किं स्यात् ॥ ४.१६ ॥

तदुपरागापेक्षित्वाच्चित्तस्य वस्तु ज्ञाताज्ञातम् ॥ ४.१७ ॥

सदा ज्ञाताश्चित्तवृत्तयस्तत्प्रभोः पुरुषस्यापरिणामित्वात् ॥ ४.१८ ॥

न तत्स्वाभासं दृश्यत्वात् ॥ ४.१९ ॥

एकसमये चोभयानवधारणम् ॥ ४.२० ॥

चित्तान्तरदृश्ये बुद्धिबुद्धेरतिप्रसङ्गः स्मृतिसंकरश्च ॥ ४.२१ ॥

चितेरप्रतिसंक्रमायास्तदाकारापत्तौ स्वबुद्धिसंवेदनम् ॥ ४.२२ ॥

द्रष्टृदृश्योपरक्तं चित्तं सर्वार्थम् ॥ ४.२३ ॥

तदसंख्येयवासनाभिश्चित्रमपि परार्थं संहत्यकारित्वात् ॥ ४.२४ ॥

विशेषदर्शिन आत्मभावभावनानिवृत्तिः ॥ ४.२५ ॥

तदा विवेकनिम्नं कैवल्यप्राग्भारं चित्तम् ॥ ४.२६ ॥

तच्छिद्रेषु प्रत्ययान्तराणि संस्कारेभ्यः ॥ ४.२७ ॥

हानमेषां क्लेशवदुक्तम् ॥ ४.२८ ॥

प्रसंख्याने ऽप्यकुसीदस्य सर्वथा विवेकख्यातेर्धर्ममेघः समाधिः ॥ ४.२९ ॥

ततः क्लेशकर्मनिवृत्तिः ॥ ४.३० ॥

तदा सर्वावरणमलापेतस्य ज्ञानस्यानन्त्याज्ज्ञेयमल्पम् ॥ ४.३१ ॥

ततः कृतार्थानां परिणामक्रमसमाप्तिर्गुणानाम् ॥ ४.३२ ॥

क्षणप्रतियोगी परिणामापरान्तनिर्ग्राह्यः क्रमः ॥ ४.३३ ॥

पुरुषार्थशून्यानां गुणानां प्रतिप्रसवः कैवल्यं स्वरूपप्रतिष्ठा वा चितिशक्तिरिति ॥ ४.३४ ॥

Appendix D

THE VIBHŪTI-S

Powers from Practicing Saṃyama

This list is just a sampling of what can be accomplished when the heart-mind is completely focused on a specific object or region. Each row is a translation of the sūtra in the first column. Most of the rows show the results of saṃyama (focusing inward) on an object or location. The last column gives a bit more information. For example, sūtra 3.16 states that if we focus completely on the three transformations (listed in sūtra 3.13), we will gain knowledge of the past and future. Displaying these extraordinary powers in table format allows for easy reference.

SŪTRA		RESULTS IN	NOTES
3.16	From saṃyama on three transformations (3.13)	Knowledge of past and future	Transformations are dharma, lakṣaṇa, avasthā (see pariṇāma)
3.17	From saṃyama on the difference between word, object, and idea	Knowledge of the sound of all beings	The confusion of word, object, and idea is because of their superimposition
3.18	From direct perception of past impressions (saṃskāra-s)	Knowledge of previous births	
3.19	From direct perception of a current thought (pratyaya)	Knowledge of another's heart-mind	Mind reading
3.20	The supporting object of that thought (of another) is not known because it was not the object of concentration		Only know the nature of the thought, not what it is based on. For example, if the other person is thinking of a tiger and is afraid, only the fright is perceived by the mind reader
3.21	From saṃyama on the form of the body	Invisibility	Disconnection of light to the eye
3.22	From saṃyama on how fast karma bears fruit, or by omens	Knowledge of time of death	Karma is either fast or slow to fructify
3.23	From saṃyama on friendship, etc. (1.33)	Strengths	Friendship, compassion, gladness, neutrality
3.24	From saṃyama on strengths	Strength of an elephant	
3.25	By projecting the light of pravṛtti (1.36)	Knowledge of objects subtle, hidden, or distant	Clairvoyance
3.26	From saṃyama on the sun	Knowledge of all worlds	Solar nāḍī, called idā
3.27	From saṃyama on the moon	Knowledge of organization of the stars	Lunar nāḍī, called pingalā

SŪTRA		RESULTS IN	NOTES
3.28	From saṃyama on the pole star	Knowledge of the motion (of other stars)	Polaris is the center of the stars, which seem to move around it
3.29	From saṃyama on the navel cakra	Knowledge of organization of the body	As Polaris is the center of the universe, the navel cakra is the center of the body
3.30	From saṃyama on the hollow in the throat	Ending of hunger and thirst	Throat cakra
3.31	From saṃyama on the tortoise nāḍī	Steadiness	This nāḍī is located below the pit of the throat, where the chin touches the chest
3.32	From saṃyama on the light at top of head	Vision of a siddha	Crown cakra
3.33	*Or* from an intuitive flash	All (knowledge)	
3.34	From saṃyama on the heart	Complete knowledge of citta (heart-mind)	Heart cakra
3.35	From saṃyama on the distinction between Puruṣa and sattva	Knowlege of Puruṣa	Bhoga (experience) has the idea that sattva and Puruṣa, which are totally different, are one and the same (see also 3.49, 3.55)
3.36	From knowledge of Puruṣa (3.35)	Flash of illumination and suprasensory hearing, touch, sight, taste, smell	All sensory organs are supernormal
3.37	These are obstacles to samādhi (though) accomplishments to a fluctuating state of mind		
3.38	From loosening the cause of bondage (to the body) and knowing (how the energy) of the heart-mind circulates	Entry into (possession of) another body	
3.39	From mastery of udāna (upward-moving energy in the body)	Not getting stuck in water, mud, thorns, etc., and the ability to die at will	The body can rise up
3.40	From mastery of samāna (energy that maintains equilibrium in the body)	Radiance	
3.41	From saṃyama on the relationship between hearing and space	Divine hearing	Space has the property of sound
3.42	From saṃyama on the relationship between body and space, and samāpatti with lightweight cotton	Travel through space	Samāpatti is a type of samādhi
3.43	From saṃyama on mahāvideha	Removing the covering of light (avidyā)	Mahāvideha occurs when the mental activity is actually external to the body

SŪTRA		RESULTS IN	NOTES
3.44	From saṃyama on all five elements' gross form, essential nature, subtle form (tanmātra), guṇa composition, and purposefulness	Mastery of the five elements	Example: gross form is water; nature is liquidity; subtle form is taste. All elements contain all three guṇa-s and exist for the purpose of Puruṣa
3.45	From mastery of the five elements (3.44)	Power to become small, etc., perfection of the body, resistance of the body to external forces	The eight powers are listed below this table*
3.46	Perfection of the body consists of beauty, grace, strength, and diamond-like firmness		
3.47	From saṃyama on all five sensory organs' process of perception, essential nature, individuality, guṇa composition, and purposefulness	Mastery of the sensory organs	
3.48	From mastery of the senses (3.47)	Speed of the mind, sensory organs working independent of the body, mastery of Prakṛti	
3.52	From saṃyama on a moment and its sequence	Knowledge born of discernment	
3.53	From that (3.51)	Ability to distinguish between two seemingly identical objects	See pariṇāma-s (transformations)

*3.45 The Eight Powers mentioned by Vyāsa, the primary commentator on the *Yoga Sūtra-s,* are

Aṇima	Can decrease in size to become as tiny as an atom
Laghimā	Can decrease in weight to become lightweight
Mahimā	Can increase in size to become huge
Prāpti	Can touch the moon with the fingertips, and so can reach any distance
Prākāmya	Can overcome obstacles, travel through solid matter
Vaśitva	Can control all objects
Īśitṛtva	Can create or destroy at will
Yatrakāmāvaśāyitva	Can transmute one element into another

Appendix E

SANSKRIT PRONUNCIATION KEY AND GRAMMAR BASICS

Sanskrit Alphabet

14 Vowels (some have 2 forms)

अ	a	another
आ / ा	ā	father (2 beats)
इ / ि	i	pin
ई / ी	ī	need (2 beats)
उ / ु	u	flute
ऊ / ू	ū	mood (2 beats)
ऋ / ृ	ṛ	macabre
ॠ / ॄ	ṝ	trill for 2 beats
ऌ / ॢ	ḷ	table
ए / े	e	etude (2 beats)
ऐ / ै	ai	aisle (2 beats)
ओ / ो	o	yoke (2 beats)
औ / ौ	au	flautist (2 beats)

Two Special Letters

अं	aṃ	hum
अः	aḥ	out-breath

33 Consonants

क	ka	paprika
ख	kha	thick honey
ग	ga	saga
घ	gha	big honey
ङ	ṅa	ink
च	ca	chutney
छ	cha	much honey
ज	ja	Japan
झ	jha	raj honey
ञ	ña	inch
ट	ṭa	borscht again
ठ	ṭha	borscht honey
ड	ḍa	shdum
ढ	ḍha	shd hum
ण	ṇa	shnum
त	ta	pasta
थ	tha	eat honey
द	da	soda
ध	dha	good honey
न	na	banana
प	pa	paternal
फ	pha	scoop honey
ब	ba	scuba
भ	bha	rub honey
म	ma	aroma
य	ya	employable
र	ra	abra cadabra
ल	la	hula
व	va	variety
श	śa	shut
ष	ṣa	shnapps
स	sa	Lisa
ह	ha	honey

Sanskrit Pronunciation Notes

i) To pronounce Sanskrit transliteration properly, I will point out the primary differences between Sanskrit and English pronunciation. Everything else can be pronounced as in English.

(1) Sanskrit syllables can be short (1 beat) or long (2 beats), giving the language a natural rhythm. A syllable is long (2 beats) if either its vowel is long (ā, ī, ū, ṝ, e, ai, o, au) or it leads into a compound consonant (two or more consonants next to each other). For example, in the word "ālasya" there are three syllables: "ā" is a long vowel, so this syllable gets 2 beats; "las" has a short vowel, but it leads into a compound consonant "sy" and so is long and takes 2 beats; "ya" has a short "a" and so takes only 1 beat.

(2) If a consonant has an "h" to its right, then a burst of breath accompanies its sound. For example, "ka" is just like in English, but "kha" is a "ka" with a simultaneous audible exhale. It is not pronounced "kaha."

(3) If a consonant has a dot below it (ṛ, ṭ, ḍ, ṇ, ṣ, excluding ṃ and ḥ), then it is pronounced further back in the mouth, where the tongue touches a smooth, round area behind and above the teeth. This mouth position in fact gives the Indian accent its distinctive sound.

(4) If an "s" has a mark above or below it (ś, ṣ), it is pronounced like the English "sh."

ii) When two vowels meet in Sanskrit, they blend into something else. For example, "a" plus "ī" becomes "e" as in svādhyāya + īśvarapraṇidhāna = svādhyāyeśvarapraṇidhāna.

iii) When two consonants meet, if their sounds are not compatible, then one or both of them will change. For example, "t" plus "v" becomes "dv" as in "tat" + "vṛtti" = "tadvṛtti."

Some Sanskrit sounds are pronounced slightly differently in North and South India. The "v" might sound like a "w" and the "ś" or "ṣ" may sound like a "sh" or a "s."

There are some differences between Sanskrit and Hindi pronunciation. In Sanskrit, when a word ends with an "a," the "a" is pronounced. In Hindi it is often dropped, even though it is written the same way in the original script. For example, the Sanskrit "āsana" sounds like "āsan" in Hindi.

SANSKRIT GRAMMAR BASICS

Only nouns and pronouns have gender, which can be masculine (M), feminine (F), or neuter (N). Adjectives that modify the noun take the same gender, number, and case ending. Most words are derived from tiny, single-syllable roots. Here is the process:

1. Convert a root into a stem-word.
   Example: The root "vid," meaning "to know, to see," can become the stem word "veda," meaning "knowledge."
   A stem word ends in a certain letter or letters (end-letters), and if it is a noun it also has a gender (M, F, or N).
   Example: "veda" is a masculine noun whose end-letter is "a."
2. Affix a case-ending to the stem-word to use the word in a sentence, creating a sentence-word. The case-ending shows where the word fits into the sentence. The exact case-ending depends upon the following:
   - The stem-word end-letter(s)
   - The gender
   - Whether used as singular, dual, or plural
   - Its function in the sentence

Below is a table showing the case endings. There is a different table for various combinations of genders and stem-word end-letters. Each blank box would have an ending in it. The outlined box would contain an ending that means by or with something singular.

Table of Case Endings

Case	Singular (sg)	Dual (du)	Plural (pl)
Subj			
Direct object			
by/with			
to/for			
from/due to			
of, 's			
in/on/upon/at			
hey!			

Example: the stem-word "veda" uses the table for masculine words whose end-letter is "a" (M-a). To say "with knowledge," the case-ending in the box "by/with" sg for table M-a is "ena," which will be affixed to "ved." So "ved" + "ena" = "vedena" meaning "with knowledge." Note that the case-ending replaces the stem-word end-letter(s).

There are also some words (indeclinables) that do not take any endings.

In summary,

1. Root becomes stem-word, which has end-letter(s) and gender (if a noun).
2. Stem-word – end-letter(s) + case-ending = sentence-word.
3. A sentence is made of several sentence-words.

Translation Grammar

In part 3, The *Yoga Sutra-s* in Translation, any grammar is denoted in square brackets [] as follows.

- Pronoun: if the word is a proper pronoun
- Ending: from Table of Case Endings, before sound blending (if any) was applied
- Case: which of eight cases from column one of Table of Case Endings
- Number: which of three numbers from the header of Table of Case Endings (sg/du/pl)
- Gender: m = masculine, f = feminine, n = neuter
- Stem Ending: end letter(s) of stem word, or "p" if a pronoun
- (Each Gender + Stem Ending combination has its own set of twenty-four endings)

For example, [aḥ subj sg m-a] indicates the ending is aḥ from the Subject Singular cell in the table for masculine stems that end in a.

Sound Blending

Sanskrit emphasizes the smooth flow of sound. If the end of one sentence-word is sound-incompatible with the beginning of the next sentence-word, then the sounds change to make them flow better. This process is called "sandhi," meaning "combination." Imagine two conflicting energies resolving their differences through compromise.

For example, when "ḥ" meets "ca" it becomes "śca." When "aḥ" meets a soft consonant, the "aḥ" changes to "o."

Compound Phrases

A compound phrase is made of several stem-words all run together, with only one case-ending. The individual stem-words will have dashes between them.

If the stem-words form a list, then the compound phrase can be read left to right. For example, sūtra 1.6 is pramāṇa-viparyaya-vikalpa-nidrā-smṛtayaḥ. There is one ending (ayaḥ), which is subject-plural, and there are no other phrases to go with it, so it must be a list.

Otherwise, the compound-phrase is read backward (right to left), inserting whatever case-endings make sense in that particular context. For example, sūtra 1.2 is yogaḥ citta-vṛtti-nirodhaḥ. The compound phrase has a singular case-ending, so it is to be read backward as "nirodha of vṛtti-s in the citta." Notice the added "of" and "in" and also how vṛtti is made plural.

Appendix F

FIGURES

Figure 1 SĀṄKHYA: PROCESS OF MANIFESTATION

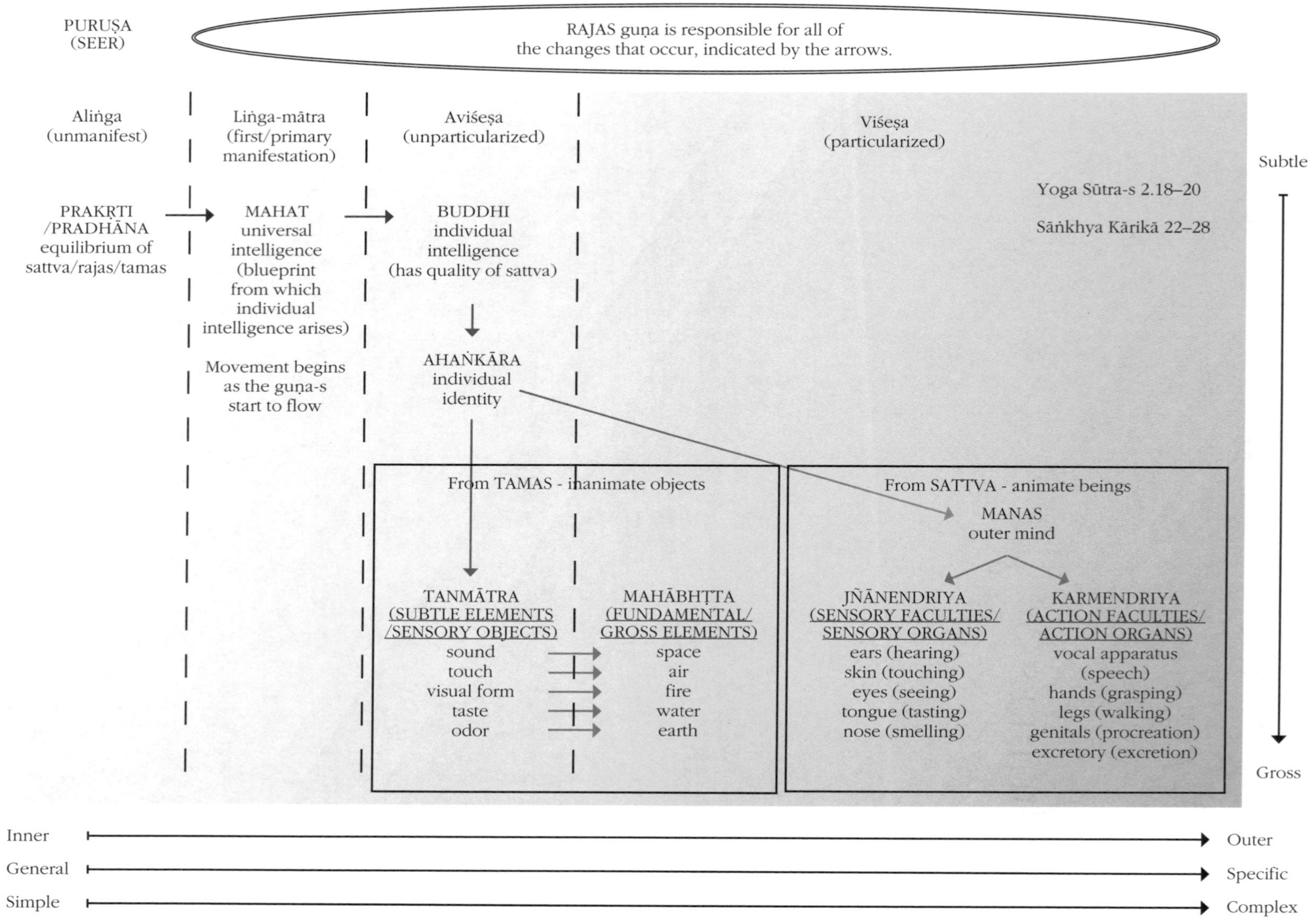

Figure 1, Cont'd SĀṄKHYA: PROCESS OF MANIFESTATION

Aliṅga or pradhāna represents the initial, unmanifest phase of Prakṛti. The guṇa-s (sattva, rajas, tamas) are in equilibrium and not moving yet. Aliṅga means "unmarked, unindicated" and indeed it has not developed into any real form yet.

Liṅga-mātra is the first manifestation of Prakṛti. The guṇa-s have begun to move and form the blueprint of intelligence behind all life (mahat). Mahat is a manifestation of Īśvara, the seed of all knowledge (1.25). Liṅga-mātra means "marked alone" or "singly indicated," used here because only one entity is manifesting. All subsequent tattva-s arise from this intelligence, which is the intelligence of life itself.

Aviśeṣa is a stage of division in which the intelligence directs the guṇa-s to fabricate the intellect, ego, and subtle elements, all that is needed to experience the remaining tattva-s of the final phase (viśeṣa). Buddhi is a person's individual intelligence (an individual form of mahat) and has the quality of sattva. Ahaṃkāra is an individual's ego, what identifies things as ourself (see citta section for more details on these). Tanmātra means "only that, a trifle" implying a small number of constituents, here only five. These are subtle forms of the five fundamental elements, which arise from them.

Viśeṣa is the final phase in which the guṇa-s form their most outer, gross manifestation. Viśeṣa means "special, particular" and indicates that the tattva-s produced are the most specialized and particular. The five fundamental elements of matter and energy are the building blocks of all that we can sense with our five sensory organs. The process of sensation occurs through the outer mind (manas). Finally, action occurs through the five action organs. (See figure 4, The Process of Perception.)

The guṇa-s always comprise Prakṛti. In terms of Prakṛti, tamas is matter or substance, rajas is the energy that transforms one tattva into another, and sattva represents the positive aspects of both and is the original quality of the buddhi.

Manifestation expands naturally from the few and simple to the many and complex in a process of complication. Yoga is the opposite, a process of refinement and simplification. From seeing the world as a myriad of objects and events, we pare our perception down by recognizing the temporal nature of existence and how it obscures (avidyā) the inner light of awareness. As the heart-mind field clears and we experience glimpses of this light, we begin to perceive the world as nothing more than the three guṇa-s working together. Eventually, through the process of pratiprasava (see that section), we experience Prakṛti in its original state and Puruṣa abiding in its own true nature (1.3, 4.34).

Figure 2 KOŚA-S: SHEATHS OF LIFE

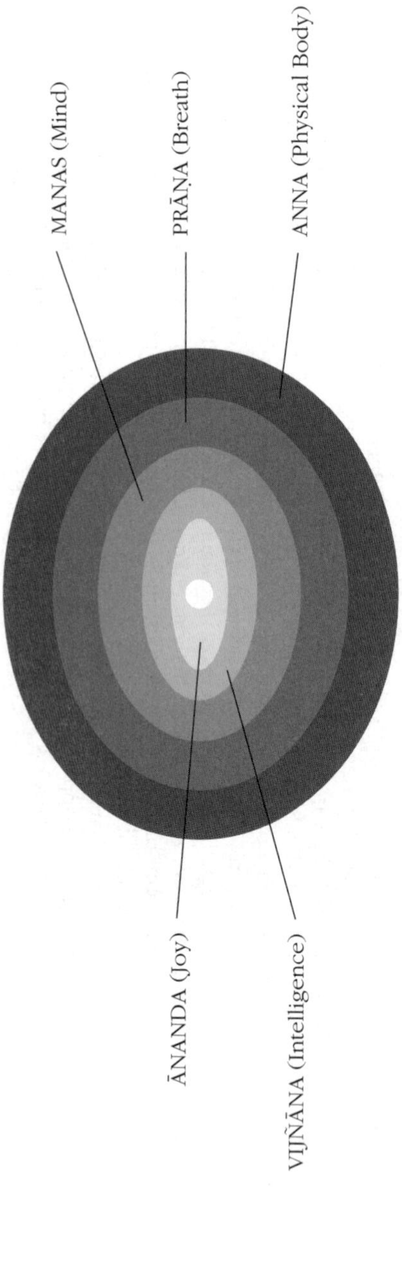

Figure 2, Cont'd KOŚA-S: SHEATHS OF LIFE

Kośa-s show us another way to view our being human, which is consistent with the outer to inner, gross to subtle paradigm. The five layers envelop the inner light of awareness, called Puruṣa, the unchanging witness behind and inside it all (white circle in the center).

The name of each kośa is structured the same: _____-maya-kośa, where _____ defines which sheath. The suffix "maya" means "consists of," and then kośa, meaning "sheath, layer, case." So each name translates to "the sheath consisting of _____."

Anna-maya-kośa is the outermost layer, representing the physical realm, all matter. In the human body this would be every actual substance. A cadaver still has this layer, but lacks the next layer (prāṇa). Anna means "food" and is the realm in which things eat and are eaten, everything transforming from one state into another. This corresponds to the mineral stage of evolution.

Prāṇa-maya-kośa is the next subtlest layer, consisting of prāṇa, the breath or life-force. Prāṇa animates (gives life to) the physical layer. Prāṇa is in fact the link among all the kośa-s, the energy behind all activity. This layer corresponds to the plant stage of evolution.

Mano-maya-kośa is the mind, even subtler than the breath, and consists of feelings, thoughts, emotions, and memory. Manas processes sensory perceptions, stores thoughts and emotions, and issues action signals. Manas is like a middle manager, taking orders from the next kośa and carrying them out without question. This corresponds to the animal stage of evolution.

Vijñāna-maya-kośa consists of the intelligence (buddhi) and ego (ahaṅkāra) parts of the heart-mind. Vijñāna means wisdom or discriminitive knowledge, which is uniquely human and allows us to judge between right and wrong, good and bad, etc. Inherently sattvic, the buddhi presents all perceptions to the inner light of awareness, the Puruṣa. This corresponds to the human stage of evolution. Animals lack this layer and the next.

Ānanda-maya-kośa is the innermost layer, consisting of pure joy. This is the subtlest sheath and closest to the inner light of awareness, the Puruṣa.

The white circle in the center represents the Puruṣa (seer) that is beyond pleasure and pain, just witnessing the activities happening in the other layers through the lens of the buddhi (vijñāna-maya-kośa). The seer provides the light of knowledge, which gets filtered through the other layers like lamplight dimmed by a series of overlapping lampshades. Just as the light itself is not affected by the lampshades, so the seer is never affected by the kośa-s that encase it.

Figure 3 CITTA: THE HEART-MIND FIELD OF CONSCIOUSNESS

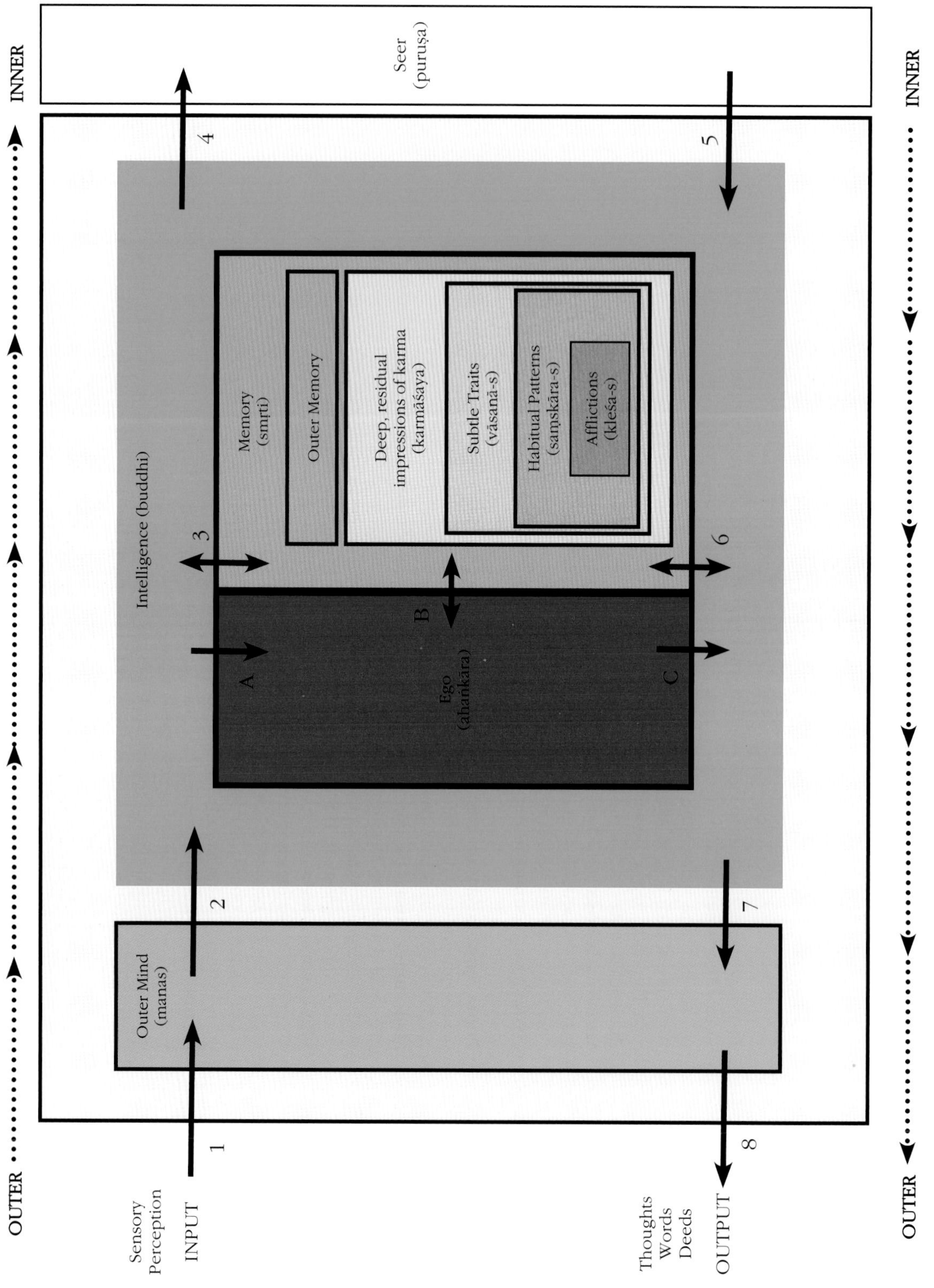

Figure 3, Cont'd CITTA: THE HEART-MIND FIELD OF CONSCIOUSNESS

INPUT

1) A perception is taken in by the outer mind (manas). If the sensory organs are defective, then the perception can be distorted here.

2) The perception is then processed by the intelligence (buddhi). Current thoughts may affect how the perception is accepted.

If one's citta is mostly clear and pure:

3) Perception is recorded accurately in the memory.
One-time or benign perceptions will store temporarily in outer memory.
Repeated or intense perceptions will form positive habitual patterns.

4) Clear, sattvic intelligence will not filter or distort the perception.
The presentation of the perception to the seer is truthful.

If one's citta is clouded by avidyā:

A) The ego makes it part of your identity, and may distort it further.

B) Distorted perception is stored in memory.
One-time or benign perceptions will store temporarily in outer memory.
Repeated or intense perceptions will form negative habitual patterns.

OUTPUT

5) Puruṣa shines all the time.

If one's citta is clear and pure:

6) The memories required to decide on an action are recalled.

If one's citta is clouded by avidyā:

A) Light cannot get through; ego takes control.

B) The ego recalls the memories it thinks are needed.

C) The ego directs the intelligence on the course of action.

7) Thought or emotion is selected to act a certain way (a pratyaya).

8) Action is carried out based on current thoughts and emotions.

Figure 4 THE PROCESS OF PERCEPTION (INPUT)

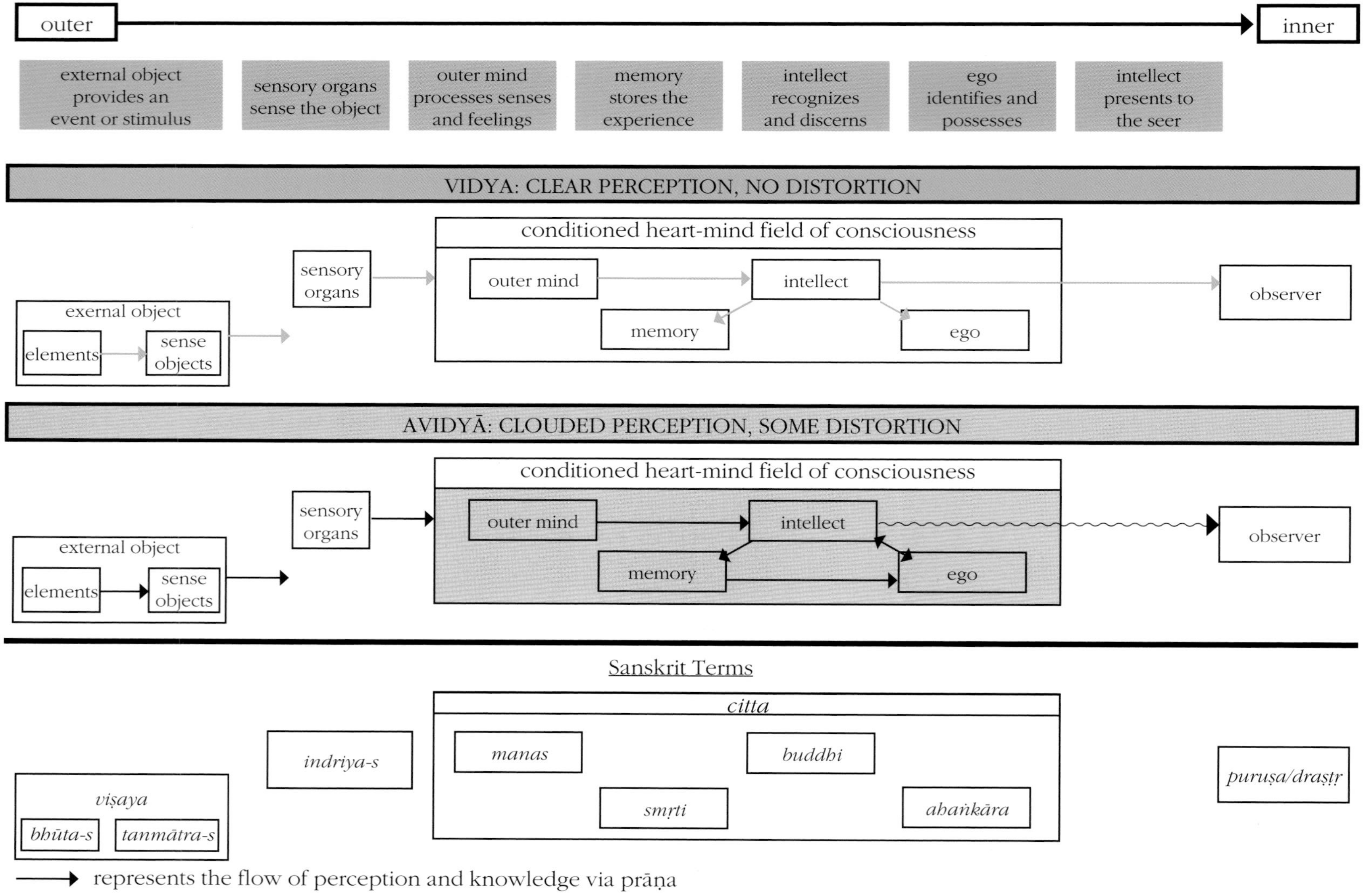

Figure 4, Cont'd THE PROCESS OF PERCEPTION (INPUT)

Perception begins when we encounter an external object. The outer mind is the door through which all sensory perceptions enter our consciousness. The intellect decides what the object is. The ego wants to own the signal, make it "ours," and likes to have control over the intellect. The observer simply sits back and notices everything. Each stage of perception can be distorted and pass on misinformation. For example, if we perceive a car, the buddhi decides "this is a car," and the ego asks, "Is this my car?"

Yoga is designed to clear impurities from every link in this chain from sensory organs through the intellect. Once tamas and rajas have been replaced by sattva in the intellect, the stage is set for moving forward toward kaivalya. When everything we perceive makes it through this process unaltered, then the channels are clear, allowing the pure light of the observer to shine through our eyes and aura. Compassion and kindness to all beings results from the understanding that inside we are all sharing the same light of awareness.

Duḥkha, internal suffering, is the best gauge of our progress. When events no longer trigger our "buttons" and our helpful habitual patterns are stronger than the harmful ones we have worked so hard to weaken, then we can act consciously, deliberately, and compassionately. On the other hand, when a situation causes us to suffer and we allow harmful past conditioning to influence our reaction, it is time to practice self-observation (svādhyāya) to find out why and work toward weeding out the underlying cause.

THE HEART-MIND FIELD IS CLEAR AND PURIFIED (GREEN)

An external object is encountered; the sensory organs accurately pick up the sound, feel, sight, taste, or smell; the correct signals pass into the outer mind, then to the intellect, which informs the ego, which records an accurate memory and presents the information in its untainted form to the observer. The ego is subservient to the intellect, and so does not cause identification with the perception. The memory recorded is unbiased by the ego. This will lead to action that is based on reality, not based on misperception.

THE HEART-MIND FIELD IS CLOUDED (GRAY)

An external object is encountered; the sensory organs pick up signals that reach the outer mind, which is filled with commotion (vṛtti-s). Because the heart-mind is not still and is caught up in busyness, the inner light of awareness is not able to illuminate the signal, and the perception becomes misinterpreted. The intellect submits to the ego, which further filters the signal by superimposing what it thinks is best for the individual's own self-interest and power, then feeds this warped information into the memory to be recorded. This will lead to action that is not based on reality, but based on misperception and even delusion.

Figure 5 THE PROCESS OF ACTION (OUTPUT)

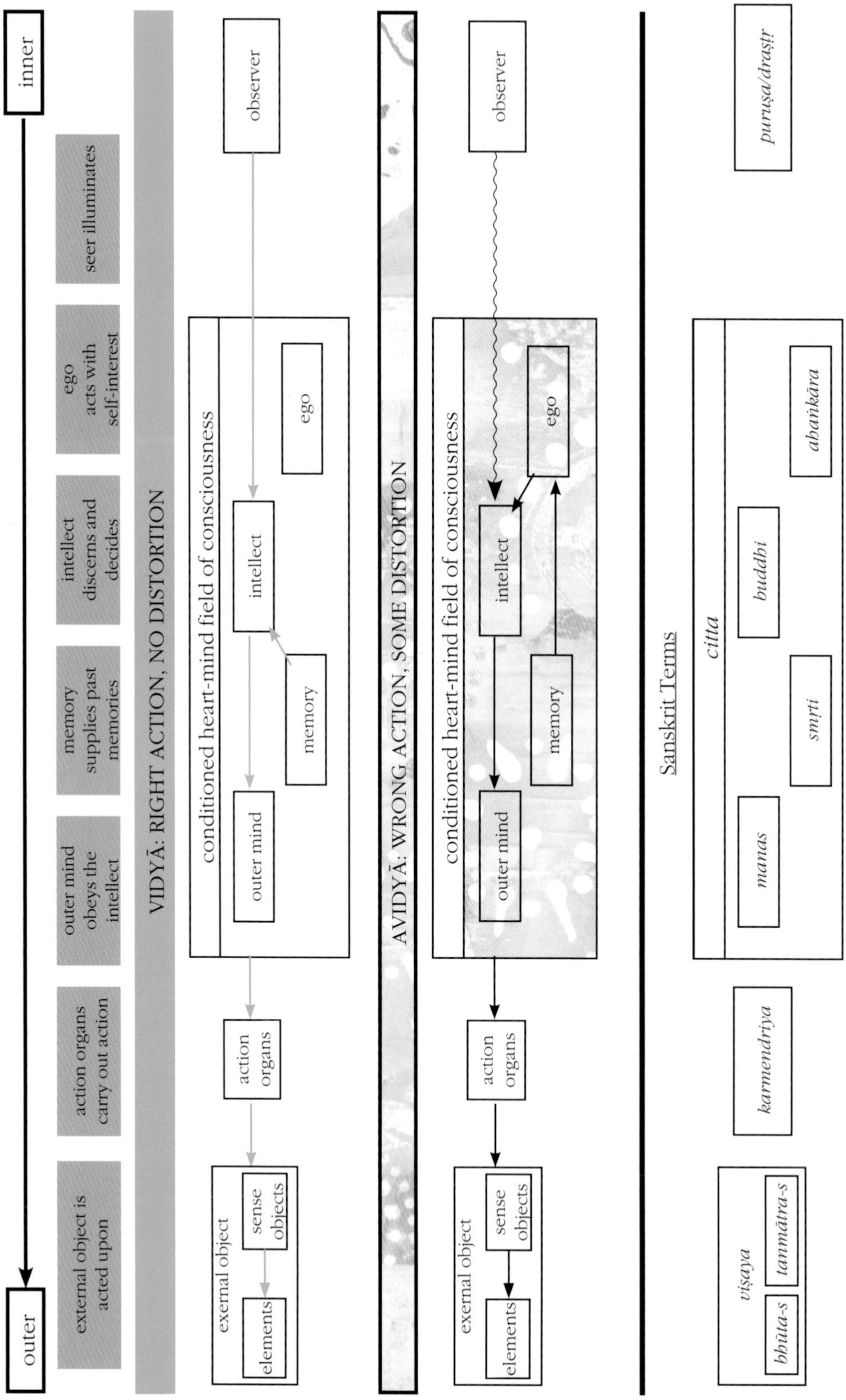

→ represents the flow of decision and action via prāṇa

Figure 5, Cont'd THE PROCESS OF ACTION (OUTPUT)

Each action issued from our being is determined by several factors, including habitual tendencies (saṃskāra-s), subtle propensities (vāsanā-s), deep emotional afflictions (kleśa-s), vṛtti-s, and the cycles of thoughts and feelings present in our consciousness (vṛtti-s). When we encounter an external stimulus, whether it be an actual sensory object or event, a sequence of rapid-fire signals race through our heart-mind, producing either an unconscious reaction, or a more discerning and conscious response.

Yoga is designed to clear impurities from every link in this chain from the intellect through the action organs, and to thereby control our actions. Once tamas and rajas have been replaced by sattva in the intellect, the stage is set for moving forward toward kaivalya. When every decision is made by a sattvic intellect, then transferred by the outer mind to the action organs, the resulting action has been influenced by the light of pure awareness. This action will always be kind and honest.

Duḥkha, internal suffering, is the best gauge of our progress. When events no longer trigger our "buttons" and our helpful habitual patterns are stronger than the harmful ones we have worked so hard to weaken, then we can act consciously, deliberately, and compassionately. On the other hand, when a situation causes us to suffer and we allow harmful past conditioning to influence our reaction, it is time to practice self-observation (svādhyāya) to find out why and work toward weeding out the underlying cause.

THE HEART-MIND FIELD IS CLEAR AND PURIFIED (GREEN)

Actions issued from a clear heart-mind are carried out with the welfare of oneself and others taken into consideration. Memory is drawn upon, but only informs the course of action; it does not determine it completely as it does below. The action reflects clear perception in the present moment. This kind of action is neither black nor white, and does not incur any karmic debt. Notice that the ego does not take part in the process; it is bypassed completely.

THE HEART-MIND FIELD IS CLOUDED (GRAY)

When the light shining from the observer is blocked or restricted, the heart-mind is filled with distractions and the flow of prāṇa is distorted. Actions tend to be more reactive and driven by habitual tendencies formed from past memories. The action reflects distorted perception in the present moment. When you react with no discernment, the saṃskāra-s determine the action, not the higher self. The ego is calling the shots, doing what it needs to do to stay in control and protect the individual. The resulting action will further strengthen the negative tendency and make it more difficult to break the pattern. The ego determines the action which then becomes biased.

Figure 6 CLARIFICATION OF THE HEART-MIND (CITTA)

AVIDYĀ

- low/self-centered awareness/knowledge
- tamas and rajas guṇa-s predominate
- narrow view based on scant knowledge of object/focus
- ego suppresses or directs the buddhi
- distorted or poor perception
- water: murky, rippled
- lens: thick layer of dirt, opaque, small openings
- crystal: no or little reflection of object
- vṛtti-s: darkened, noisy, distract completely

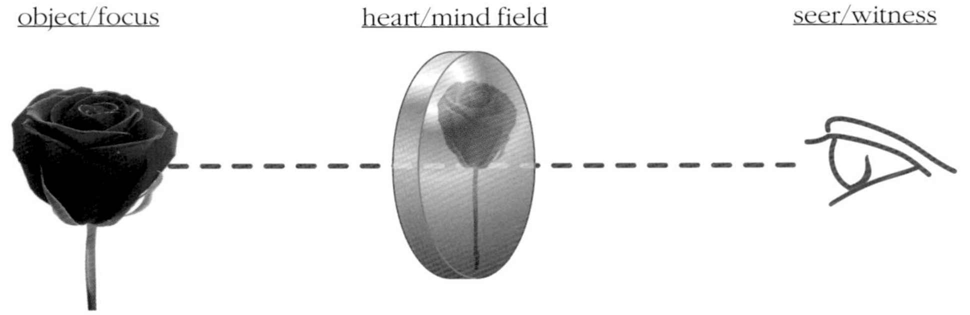

PROGRESSING FROM AVIDYĀ TO VIDYĀ USING VIVEKA, ABHYĀSA, VAIRĀGYA, YOGA/NIRODHA, CITTA-PRASĀDANA

- more awareness/knowledge/discernment
- wider view based on more knowledge of object/focus
- rajas guṇa predominates, some sattva is there
- ego and buddhi share power
- decent perception, still some distortion
- water: semi-clean, wavy
- lens: thin layer of dirt, translucent, larger openings
- crystal: partial reflection of object
- vṛtti-s: calmer, less agitated, distract less

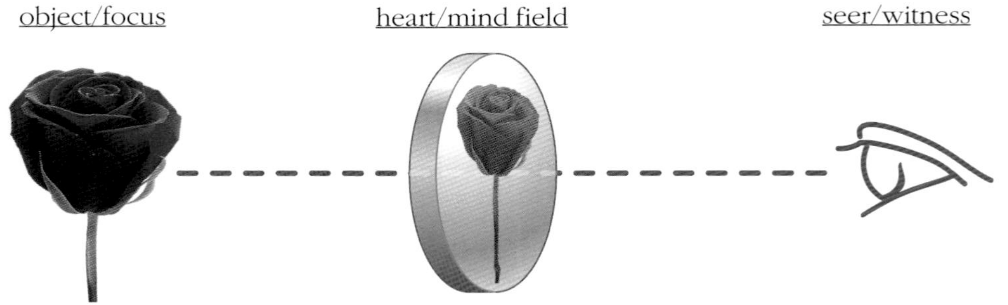

SAMĀDHI

- high awareness/knowledge/discernment
- broad view, full knowledge of object/focus
- sattva guṇa predominates
- ego serves buddhi
- clear and accurate perception, no distortion
- water is still, no movement
- lens: clean and transparent
- crystal: perfect reflection of object
- vṛtti-s: calm, do not distract anymore

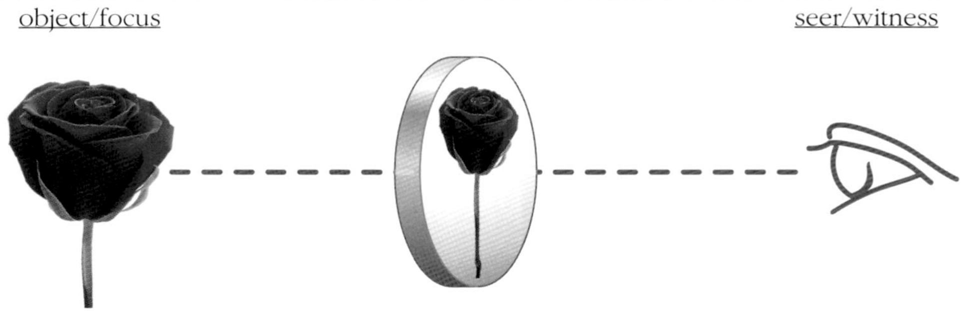

Figure 6, Cont'd CLARIFICATION OF THE HEART-MIND (CITTA)

ABHYĀSA, (VIVEKA) and VAIRĀGYA	→ (1.2)	NIRODHA of vṛtti-s	→ (1.2)	yoga
friendliness toward happy people compassion toward suffering people appreciation/gladness toward virtue caution/neutrality toward vice			→ (1.33)	clarification of citta
exhalation and retention of prāṇa			→ (1.34)	clarification of citta
developing finer sensory perception			→ (1.35)	clarification of citta
perception which is free from sorrow (duḥkha) and filled with light (sattva)			→ (1.36)	clarification of citta
object of focus is free of rāga (desirous attachment)			→ (1.37)	clarification of citta
supported by the knowledge from dreams or deep sleep			→ (1.38)	clarification of citta
continuous meditation (dhyāna) on whatever one likes			→ (1.39)	clarification of citta
when memory has been purified			→ (1.43)	object is perfectly reflected
saṃyama on the heart			→ (3.34)	complete knowledge of citta

Figure 7 THE PROCESS OF NIRODHA: SILENCING THE HEART-MIND

helpful thoughts and feelings (aklișța-vṛtti-s)

harmful thoughts and feelings (klișța-vṛtti-s)

moments of silence, the effect of yoga and nirodha

ordinary state of mind

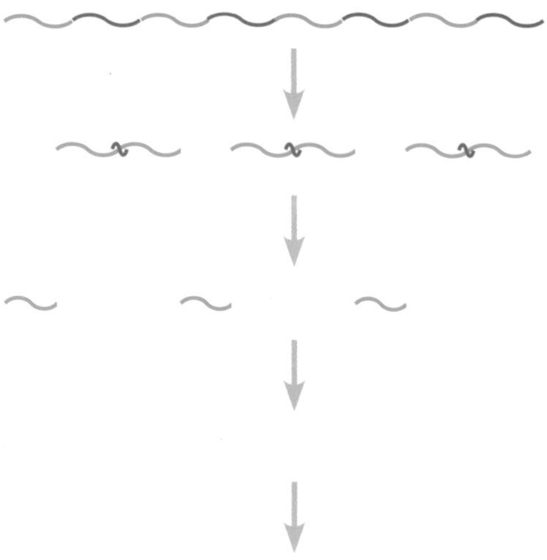

kaivalya

The heart-mind is distracted by helpful and harmful thoughts and feelings (vṛtti-s). There is a lack of awareness (avidyā) covering the inner light of consciousness. Tamas and rajas guṇa-s dominate sattva. The intellect (buddhi) obeys the ego (ahaṅkāra).

Yoga practices begin cultivating a one-pointed state of mind (ekāgra), lessening harmful vṛtti-s while increasing helpful vṛtti-s. Positive behavioral patterns (saṃskāra-s) begin to take hold, and negative ones weaken. Glimpses of silence are present due to the effect of nirodha. The onset of the nirodha saṃskāra begins.

As the attention turns inward via saṃyama, the distracting vṛtti-s are further superseded by moments of silence. Kleśa-s are too weak to manifest as harmful vṛtti-s. The nirodha saṃskāra has overtaken other saṃskāra-s, which weaken, building momentum toward kaivalya.

Yoga as a continuous state of samādhi. Neither helpful nor harmful vṛtti-s affect the attention. A one-pointed state of mind (ekāgra) is present. Only the nirodha saṃskāra exists.

The effect of viveka-khyāti and pratiprasava. The nirodha saṃskāra goes away with the complete nirodha of all citta-vṛtti-s and all saṃskāras, as Puruṣa rests in its own nature, which is kaivalya.

Figure 8 VṚTTI-S: DISTRACTING THOUGHTS AND FEELINGS (1.6–11)

VṚTTI	SŪTRA	MEANING	DEFINITION	KLIṢṬA (HARMFUL)	AKLIṢṬA (HELPFUL)
pramāna	1.7	correct means of evaluation	pratyakṣa (direct observation) anumāna (inference) āgama (testimony from a reliable secondhand source)	see something but not ready for it idea or label interferes with perception	see object as it really is reflection based on reliable info
viparyaya	1.8	misperception	erroneous knowledge based on form which is not that	delusion (think one thing, reality is another thing)	adjust knowledge to fit reality verification, asking questions admitting you are wrong
vikalpa	1.9	conceptualization imagination, fantasy, our fictional creation	without an object, relying on knowledge from words or language	fantasies from which you make decisions; daydreaming	high-level abstract thinking; compositions: art, music, math . . . tool=bhāvana (realistic intention)
nidrā	1.10	sleep	tamasic activity supported by the absence of presented thoughts	drowsiness, absence of attention; e.g., nod off during an important meeting	deep, dreamless sleep e.g., want to sleep at 6:00, fall asleep at 6:15
smṛti	1.11	memory	mental retention of a (previously) experienced object	see disturbing images, have nightmares about them OR rāga/dveṣa (past pleasure/ pain) causes action without discrimination	memorize a helpful verse or saying OR remember to step back from situation so as to weaken rāga/dveṣa

Figure 9 ANTARĀYA-S: OBSTACLES THAT DISTRACT (1.30)

ANTARĀYA	MEANING	NOTES
vyādhi	disease, imbalance	only one that does not involve the kleśa-s
styāna	apathy, mental dullness, lack of interest	can have an external cause
saṃśaya	doubt, indecision	like fire, consumes everything in its path
pramāda	carelessness, intoxication, inattention	action without reflection
ālasya	lethargy, fatigue, lack of enthusiasm	disinclination to act
avirati	sexual preoccupation, temptation	over-indulgence of sense organs
bhrānti-darśana	erroneous perception, mistaken view	think we know what we do not know
alabdha-bhūmikatva	cannot get grounded, lack of perseverance	cannot hold on to what is achieved, thus cannot progress further
anavasthitatva	instability, regression	cannot stabilize at current level, fall backward into a previous stage

Accompanying Symptoms (1.31)

duḥkha	pain, mental discomfort, constricted space in head/heart; grief, distress
daurmanasya	"mental pain" depression, negative thinking, pessimism
aṅgamejayatva	restlessness, trembling of body; inability to sleep when body needs to
śvāsa	inhalation: disturbed, inability to control
praśvāsa	exhalation: disturbed, inability to control

Figure 10 KLEŚA-S: CAUSES OF SUFFERING (2.3–9)

2.4 All can be dormant, weakened, intermittent, or active

KLEŚA	SŪTRA	MEANING	NOTES
avidyā	2.5	lack of awareness, ignorance	the field in which the other kleśa-s exist breeds fear, which the other kleśa-s are based upon
asmitā	2.6	"I am-ness," identifying the seer and instrument of seeing as the same	identification with the ego self; thinking you are more than you are (puffed up) or less than you are (failure/insecure); afraid of losing control of the organism
rāga	2.7	attachment to past pleasure	opposite of vairāgya product of asmitā, which is destroyed by vairāgya
dveṣa	2.8	attachment to past suffering	repress/shun a bad experience; past suffering negatively affects current actions; product of asmitā, which is destroyed by vairāgya
abhiniveśa	2.9	survival instinct, fear of death	only kleśa we are born with; most difficult one to remove; fear of losing something product of asmitā, which is destroyed by vairāgya

Figure 11 OUTER LIMBS OF YOGA (BAHIRAṄGĀṆI)

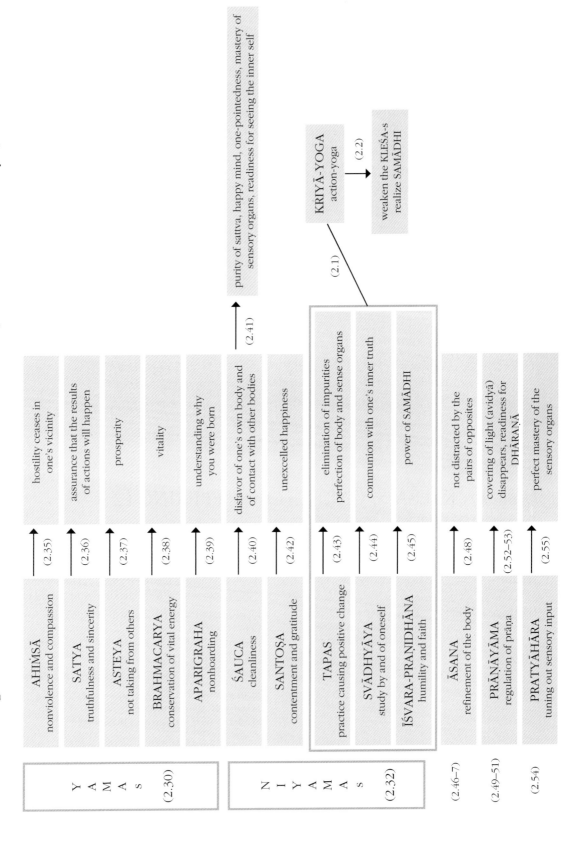

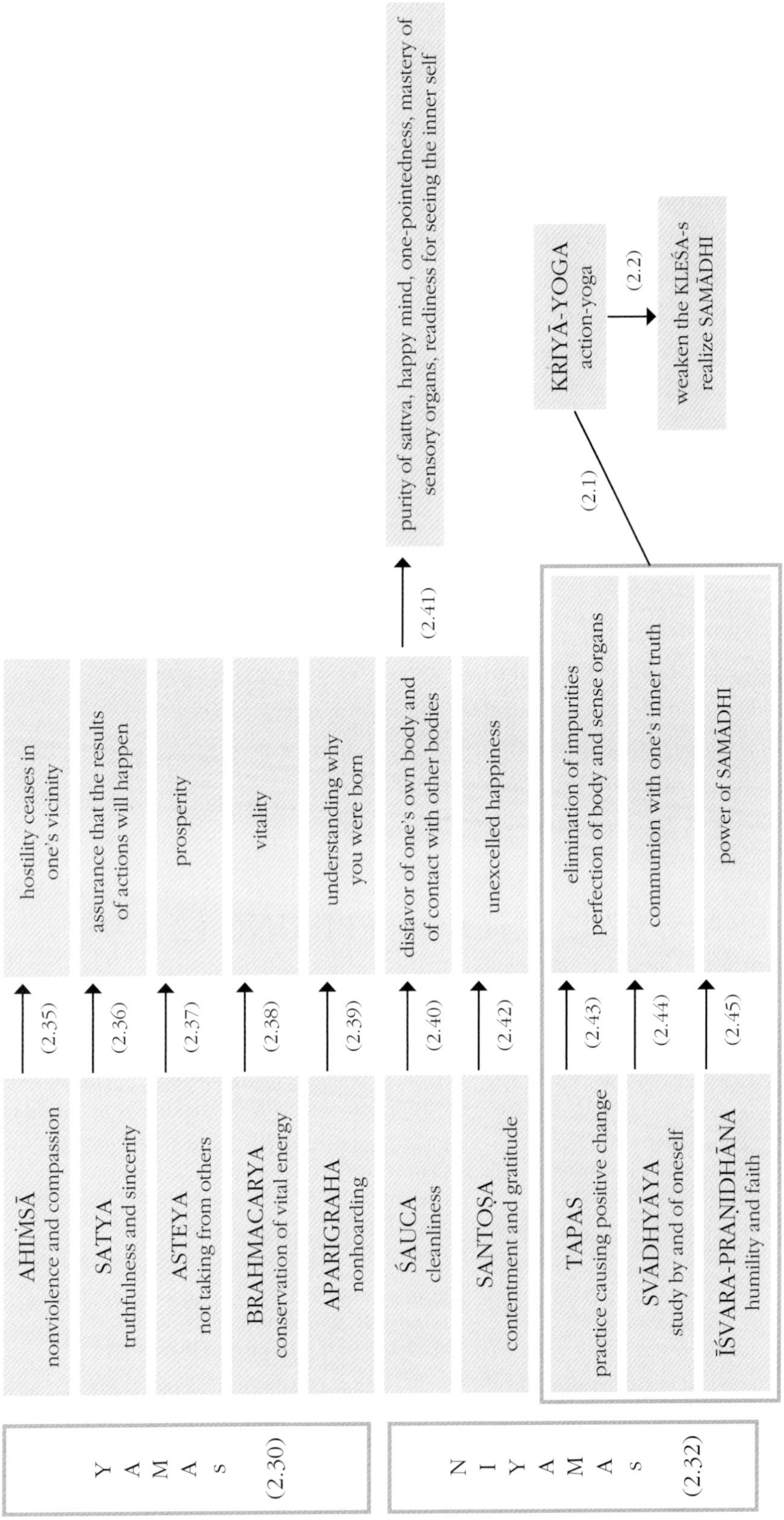
YAMAs (2.30)
AHIṀSĀ nonviolence and compassion
(2.35)
hostility ceases in one's vicinity
SATYA truthfulness and sincerity
(2.36)
assurance that the results of actions will happen
ASTEYA not taking from others
(2.37)
prosperity
BRAHMACARYA conservation of vital energy
(2.38)
vitality
APARIGRAHA nonhoarding
(2.39)
understanding why you were born
NIYAMAs (2.32)
ŚAUCA cleanliness
(2.40)
disfavor of one's own body and of contact with other bodies
(2.41)
purity of sattva, happy mind, one-pointedness, mastery of sensory organs, readiness for seeing the inner self
SANTOṢA contentment and gratitude
(2.42)
unexcelled happiness
TAPAS practice causing positive change
(2.43)
elimination of impurities perfection of body and sense organs
SVĀDHYĀYA study by and of oneself
(2.44)
communion with one's inner truth
ĪŚVARA-PRAṆIDHĀNA humility and faith
(2.45)
power of SAMĀDHI
(2.1)
KRIYĀ-YOGA action-yoga
(2.2)
weaken the KLEŚA-s realize SAMĀDHI
(2.46–7)
ĀSANA refinement of the body
(2.48)
not distracted by the pairs of opposites
(2.49–51)
PRĀṆĀYĀMA regulation of prāṇa
(2.52–53)
covering of light (avidyā) disappears, readiness for DHĀRAṆĀ
(2.54)
PRATYĀHĀRA tuning out sensory input
(2.55)
perfect mastery of the sensory organs

Figure 12 INNER LIMBS OF YOGA (SAṂYAMA)

	DHĀRAṆĀ	DHYĀNA	SAMĀDHI
Definition	3.1 choosing a focus and directing the attention there	3.2 the continuous flow of attention on a single focus	3.3 the object alone shines forth (in the citta) as if devoid of its own form
Type of focus	choosing and holding a focus focusing is intermittent	holding and maintaining a focus focusing is continuous	focus is inseparable from the perceiver
State of attention	developing the power of attention	exercising the power of attention	total control of attention
Distractions	peripheral distractions still exist (squiggles) pratyāhāra is partial	peripheral distractions are controlled pratyāhāra is in place now	nothing else seems to exist except the focus, the sense of individual self disappears
Object	object is a prop	object is to be understood feels closer, more known	object is completely understood
Example	Choose a rose among all other flowers as the object of focus. Other objects still distract, but we keep bringing our attention back to the rose.	Only the rose is seen, no other flowers or objects distract the attention. The heart-mind is continuously focused on the rose alone.	The heart-mind is like a crystal, reflecting the rose perfectly, appearing to take on its form. The rose seems no different than the heart-mind.

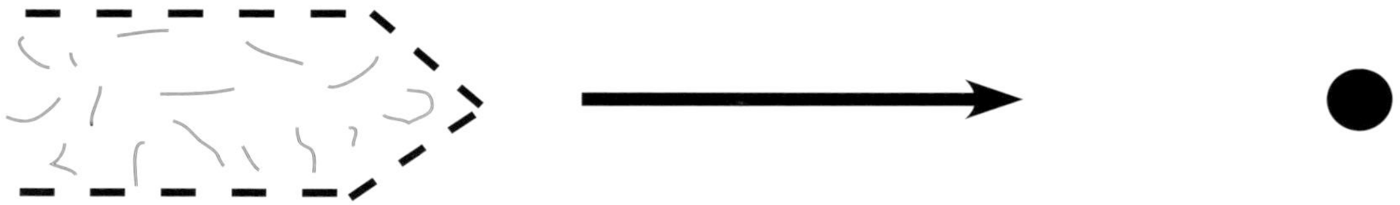

Figure 13 PATHWAYS OF YOGA:
MOVING FROM NEGATIVE TO POSITIVE

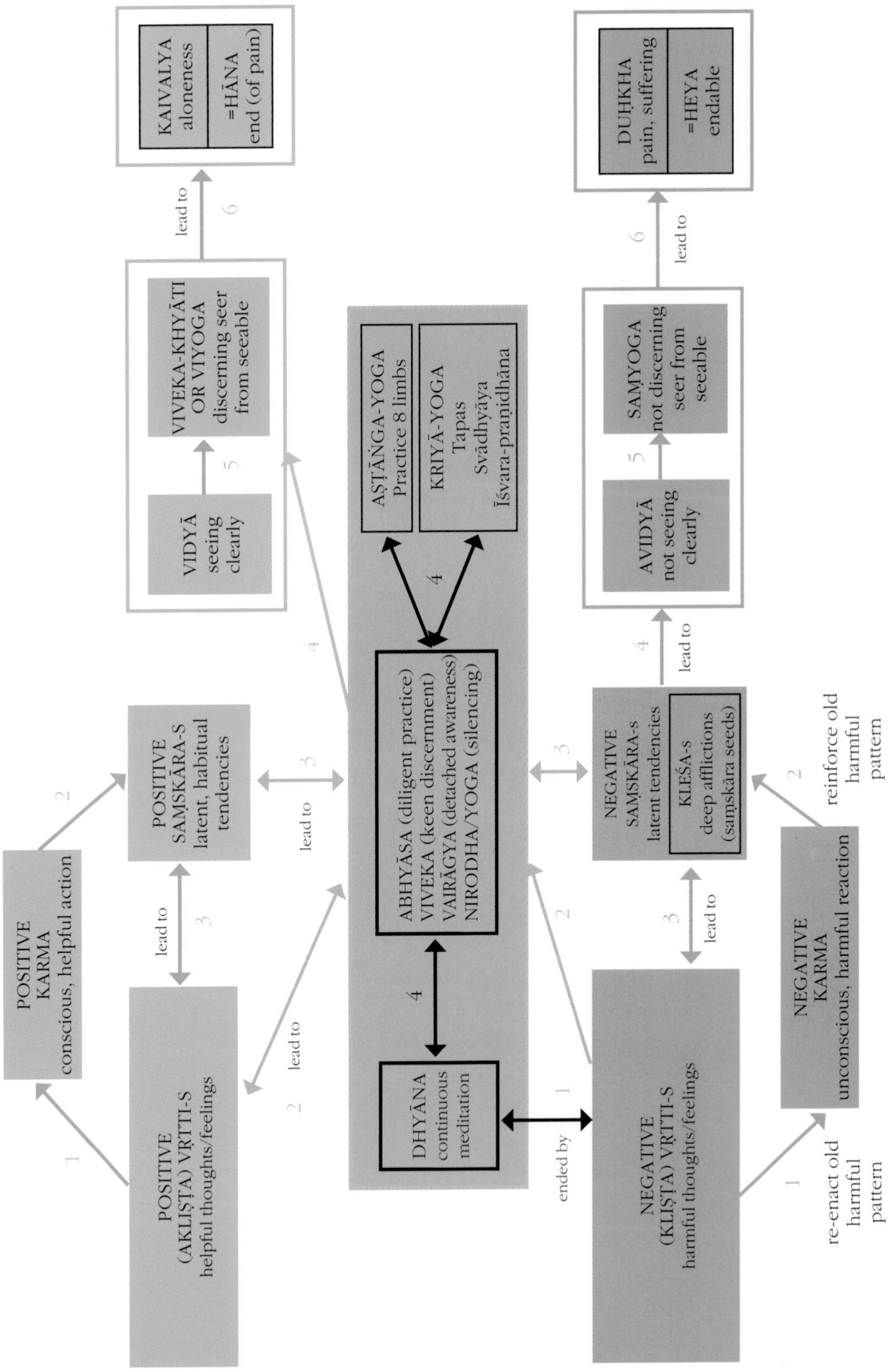

Figure 13, Cont'd PATHWAYS OF YOGA: MOVING FROM NEGATIVE TO POSITIVE

CYCLE OF POSITIVE ACTION

1 Helpful thoughts and feelings (aklişṭa-vṛtti-s) lead to positive, conscious action.
2 Positive, conscious action creates positive habitual tendencies.
3 These helpful habitual tendencies in turn cause more helpful thoughts and feelings.

POSITIVE FLOW TOWARD KAIVALYA

4 Yoga practices clarify the heart-mind, disintegrating the dark covering of ignorance (avidyā) and leading to clear perception (vidyā).
5 With awareness comes discriminating perception (viveka-khyāti).
6 Discerning what changes (seeable) from what does not change (seer) eventually leads to the full experience of the inner light of awareness, and liberation (kaivalya).

PRACTICES TO TRANSFORM NEGATIVE ATTITUDES INTO POSITIVE ATTITUDES

1 Negative thoughts and feelings can be ended by dhyāna (2.11).
2 Yoga practices can transform negative, harmful thoughts and feelings into positive, helpful thoughts and feelings.
2 Helpful practices lead to helpful thoughts and feelings (klişṭa-vṛtti-s).
3 Negative tendencies (saṃskāra-s) can be replaced with positive tendencies by the practices of yoga.
The afflictions (kleśa-s), strengthened by negative tendencies, are weakened by kriyā-yoga (2.2).
Positive tendencies further encourage the practices of yoga.
4 All of the yoga practices in the blue box reinforce each other.

CYCLE OF NEGATIVE ACTION

1 Negative thoughts and feelings (klişṭa-vṛtti-s) lead to negative, unconscious actions.
2 Negative, unconscious actions create new or reinforce old negative, harmful habitual tendencies that worsen the afflictions (kleśa-s).
3 Negative habitual tendencies (saṃskāra-s) strengthen the deep affflictions (kleśa-s), which cause negative thoughts and feelings (klişṭa-vṛtti-s).

NEGATIVE FLOW TOWARD SUFFERING

4 Negative tendencies reduce awareness and lead to ignorance (avidyā).
5 Lack of awareness (avidyā) is the cause of falsely identifying what changes with what never changes (saṃyoga - 2.24).
6 This confusion (saṃyoga) is the cause of suffering (duḥkha - 2.17) which is endable (2.16).

Glossary of Terms

Bold terms are the concepts in part 2. Numbers reference sutras (chapter, sutra number).

abhāva Absence, disappearance (1.10, 29; 2.25; 4.11)

abhibhava Subduing (3.9)

abhijāta Perfect, flawless (1.41)

abhimata Conceived, thought-up (1.39)

abhiniveśa A kleśa: inclination to live, fear of death (2.3, defined in 2.9)

abhivyakti Manifestation (4.8)

abhyantara Internal (2.50–51)

abhyāsa Diligent and continuous practice, vigilance (1.12, def 1.13–14, 1.18, 32)

ādara Respect, honor; eagerness, regard, attention, care (1.14)

ādarśa Enhanced seeing, clairvoyance (3.36)

adhigama Obtaining (1.29)

adhimātrā Strong, intense (1.22; 2.34)

adhva Path, journey, course, way (4.12)

adhyāsa False attribution, wrong assumption (3.17)

adhyātman Inner instrument, individual self (1.47)

ādi Etc., beginning with (2.34; 3.23–24, 39, 45)

āgama Testimony, secondhand knowledge based upon hearing or reading (1.7)

ahiṃsā A yama: nonviolence (2.30, results of 2.35)

ajñāna Lack of knowledge, ignorance (2.34)

akalpitā Real, unimagined (3.43)

ākāśa Space, the subtlest element (3.41–42)

ākṣepin Transcending, going beyond (2.51)

akusīda Disinterest (4.29)

alabdha-bhūmikatva An antarāya: ungroundedness, inability to progress (1.30)

ālambana Support (1.10, 38; 4.11)

ālasya Lethargy, fatigue (1.30)

aliṅga Unmarked, unmanifest (1.45; 2.19)

āloka Brilliance, radiance (3.25)

alpa Little, small (4.31)

anabhighāta Not distracted or disturbed; unaffected; invulnerable (2.48; 3.45)

anāditva Beginninglessness (4.10)

anāgata Not come yet, future (2.16; 3.16; 4.12)

ānanda Extreme happiness, bliss, joy (1.17)

ananta Endless, infinite (2.34, 47)

ānantarya Continuity, being endless (4.9)

ānantya Eternality (4.31)

anāśaya Absence of saṃskāra-s (4.6)

anātman Nonself (2.5)

anavaccheda Unlimited (1.26; 3.53)

anavacchinna Not limited (2.31)

anavadhāraṇa Not cognized (4.20)

anavasthitatva An antarāya: instability, regression (1.30)

aneka Many (4.5)

aṅga Limb, part (2.28–29, 40; 3.7–8)

aṅgamejayatva Agitation, restlessness (1.31)

añjanatā Characteristics (1.41)

aṇiman Miniaturization (3.45)

anta End, limit (1.40; 4.33)

antara Other; interior (4.2)

antaraṅga Internal limb, the last three inner limbs of yoga comprising saṃyama (3.7)

antarāya Obstacle (1.29–30)

antardhāna Invisibility (3.21)

anubhūta Experienced (1.11)

anugama Following, comprehending (1.17)

anuguṇa Following the guṇa-s, appropriate (4.8)

anukāra Resemblence, following the form (2.54)

anumāna Inference, secondhand knowledge based on assumption (1.7, 49)

anumodita Approved, consented to (2.34)

anupaśya "Watching after" (2.20)

anupātin Relying, formed (1.9; 3.14)

anuśāsana Teaching that follows (1.1)

anuśayin Following as a consequence, attached to (2.7–8)

anuśravika Heard after (1.15)

anuṣṭhāna Practicing, executing (2.28)

anuttama Highest, unexcelled (2.42)

anvaya Relationship, guṇa composition (3.44, 47)

anya Other (1.18, 49–50; 2.22)

anyatā Otherness, difference (3.49, 53)

anyatva Otherness, difference (3.15)

apara Nothing higher; other (4.33)

aparāmṛṣṭa Untouched by (1.24)

aparānta Culmination, final, highest ending (3.22)

aparigraha A yama: nonpossessiveness (2.30, results of 2.39)

apariṇāmitva Unchangeableness (4.18)

āpatti Appearance, occurrence, attainment (4.22)

apavarga Completion, emancipation (2.18)

apekṣitva Necessity (4.17)

apeta Removal, departed, withdrawal (4.31)

apramāṇaka Not depending on, not relying on a pramāṇa (4.16)

apratisaṅkrama Unchanging, lacking sequential changes (4.22)

aprayojaka Inoperative, nonmotivator (4.3)

apuṇya Vice, impurity (1.33; 2.14)

āpūra Overflowing (4.2)

ariṣṭa Omen, sign (3.22)

artha Object, meaning, purpose, aim (1.28, 32, 42–43, 49; 2.2, 18, 21–22; 3.3, 17; 4.32, 34)

arthavattva Sense of purpose (3.44, 47)

asaṃprajñāta-samādhi (See samādhi)

asaṃpramoṣa Nonescaping, retention (1.11)

asaṃprayoga Disconnecting, not contacting, separating (2.54; 3.21)

asaṃsarga Noncontact (2.40)

āsana Posture, physical positions to loosen up the body (2.29, def 2.46–47, results of 2.48)

asaṅga Nonattached, unaffected (3.39)

asaṅkīrṇa Distinct, "not mixed together" (3.35)

asaṅkhyeya Innumerable, countless (4.24)

āsanna Near (1.21)

āśaya Reservoir, storehouse, container (1.24; 2.12)

āsevita Attended to, nourished (1.14)

āśis Instinct to live, survive (4.10)

asmitā A kleśa: egotism; the ego (1.17; 2.3, def 2.6; 3.47; 4.4)

āśraya Substratum, resting place (4.11)

āśrayatva Confidence, surity (2.36)

aṣṭa Eight (2.29)

asteya Nonstealing (2.30, def 2.37)

āsvāda Enhanced/suprasensory taste (3.36)

atha Here begins (1.1)

atiprasaṅga Infinite regression (4.21)

atīta Past, "way gone" (3.16; 4.12)

ātmaka Having the nature of, consisting of (2.18)

ātman Inner self (see also Puruṣa); composed of, having the nature of (as a suffix) (2.5, 21, 41; 4.13, 25)

ātmatā Identity, "self-ness" (2.6)

atyanta Absolutely (3.35)

āvaraṇa Covering, shroud (2.52; 3.43; 4.31)

avasthā State at any moment; current situation or condition (3.13)

avasthāna Resting, dwelling (1.3)

āveśa Entry into, possession (3.38)

avidyā A kleśa: lack of awareness, shroud of ignorance (2.3, def 2.4–5, 2.24)

aviplava Flowing continuously, uninterrupted (2.26)

aviṣayin Without object (3.20)

aviśeṣa Nonspecific (2.19; 3.35)

avirati An antarāya: sexual preoccupation, temptation (1.30)

avyapadeśya The future (3.14)

āyus Longevity, life (2.13)

bādhana Binding; troubling, disturbing (2.33)

bahiraṅga External limb (3.8)

bahis External (3.8, 43)

bala Strength (3.23, 24, 46)

bandha Bond, lock, fixation (3.1; 38)

bāhya External (2.50, 51)

bīja Seed (1.25; 3.50)

bhara Bearing, supporting, holding (1.48)

bhauma Earth, ground (2.31)

bhāva Existing, state, mood (1.19; 3.48)

bhāvana Feeling, attitude, disposition; intention; cultivation (1.28, 33; 2.2, 33, 34; 4.25) bheda Division, separation, parting; difference (4.3, 5, 15)

bhoga Life experience, enjoyment (2.13, 18, def 3.35)

bhrānti-darśana An antarāya: erroneous perception (1.30)

bhūmi Ground (1.14; 3.6)

bhūta Fundamental element (earth, water, fire, air, and space) (2.18; 3.13, 44); being (3.17)

bhūtatva Existence, nature of being, "being-ness" (3.20)

bhuvana World, realm, plane of existence (3.26)

brahmacarya A yama: conservation of vital energy (listed 2.30, results of 2.38)

buddhi Intellect; decision-making part of the heart-mind (4.21) (see citta)

cakra Wheel, energy center (3.29)

cakṣus Eye (3.21)

candra Moon (3.27)

caturtha Fourth (2.51)

cetana Consciousess, perception (1.29)

chidra Break, gap, interval (4.27)

citi Unconditioned heart-mind field (4.22, 34)

citra Manifold, variegated, varicolored (4.24)

citta Heart-mind field of consciousness (1.2, 30, 33, 37; 2.54; 3.1, 9, 11, 12, 19, 34, 38; 4.4, 5, 15–18, 23, 26)

darśana Seeing, perceiving, point of view (1.30; 2.6, 41; 3.32)

darśin One who perceives (4.25)

daurmanasya "Negative minded"; mental pain, depression, negativity (1.31)

deśa Place, location, locus (2.31, 50; 3.1, 53; 4.9)

devatā Deity (2.44)

dhāraṇā Choosing a focus and directing our attention there (2.29, 53; def 3.1)

dharma "That which upholds"; orderly structure/function; virtue; characteristic form (3.13, 14, 45; 4.12, 29)

dharmin Substratum (3.14)

dhruva Pole star, unmoving center of the universe (3.28)

dhyāna Focused and uninterrupted attention on a single place (1.39; 2.11, 29; def 3.2; 4.6)

dīpti Radiance, light (2.28)

dīrgha Long, protracted (1.14; 2.50)

divya Divine (3.41)

doṣa Defect (3.50)

draṣṭṛ The seer, witness, observer (1.3; 2.17, 20; 4.23)

dṛḍha Firm (1.14)

dṛk One who sees, perceives (2.16)

dṛśi Seeing (2.25)

dṛṣṭa Seen (1.15; 2.12)

dṛśya Seeable (2.17, 18, 21; 4.23)

duḥkha "Bad/negative space"; suffering, pain, discomfort (1.31, 33; 2.5, 8, 15, 16, 34)

dvandva Duality, pair (of opposites) (2.48)

dveṣa A kleśa: aversion to past painful experiences (listed 2.3, def 2.8)

eka One, single (1.32; 2.6; 4.5, 16)

eka-rūpatva Affinity, uniformity (4.9)

eka-tānatā Continuous flow, extension (3.2)

ekatra One place, single point (3.2)

ekatva Oneness, unity (4.14)

ekāgratā One-pointedness (3.11, 12)

ekāgrya One-pointedness (2.41)

gati Movement, gait (2.49; 3.28)

grahaṇa Process of perception (1.41; 3.47)

grāhya An object perceived, "graspable" (1.41; 3.21)

guṇa Quality of nature, there are three: sattva, rajas, and tamas "strand" (1.16; 2.15, 19; 4.13, 32, 34)

guru Teacher, guide (1.26)

hastin Elephant (3.24)

hāna End, death, cessation (2.25, 26; 4.28)

heya Endable, avoidable (2.10, 11, 16, 17)

hetu Cause (2.17, 23, 24; 3.15; 4.11)

hetutva Causality (2.14)

hiṃsā Violence, harming (2.34)

hlāda Joy, gladness (2.14)

hṛdaya Heart (3.34)

indriya Sensory organ of perception (2.18, 41, 43, 54, 55; 3.13, 47)

iṣṭa Desired, chosen (2.44)

itaratra Otherwise (1.4)

itara Other (1.20; 4.7)

iti Thus (2.34; 3.54; 4.34)

Īśvara The teachings, universal teacher, eternal teacher, omniscience (1.23, def 1.24, expl 25–27)

īśvara-praṇidhāna Honoring the divine inner teacher (2.1, 32, results of 2.45)

jala Water (3.39)

janma Birth (2.12, 39; 4.1)

japa Repetition (1.28)

javitva Swiftness, speed (3.48)

jaya Victory, conquest, mastery (2.41; 3.5, 39, 40, 44, 47, 48)

jāti Birth class/condition/status; caste; category of existence (2.13, 31; 3.18, 53; 4.2, 9)

jñāna Knowledge (1.8, 9, 38, 42; 2.28; 3.16–19, 22, 25–29, 35, 52, 54; 4.31)

jñāta Known (4.17, 18)

jñeya To be known (4.31)

jugupsā Disgust (2.40)

jvalana Radiance (3.40)

jyotis Light (3.32)

jyotiṣmatī Luminous (1.36)

kaivalya Final emancipation; permanent oneness; independent simplicity; topic of fourth chapter (2.25; 3.50, 55; 4.26, 34)

kāla Time (1.14, 26; 2.31, 50; 4.9)

kaṇṭaka Thorn (3.39)

kaṇṭha Throat, neck (3.30)

karaṇa Act, doing, cause (2.2)

kāraṇa Cause (3.38)

kārita Caused (2.34)

kāritva Activity (4.24)

karma Action (1.24; 2.12; 3.22; 4.7, 30)

karmāśaya Collection/reservoir of saṃskāra-s stored in the memory of the heart-mind (see āśaya)

karuṇā Compassion (1.33)

kathaṃtā How, reason for (2.39)

kāya Body (2.43; 3.21, 29, 42, 45, 46)

khyāti Reknown, fame, glory; awareness, realization, understanding, identification (1.16; 2.5, 26, 28; 3.49; 4.29) (see viveka-khyāti)

kim What? (4.16)

kleśa Deep emotional affliction (1.24; 2.2, five listed 2.3, 2.12; 4.30); cause of kliṣṭa-vṛtti-s

kliṣṭa Afflicted, not helpful, harmful, producing suffering

krama Sequence, succession, sequential progression (3.15, 52; 4.32, 33)

kriyā Work, action (2.36); type of yoga composed of the last three niyama-s (2.1); activity (2.18)

krodha Anger (2.34)

kṛta Done, accomplished, realized (2.22, 34; 4.32)

kṣaṇa Moment of time, an instant (3.9, 52; 4.33)

kṣaya Destruction, elimination (2.28, 43; 3.11, 43, 50)

kṣetra Field, area (2.4)

kṣetrika Farmer (4.3)

kṣīṇa Reduced, diminished (1.41)

kṣudh Hunger (3.30)

kūpa Hole, cavity, hollow (3.30)

kūrma Tortoise (3.31)

lakṣaṇa Temporal characteristic, feature, marker (3.13, 53) (see pariṇāma)

laghu Lightweight (3.42)

lābha Gain, obtaining (2.38, 42)

lāvanya Gracefulness (3,46)

liṅga-mātrā Primary manifestation (2.19) (see Sāṅkhya diagram in appendix F, figure 1)

lobha Greed (2.34)

loka Light, realm (3.5)

madhya Medium, middle (1.22; 2.34)

mahā Great, large (2.31)

mahattva Greatness, largeness (1.40)

maitrī Friendship (1.33; 3.23)

mala Impurity, waste (4.31)

manas Outer mind which functions to accept sensory perceptions (1.35; 2.53; 3.48)

mani Gemstone, jewel (1.41)

mantra Sound causing a specific effect (4.1)

mātrā Suffix: alone, only (1.43; 3.3, 49; 4.4)

megha Cloud (4.29)

mithyā Mistake, false (1.8)

moha Delusion (2.34)

mṛdu Soft, mild (1.22; 2.34)

mudita Joy, elation (1.33)

mūla Root, basis, foundation (2.12, 13)

mūrdhan Top apex (crown) of the head (3.32)

na No, not (3.20; 4.16, 19)

nairantarya Uninterrupted, continuous (1.14)

naṣṭa Lost, vanished (2.22)

nābhi Navel (3.29)

nāḍī Energy channel, meridian (3.31)

nibandhinī Bound down (1.35)

nidrā A vṛtti: sleep (1.6, def 1.10, 1.38)

nimitta Primary cause, catalyst (4.3)

nimna Deep, slope, incline, oriented toward (4.26)

niratiśaya Beyond compare (1.25)

nirbhāsa Beyond brilliance (1.43; 3.3)

nirbīja Without seed, without object; a kind of samādhi (1.51; 3.8)

nirgrāhya Beyond understanding (4.33)

nirmāṇa Fabricating, constructing, shaping, forming (4.4)

nirodha Process of stilling, settling, calming, breaking (1.2, 12, 51; 3.9)

nirupakrama Without momentum, not started yet, slow (3.22)

nirvicāra Beyond reflection; a stage of samāpatti/samādhi (1.44, 47)

nirvitarka Beyond analysis; a stage of samāpatti/samādhi (1.43)

nitya Eternal, permanent (2.5)

nityatva Eternality, permanence

nivṛtti Inactivating, stopping activity (4.25, 30)

niyama Personal observances (2.29, 32)

nyāsa Projection (3.25)

oṣadhi Herb, medicine, plant (4.1)

pāda Leg, quarter, part, chapter

paṅka Mud (3.39)

pañcatayī Fivefold (1.5)

panthan Path, way, method (4.15)

para Other; supreme (1.16; 2.40; 3.19, 38)

parama Supreme, highest, extreme (1.40; 2.55)

paramāṇu Extremely small (1.40)

parārthatva Having the purpose of another (3.35)

paridṛṣṭa Observed completely, seen from all angles (2.50)

pariṇāma Transformation, change, mutation (2.15, 3.11–13, 15, 16; 4.2, 14, 32, 33)

pariśuddhi Complete purification (1.43)

paritāpa Sorrow (2.14)

parvan Stage, phase (2.19)

paryavasāna Extending, ending up (1.45)

phala Fruit, result (2.14, 34, 36; 4.11)

pipāsā Thirst (3.30)

prabhū Master, lord (4.18)

pracāra Movements forward, onward (3.38)

pracchardana Exhaling (1.34)

pradhāna See Prakṛti (3.48)

prādurbhāva Arising, emergence; attainment (3.9, 45)

prāgbhāra Gravitation, "weighted in the front" (4.26)

prajñā Deep intuitive insight, wisdom with discernment (1.20, 48, 49; 2.27; 3.5)

prakāśa Radiance—a characteristic of sattva guṇa (2.18, 52; 3.21, 43)

Prakṛti Nature, the manifest, changing world (4.2, 13)

prakṛtilaya Absorbed back into nature (1.19)

pramāda Carelessness—one of nine obstacles called antarāya-s (1.30)

pramāṇa A vṛtti: correct way to evaluate something (there are three: pratyakṣa, anumāna, āgama) (1.6, 7)

prāṇa Life-force, breath, chi (1.34) (see prāṇāyāma)

praṇava The original sound that began the manifest world; Om (1.27)

prāṇāyāma Regulation of breath, control of life-force (2.29, def 2.49)

pranidhāna Devotion, surrender, faith, "placing beneath and in front of" (1.23)

prāntabhūmi Ultimate, final (2.27)

prasāda Purity, clarity (1.47)

prasādana Purification, clarification (1.33)

prasaṅga Possibility of attachment, opportunity (3.51)

prasaṅkhyāna Higher state (4.29)

praśānta Quieted (3.10)

prasupta Dormant, latent (2.4)

praśvāsa Exhalation, "forward breath" (2.49)

prati Prefix opposing, contra-; regarding (2.22)

pratibandhin Inhibition (1.50)

prātibha Intuitive flash (3.33, 36)

pratipakṣa-bhāvana Cultivating the opposite side (2.33–34)

pratipatti Ascertainment, ability to perceive (3.53)

pratiprasava Returning back to the origin (2.10; 4.34)

pratiṣedha Prevention, counteracting (1.32)

pratiyogin Corresponding (4.33)

pratyāhāra Tuning out sensory input (2.29, def 2.54, results 2.55)

pratyak Inward (1.29)

pratyakṣa Direct, firsthand perception—first of three pramāṇa-s (1.7)

prayatna Effort forth, appropriate effort (2.47)

pratyaya A presented thought, current vṛtti directed toward an object (1.10, 18, 19; 2.20; 3.2, 12, 17, 19, 35; 4.27)

pravibhāga Difference, distinction (3.17)

pravṛtti Activity, development (1.35; 3.25; 4.5)

prayojaka Initiator, motivator, director (4.5)

punar Again (3.12, 51)

puṇya Virtue, goodness (1.33; 2.14)

Puruṣa The inactive, inner light of awareness; the conscious observer (1.16, 24; 3, 35, 49, 55; 4.18, 34)

pūrva Previous (1.18, 26; 3.7, 18)

pūrvaka Preceded by (1.20, 34)

rāga A kleśa: desire for past pleasurable experiences (2.3, def 2.7)

rajas Guṇa (quality) of activity, stimulation, motivation

rasa Essence, juice (2.9)

ratna Gemstone, jewel (2.37)

ṛta Fact, natural law (1.48)

ruta Sound, vocalization (3.17)

rūpa Form (1.17; 3.21, 46)

sabīja "With seed"; samādhi with a point of focus (1.46)

sādhana Accomplishing, practicing; topic of second chapter

sādhāraṇatva Commonness (2.22)

sākṣāt Witnessing, viewing firsthand (3.18)

sālambana With support (3.20)

samādhi State in which the heart-mind reflects the object perfectly so the two seem as one (def 3.3), complete absorption of the heart-mind in the focus (1.20, 46, 51; 2.2, 29, 45; 3.3, 11, 37; 4.1, 29), name of first chapter

samāna Bodily energy of homeostasis, equilibrium (3.40)

samāpatti Saturation of the heart-mind with the focus; stages of samādhi (1.41, 42; 2.47; 3.42)

samāpti Finished (4.32)

samārūḍha Grown or developed completely (2.9)

samaya Time, circumstance (2.31)

saṃbandha Relationship (3.41, 42)

saṃbodha Complete knowledge/ understanding (2.39)

saṃhananatva Firmness (3.46)

saṃhatya Collaboration (4.24)

saṃjñā Complete knowledge/awareness (1.15)

saṃkhyā Number, count (2.50)

saṃnidha Proximity, nearness (2.35)

saṃpad Abundance (3.45, 46)

saṃprajñāta-samādhi Complete comprehension of the focus of samādhi (1.17) (see samādhi)

saṃprayoga Communion (2.44)

saṃśaya Doubt, indecision—one of 9 obstacles called antarāya-s (1.30)

saṃskāra Deep impression stored in memory from a strong or repeated perception or action, and its resulting habitual tendency (1.18, 50; 2.15; 3.9, 10, 18; 4.9, 27) (see karma and saṃskāra)

saṃvedana Complete experience/feeling/ knowledge (3.38; 4.22)

saṃvega Impulse, momentum (1.21)

saṃvid Complete knowledge (3.34)

sāmya Same, identical (3.55; 4.15)

saṃyama "Complete control"; turning the attention inward toward a focus. Comprises dhāraṇā, dhyāna and samādhi (def 3.4, expl 3.5–8, results of 3.16; occurs in 3.4, 16, 17, 21, 22, 26, 35, 41, 42, 44, 47, 52)

saṃyoga "Joining, unification, confusion"; here mistakenly identifying the seer as the seen (2.17, def 2.23, expl 2.24–25)

saṅga Attachment, contact (3.51)

saṅgṛhītatva "Held-together-ness" (4.11)

saṅkara Mixed up, confused (3.17; 4.21)

Sāṅkhya Name of a system of philosophy. See appendix F, figure 1.

saṅkīrṇa Completely mixed up (1.42)

santoṣa A niyama: contentment (2.32, results of 2.42)

saptadhā Sevenfold (2.27)

sārūpya Conformity, identification (1.4)

sarva All, everything (1.51; 2.15, 37; 3.17, 33; 4.31)

sarvajña All-knowing, omniscient (1.25)

sarvajñātṛtva All-knowingness, omniscience (3.49)

sarvathā In all ways, in every way (3.54; 4.29)

sarvārthatā Multidirectional, "all objectness" (3.11)

satkāra Acting truthfully, sincerity (1.14)

sattva Guṇa of light, intelligence, purity, goodness, etc. (1.16; 2.41; 3.35, 49, 55)

satya A yama: truthfulness (2.30, results of 2.36)

śauca A niyama: cleanliness, purity of body, mind, and surroundings; personal hygiene (2.40–41)

saumanasya Delight, positive-minded (2.41)

savicāra Reflective stage of samāpatti/samādhi (1.44)

savitarka Cognitive/analytical stage of samāpatti/samādhi (1.42)

siddha Accomplished; one who has acquired power (3.32, 37; 4.1)

siddhi Power, accomplishment (2.43, 45)

smaya Amazement; pride (3.51)

smṛti A vṛtti: memory of the citta that holds saṃskāra-s and kleśa-s (1.6, def 1.11; 1.20, 43; 4.9, 21)

sopakrama With momentum, already started, fast (3.22)

stambha Suspension (2.50; 3.21)

sthairya Stability (2.39; 3.31)

sthānin Elevated being, astral energy (3.51)

sthira Stable, structured (2.46)

sthiti Staying, stability—a characteristic of tamas guṇa (1.13, 35; 2.18)

sthūla Gross, coarse (3.44)

styāna Apathy—one of nine obstacles called antarāya-s (1.30)

sukha Pleasure, ease, relaxation (1.33; 2.5, 7, 42, 46)

sūkṣma Subtle (1.44, 45; 2.10, 50; 3.25, 44; 4.13)

śūnya Empty, devoid, zero (4.34)

sūrya Sun (3.26)

sva One's own, belonging to oneself (2.9, 23, 40, 54)

svābhāsa One's own inner radiance (4.19)

svādhyāya A niyama: self-study, self-observation (2.1, 32, results of 2.44); part of kriyā-yoga.

svāmin Master, "having oneself" (2.23)

svapna Dream (1.38)

svārtha "Own-purpose" (3.35)

svarūpa Own nature, own form/shape (1.3, 43; 2.23, 54; 3.3, 44, 47; 4.12, 34)

tad/tat That, it

tadā Then . . .

tamas Guṇa (quality) of inertia, darkness, negativity (1.10, 16)

tantra Depending on (4.16)

tanu Weak, feeble (2.2, 4)

tāpa Discomfort caused by tapas (2.15)

tapas A niyama: practice causing positive change (2.1, 32, results of 2.43; 4.1), part of kriyā-yoga.

tārā Star (3.27)

tāraka Crossing over, transcending (3.54)

tatra There, in that case (1.13, 25, 42, 48; 3.2; 4.6)

tatstha Established in that (1.41)

tattva Thing, part of the manifest world, building block of nature (1.32; 4.14)

tīvra Intense, serious, ardent (1.21)

traya Threefold, triad (3.4, 7, 16)

trividha Of three kinds (4.7)

tūla Cotton (3.42)

tulya Same, similar (3.12, 53)

tyāga Abandonment (2.35)

ubhaya Both (4.20)

udāna Upward moving prāṇa (3.39)

udāra Aroused, active (2.4)

udaya Emergence, appearance (3.11)

udita Arisen; present time (3.12, 14)

ukta Said (4.28)

upalabdhi Acquisition (2.23)

upaṇimantrana Invitation, admiration, beckoning, temptation (3.51)

uparāga Reflected color (4.17)

uparakta Colored through reflection (4.23)

upasarga Obstacle (3.37)

upasthāna Approaching (2.37)

upāya Way, means, method (2.26)

upekṣa Neutrality, indifference (1.33)

utkrānti Rising up, ascension; ability to die at will (3.39)

utpannā Development, arising (1.35)

uttara Other, subsequent (2.4)

vā Or

vācaka Expression, speech (1.27)

vāhin That which carries (2.9)

vāhitā Flow, current (3.10)

vaira Hostility, animosity, hatred (2.35)

vairāgya Unattached awareness, noninvolvement, noninterference (1.2, def 1.15–16; 3.50)

vaiśāradya Maturity, proficiency (1.47)

vaitṛṣṇya Nonclinging (a more subtle and higher form of vitṛṣṇa) (1.16)

vajra Diamond, thunderbolt (3.46)

varaṇa Choice; covering; obstacle (4.3)

vārta Suprasensory smell

vāsanā Subtle residue of a perception or action; subtle saṃskāra, propensity or trait (4.8, 24) (see karma and saṃskāra discourse)

vaśīkāra Mastery (1.15, 40)

vastu Object (1.9; 4.14–17)

vaśyatā Mastery (2.55)

vedana Suprasensory touch (3.36)

vedanīya Experienced, come to be known (2.12)

vibhakta Distinct, different (4.15)

vibhūti Power, accomplishment; ash; topic of chapter 3

viṣaya Object perceived by the sensory organs

vicāra Analysis (1.17)

viccheda Interruption, disturbance (2.49)

vicchinna Interrupted, intermittent (2.4)

videha Out-of-body, discarnate (1.19)

vidhāraṇa Extending, holding (1.34)

vidvas Wise person, one who has knowledge (2.19)

vikalpa Imagination (1.6, def 1.9, 1.42)

vikaraṇa Independent of instruments (sensory organs) (3.48)

vikṣepa Disruption, distraction (1.30, 31)

viniyoga Application (3.6)

vipāka A ripening, result, consequence (1.24; 2.13; 4.8)

viparyaya A vṛtti: misperception, erroneous perception (1.6, def 1.8)

viprakṛṣṭa Distant (3.25)

virāma Stopping, arresting (1.18)

virodha Conflict, obstruction (2.15)

vīrya Courage, virility (1.20; 2.38)

viṣaya Sensory object (1.11, 15, 33, 37, 44, 49; 2.51, 54; 3.54)

viṣayatva Objectness (1.45)

viṣayavatī Having a sensory object (1.35)

viśeṣa Specific, distinct (1.22, 24, 49; 2.19; 4.25)

viśoka Sorrowless (1.3)

vītarāga Without rāga (attachment to pleasure) (1.37)

vitarka Cognitive analysis (1.17, 2.33–34)

vitṛṣṇa Noncraving, nonclinging, absence of desire (1.15)

viveka Wise discernment, ability to insightfully discriminate (2.26, 28; 3.52, 54; 4.26, 29)

vivekaja Born of/produced by wise discernment (3.52, 54)

viveka-khyāti Discriminating perception; identification with viveka; integration of viveka (2.26, 28; 4.29)

vivekin One who has viveka (2.15)

vrata Vow, promise (2.31)

vṛtti "Fluctuation, activity"; here a citta-vṛtti is a fluctuation or activity in the heart-mind; the current vṛtti directed toward an object is called a pratyaya (1.2, 4, 5, five listed 1.6, 1.10, 41; 2.11, 15, 50; 3.43; 4.18)

vyādhi An antarāya; disease (1.30)

vyākhyātā Explained (1.44; 3.13)

vyakta Manifested (4.13)

vyavahita Hidden, concealed, obscure; separated by anything intervening, "placed apart" (3.25; 4.9)

vyūha Arrangement (3.27, 29)

vyutthāna Activity, externalization (3.9, 37)

yama Social ethics (2.29, 30)

yathā As (1.39)

yatna Effort (1.13)

yoga "Connection, conjunction, relationship"; process of calming the fluctuations in the heart-mind (1.1, def 1.2, 2.28). Also, the state of samādhi.

yogin One who practices yoga

yogyata Readiness, aptitude (2.53)

yogyatva Fitness, readiness (2.41)

Prefixes

a/an Not, without

ā Enhances meaning of word, up to, until; reverses direction of movement

abhi Toward

anu After

ni Beneath, into

nir/niḥ/niṣ Without, beyond

pra Toward, forth, in front

sa With, together

sam Completely, fully, together

upa Near

vi Separating, cutting through, discriminating

Suffixes

ja Born of

ga Going

Bibliography

The dictionary referenced in the book is *The Practical Sanskrit-English Dictionary* by Principal Vaman Shivaram Apte. Kyoto, Japan: Rinsen Book Company, 1992, reprinted from the 1957 edition, Poona, India.

Bouanchaud, Bernard. *The Essence of Yoga; Reflections on the Yoga Sutra-s of Patañjali.* Portland, Oregon: Rudra Press, 1997 (RT, ET, DEF). Refined and practical interpretation. One sūtra per page with reflections to contemplate on each sūtra. Full index of terms in the back.

Desikachar, T. K. V. *The Heart of Yoga.* Rochester, Vermont: Inner Traditions International, 1995 (SS, RT, ET). Loose yet practical interpretation with brief commentary. Book includes much more than the sūtra-s.

Hariharananda Aranya, Swami. *Yoga Philosophy of Patañjali.* Albany: State University of New York Press, 1983 (SS, ET, VV, COM). The most comprehensive, with long commentaries on each sūtra and on Vyās's commentary. A very traditional interpretation.

Hartranft, Chip. *The Yoga-Sūtra of Patañjali.* Boston, Massachusetts: Shambhala Publications, Inc., 2003, arlingtoncenter.org (ET, COM). Smooth and clear explanation in English, with a slightly Buddhist leaning.

Houston, Vyaas. *The Yoga Sūtra Workbook: The Certainty of Freedom.* Warwick, New York: American Sanskrit Institute, 1995, americansanskrit.com (SS, RT, ET, DEF, GR). Translation is literal with no commentary. One sūtra per letter-size page with plenty of room for notes.

Iyengar, B.K.S. *Light on the Yoga Sūtra-s of Patañjali.* San Francisco, California: Aquarian/Thorsons (Harper Collins), 1993 (SS, RT, ET, DEF, COM). Excellent reference, includes many tables, great indices in the back. A very traditional interpretation.

Virupakshananda, Swami. *Sāṁkhya Kārikā of Īśvara Kṛṣṇa.* Mylapore, Madras: Sri Ramakrishna Math, 1995 (SS, ET).

Zambito, Salvatore. *The Unadorned Thread of Yoga.* Poulsbo, Washington: The Yoga Sūtra-s Institute Press, 1992 (SS, RT, ET, DEF). Shows twelve different translations of each sūtra.

SS = Sanskrit Script

RT = Romanized Transliteration

ET = English Translation

VV = Veda Vyaas's commentary on the *Yoga Sūtra-s*

DEF = Definitions of each individual word

GR = Grammatical endings

About the Author

Nicolai Bachman has been teaching Sanskrit, yoga philosophy, and Ayurveda nationally since 1994. His studies with individual teachers in one-on-one or small-class settings form the core of his education. He began learning Sanskrit in 1992 while studying Ayurveda (East Indian medicine) with Dr. Vasant Lad at the Ayurvedic Institute in Albuquerque, New Mexico. The following summer he completed a six-week Sanskrit intensive given by Vyaas Houston at the American Sanskrit Institute (ASI). From there he traveled to India for over a year, studying with Dr. Vagish Shastri, director of the Sampurnand Sanskrit University in Varanasi. Upon returning he worked for ASI while learning one-on-one with Vyaas Houston for one year. From there he moved to Santa Fe and completed an M.A. in Eastern Classics at St. John's College in 1996. From 1996 to 2014 he studied regularly with David Frawley (American Institute of Vedic Studies) and Sonia Nelson (Vedic Chant Center), and he completed another masters degree (nutrition) in 2005.

Nicolai's passion for Sanskrit, Ayurveda, and yoga philosophy infuse every class he teaches, and he has a knack for organizing complex scientific and philosophical concepts into a clear and understandable format. He travels nationally to share the deeper wisdom of yoga and to inspire students on their paths.

For more information, visit SanskritSounds.com.

About Sounds True

Sounds True is a multimedia publisher whose mission is to inspire and support personal transformation and spiritual awakening. Founded in 1985 and located in Boulder, Colorado, we work with many of the leading spiritual teachers, thinkers, healers, and visionary artists of our time. We strive with every title to preserve the essential "living wisdom" of the author or artist. It is our goal to create products that not only provide information to a reader or listener but also embody the quality of a wisdom transmission.

For those seeking genuine transformation, Sounds True is your trusted partner. At SoundsTrue.com you will find a wealth of free resources to support your journey, including exclusive weekly audio interviews, free downloads, interactive learning tools, and other special savings on all our titles.

To learn more, please visit SoundsTrue.com/freegifts or call us toll-free at 800.333.9185.

sounds true
WAKING UP THE WORLD